GEORGE A. BRAY, M.D.

Professor of Medicine, University of California
at Los Angeles, and Director of the Clinical Study Center,
Harbor General Hospital, Torrance, California

THE
OBESE
PATIENT

VOLUME

IX

IN THE SERIES

MAJOR PROBLEMS IN INTERNAL MEDICINE

Lloyd H. Smith, Jr., M.D., *Editor*

W. B. SAUNDERS COMPANY · PHILADELPHIA · LONDON · TORONTO · 1976

W. B. Saunders Company: West Washington Square
                            Philadelphia, Pa.   19105

                            1 St. Anne's Road
                            Eastbourne, East Sussex BN21 3UN, England

                            833 Oxford Street
                            Toronto, M8Z 5T9, Canada

Library of Congress Cataloging in Publication Data

Bray, George A
  The obese patient.

  (Major problems in internal medicine; v. 9)
  Bibliography: p.
  Includes index.
  1. Obesity.   I. Title.
RC628.B653   616.3′98   75-20798
ISBN 0-7216-1931-2

The Obese Patient   ISBN   0-7216-1931-2

Last digit is the print number: 9   8   7   6   5   4   3   2   1

This book is dedicated to my mentors.

D. H. FUNKENSTEIN
R. W. BERLINER
R. PITT-RIVERS
E. B. ASTWOOD

FOREWORD

Fat in the form of the various triglycerides is one of the basic chemical constituents of the body. The formation of fat is an admirable evolutionary development, allowing for compact (virtually anhydrous) storage of energy reserves, cushioning, insulation and even aesthetic appeal. Marvelously adapted to the energy needs of the body, fat molecules flow into and out of the adipocytes under the constant titration of hormones and enzymes and are often tucked away in complex macromolecules which allow rapid transport in an aqueous environment. This disposal system is usually finely tuned to the appetite; in a society of abundance such as our own, an adult's weight may vary only a few pounds or not at all over a decade despite the production of energy totalling some millions of kilocalories. Perhaps it is surprising that obesity is not more frequent, considering the exquisite balance between food ingestion and energy output which must be maintained over years during which both activities tend to be somewhat casually controlled.

But obesity is common enough; it has been called the main public health problem in the United States. Beyond the toll which it exacts in morbidity and premature death (fully documented by actuarial analysis), obesity leads to loss of self esteem and social stigma in an era when Twiggy has been hailed as a model. Medical records are real enough when they report an alarmingly high incidence of hypertension, diabetes, atherosclerosis, arthritis and multiple disabilities in performing many of life's ordinary activities. Too much stored energy, whether in hypertrophied adipocytes or in increased (hyperplastic) adipocytes, may be more dangerous and debilitating than moderate malnutrition.

What is the pathogenesis and treatment of obesity? The explanation should be easy since this was one of the first of the great medical discoveries, made by Sir Isaac Newton some centuries ago. We believe that the tissues of the obese patient are incapable of "fixing" atmospheric nitrogen or carbon, and therefore the patient must have an imbalance between food ingested and energy released. Unfortunately, the mere recitation of the first law of thermodynamics has rarely been persuasive in medical practice relating to obesity. A greater understanding of the variables at work is required, for hypertrophy or hyperplasia of the fat organ is a serious matter.

In a relatively thin book Dr. George A. Bray has managed to summarize most of the salient features now known about the obese patient, including pathogenesis, complications, treatment and prognosis. At least one third of our patients might be classified as obese; it therefore behooves the internist to take an interest in this frequent and debilitating disorder. Dr. Bray's monograph offers an authoritative and scholarly treatment of this important subject, to which he himself has made many signal contributions.

LLOYD H. SMITH, JR., M.D.

PREFACE

Leave gourmandizing. Know the grave doth gape
For thee thrice wider than for other men.
William Shakespeare
HENRY IV, part II; V, v, 54-55.

Obesity is a subject of universal interest. It affects a substantial number of people in most affluent nations and its long and interesting history has even left its mark on the literary world. In a recent review (Ayers, 1958), the changing attitudes towards overweight and obesity were traced from Greco-Roman times through the twentieth century. There has been a gradual shift away from acceptance of obesity. Indeed, the form of idolatry seen in the curvaceous nudes of Rubens' paintings has been replaced by a rejection of obesity most clearly shown in the predominance of the very lean body types of most modern fashion models. To quote from Ayers (1958), "Practically everyone will agree that obesity is the number one health problem today and that, willy-nilly, the fat person must undergo therapy of some kind. Imprisoned in every fat man, a thin one is wildly signalling to be let out: and though—as Omar claimed—fat people may die happy, they nevertheless die sooner than their lean brothers." Herein lies the fundamental difference which distinguishes our modern attitude toward obesity from that of former years. This volume is an attempt to place some of the current information about obesity in perspective.

The problem of obesity has been with us for centuries. The Venus of Willenbach is a Stone Age carving of a fat woman which is on display in the Kunstmuseum in Vienna. The figure dates from Neolithic time. Today obese people are rarely the object of artistic representation and are more likely to be the subject of ridicule and caricature. A wonderful cartoon from 1777 depicts a man carrying his panniculus in a wheelbarrow while his lean servant follows at an appropriate distance carrying the man's belongings on his head (British Museum Print Collection No. 1777–5433).

Obesity has received serious consideration over the past 200 years. In 1829 William Wadd published his *Comments on Corpulency*. In this book he depicts a number of grossly obese people and documents the characteristics of this problem in detail. The fat boy named Joe in Dickens' *Pickwick Papers* has been used as a literary illustration of the syndrome of respiratory insufficiency and hypoventilation in obesity. The syndrome was described in great detail by Burwell and his associates in 1956, and will be discussed subsequently in Chapter 6 of this volume.

In addition to these scientific and literary contributions, the nineteenth century also saw the introduction of methods for treating obesity. Among these, a high fat diet prescribed by Dr. Harvey was the most long lasting. In "A Letter of Corpulence" published in 1863, Banting described the wonders of this diet. The apparent effectiveness of this method has been called forth from time to time in popular books on dieting, of which *Dr. Atkins' Diet Revolution* is one of the most recent.

Little scientific attention was paid to obesity until the beginning of the twentieth century. In the classic textbook *Principle and Practice of Medicine* published in 1892 by Osler, the subject of obesity occupies only a page and three quarters. In it, the author describes the use of dietary methods of treatment and notes that genetic factors interact with environmental problems of overeating and low levels of exercise to produce the corpulence which is so common in the middle years of life. The most extensive early account of obesity was written by von Noorden, who published a systematic treatise on the subject in 1900. The important concept presented in this work was the distinction between obesity due to overeating (exogenous obesity) and obesity due to glandular disorders (endogenous obesity). In addition, his treatise provided a description of appropriate body weight as an approach to treatment.

In 1940 Rony provided a second systematic attempt at presenting information about obesity. In his well written little book he describes many clinical forms and therapeutic approaches to obesity. More recently there have been several other individual attempts to provide a cohesive picture of clinical problems of obesity (Rynearson and Gastineau, 1948; Mayer, 1968; Craddock, 1973; Garrow, 1974), and a larger number of works with multiple authors.

Why, then, another book on obesity? First, after reviewing the literature, it is my belief that a coherent scientific review of the problem of obesity is not now generally available. All of the books described above have a specific point of view. In addition, they sometimes omit areas which I consider important. Second, it is my hope that by distilling the vast literature about obesity into a small readable volume, I may provide some insights into the problem for direction of my own research and that of others. Third, there is an enormous interest in obesity and weight control among the public. Several of the popular diet books have sold over one million copies. In 1973, *Newsweek* estimated that the diet industry consumed ten billion dollars. Moreover, there is an ever growing number of books on diet available to the public, and a large amount of information appears almost monthly in popular magazines. In a survey of public opinion conducted in Southern California in late March, 1974 by the Field Research Corporation for television station KNXT, 505 individuals from a random sample were polled. Thirty two percent of the men and 46 percent of the women described themselves as too heavy. Of those who considered themselves too heavy, over 70 percent were actively trying to do something about it, and 27 percent were actually on a diet. This volume is an effort to provide a factual background for physicians and interested laymen who wish to obtain a unified perspective into the problems and information about obesity.

The effort in preparing this book has been sustained by several important people. First of all, my wife has had the patience and forbearance to let me undertake this work and has provided the consideration and support to keep me going when it often seemed a hopeless task. Second, I have been most ably assisted by my secretary, Ms. Josie Martinez and by the excellent typographical work of Ms. Beverly Fisher and Ms. Ruby Belegrin. Ms. Debbie Boyd has provided valuable editorial assistance. The nurses and dietitians in the Clinical Study Center at the Harbor General Hospital and at Tufts New England Medical Center have provided the support for many of the original studies described in this volume. Finally, my colleagues at the Harbor General Hospital have reviewed and helped to improve many aspects of this manuscript. The original scientific investigations have been supported by grants from the National Institutes of Health (AM 15165, RR 00425, AM 09897) and the Diabetes Association of Southern California.

GEORGE A. BRAY

REFERENCES

Atkins, R. C.: Dr. Atkins' Diet Revolution. New York, David McKay Co., 1972.
Ayers, W. M.: Changing attitudes toward overweight and reducing. J. Am. Dietetic Assoc., 34:23–29, 1958.
Banting, W.: Letter on Corpulence. Addressed to the Public. London, Harrison, 1863.
Burwell, C. S., Robin, E. D., Whaley, R. D. and Bickelman, A. G.: Extreme obesity associated with alveolar hypoventilation—A 'Pickwickian' syndrome. Am. J. Med. 21:811–818, 1956.
Craddock, D.: Obesity and its Management. Baltimore, The Williams & Wilkins Co., second edition, 1974.
Garrow, J.: Energy Balance and Obesity in Man. London, North-Holland Publishing Company Ltd., 1974.
Mayer, J.: Overweight: Causes, Cost and Control. Englewood Cliffs, Prentice-Hall, Inc., 1968.
Rony, H. R.: Obesity and Leanness. Philadelphia, Lea and Febiger, 1940.
Rynearson, E. H. and Gastineau, C. F.: Obesity. Springfield, Charles C Thomas, 1949.
von Noorden, K.: Die Fettsucht. Nothnagel Specielle Pathologie und Therapie, 7:1–156, 1900.
Wadd, W.: Comments on Corpulency, London, John Ebers and Co., 1829.

CONTENTS

CHAPTER 1

WHO ARE THE OBESE?

To answer the question, who are the obese, the term obesity must be defined. This would seem to be simple and in many instances it is, particularly when the individual in question is massively obese. Such people require no sophisticated criteria to indicate this diagnosis. The heaviest reported body weight according to the Guinness Book of Records was 1069 pounds (Guinness Book of Records, 1974). Table 1–1 summarizes the data on this and other cases of massively obese individuals weighing over 700 pounds. It is apparent that the maximal weight was usually achieved in or before the fourth decade of life, and that survival beyond this age was unusual.

TABLE 1–1. *Cases of Extraordinary Obesity*

NAME	SEX	AGE AT DEATH	MAXIMUM WEIGHT LB.	KG
Lambert†	M	39	739	335
Darden°	M	59	1020	462
Campbell	M	22	732	332
Valenzuela°	M	39	850	385
Titman*	–	36	700	318
Zadina*	M	29	732	332
Raggio*	M	27	701	318
Maguire*	M	31	810	367
Karns*	F	28	745	338
Nunez*	F	23	756	343
Hall*	M	37	700	318
Pontico*	F	35	772	350
Hughes°	M	32	1069	485
Craig°	M	38	907	411
Knorr°	M	46	900	408
King°	F	35	840	381

†Bowmer (1969)
*Willoughby (1942)
°Guinness Book of Records (1974)

1

The rarity of individuals with extreme obesity points up the need for careful definitions of obesity and excess body weight when dealing with less obvious situations. The distinction between overweight and obesity is very important; for example, some athletes are heavier than nonathletes of comparable height, although the nonathletes may be fatter. Also, in studies of populations, it is important to have clear definitions of the criteria to be used for designating obesity.

DEFINITION OF TERMS

Obesity

Obesity is an excess of body fat. To establish whether an individual is obese requires first a measurement of body fat. It is then necessary to relate body fatness to some standard or range of acceptable degrees of fat for the particular population under study. As obesity varies in relation to age, sex and degree of physical activity, an accurate definition must also take these variables into account.

Overweight

Overweight is used to denote a body weight which is higher than some standard weight. Generally the standard weights are obtained from tables which provide appropriate, desirable or satisfactory weights in relation to height. A person is overweight when his or her body weight exceeds the limits provided by these standards. A discussion of some of the standards and their derivation is presented below. In most studies which have dealt with populations, the measurement obtained is body weight in relation to height. This relationship cannot be used satisfactorily to define cases of obesity.

Relative Weight

Relative weight refers to the deviation of body weight in relation to some arbitrary standard. These relative weights are usually expressed as a percentage deviation above or below the standard weight. Thus individuals with relative weights above the "ideal" or "desirable" weight are overweight, while those individuals with weights below the standard are said to be underweight.

Body Compartments

To provide a more accurate and complete description of the various components which comprise the body and the methods whereby they may be measured, the schematic diagram shown in Figure 1–1

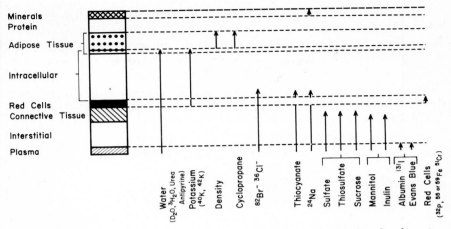

Figure 1–1. Body compartments as measured by various chemical and radioactive substances.

has been provided. The components of the body are divided into several groups including minerals, protein, adipose tissue, intracellular water, red cell mass, connective tissue, interstitial fluids and plasma. Each of these components of the body shall be defined and some of the techniques which can be used to measure them shall be discussed. Figure 1–1 also contains several techniques for measuring other components of body space which will not be dealt with here (details on these methods may be found in Moore et al., 1963; Brozek, Grande, Anderson and Keys, 1963; Brozek, 1965; the National Academy of Sciences Body Composition in Animals and Man, 1968; Behnke and Wilmore, 1974).

Body fat is the quantity of triglyceride and other fats which the body contains. This is indicated in Figure 1–1 as the major component of adipose tissue.

Body water refers to the total amount of water in the body. As indicated by Figure 1–1, this includes the water in plasma, in interstitial fluid, red cells, connective tissues, intracellular water and the part of the adipose tissue volume occupied by water. In this diagram, minerals, protein and triglycerides are excluded from body water compartments. The measurement of body water provides a volume by which lean body mass may be estimated by the appropriate correction. Figure 1–2 compares the fractionation of body water, fat and fat free solids by compartments obtained by measuring body density, body water (by ^3H_2O or H_2O) or body potassium (^{40}K or ^{42}Ke).

Lean body mass is that fraction of body weight which is required to contain total body water at the percentage normally found in lean tissues such as muscle and liver. This calculation, based on studies of animal tissues (Pace and Rathbun, 1945), is obtained by dividing total body water by 0.72.

Intracellular water is the fraction of body water which is contained within the cells. As indicated in Figure 1–1, it can be determined by calculating total body water and subtracting the water in the interstitial space and the water contained in connective tissue.

Extracellular water is the body water located outside of cells. This can be measured by a number of methods indicated in Figure 1–1.

Cell mass refers to the weight of the cellular components of the body. Since the principal inorganic constituent of cells is potassium, measurement of ^{40}K, a naturally occurring isotope of potassium or exchangeable potassium (Ke) determined by injecting the radioactive isotope ^{42}K, provides an estimate of cell mass. The distribution of potassium in body constituents is shown in Figure 1–1 and the calculation of cell mass from potassium is shown in Figure 1–2.

Fat free body is a term used to designate the nonfat fraction of body weight. This can be measured by determining density or using fat soluble chemicals such as cyclopropane. The fat free body is assumed to have a density of 1.10 (Keys and Brozek, 1953). A comparison of the amount of the body water, fat and fat free solids as measured by density, isotopic water or isotopic potassium is shown in Figure 1–2.

The *inorganic constituents* of the body include calcium, potassium, sodium, magnesium, phosphorus, iron and other salts and minerals. A list of the major inorganic constituents in the body and their

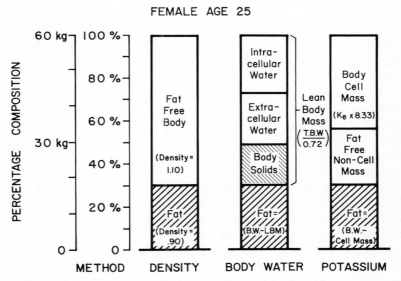

Figure 1–2. Comparison of the body compartments as determined by measuring density, the distribution of radioactive water, and the quantity of body potassium. (T.B.W.=Total body water; Ke=Exchangeable potassium; B.W.=Body Weight; L.B.M.=Lean body mass.)

TABLE 1–2. *Body Constituents in a 70 kg Man*

CONSTITUENT	MASS (KG)	PERCENTAGE
Major constituents		
Water	42.0	60
Fat	14.0	20
Protein	10.5	15
Minor constituents		
Calcium	1.00	
Magnesium	.0025	
Iron	.005	
Zinc	.002	5
Copper	.001	
Iodine	.0002	
Manganese	.0002	
Molybdenum	.0002	

relative proportions in comparison with the organic constituents is shown in Table 1–2.

METHODS OF DETERMINING BODY COMPOSITION

Direct Methods

The only direct method is analysis of carcass composition. This has been performed on cadavers of 8 adults within the past 50 years (Mitchell et al., 1945; Widdowson, McCance and Spray, 1951; Forbes, Cooper and Mitchell, 1953; Forbes, Mitchell and Cooper, 1956; Forbes and Lewis, 1956). The results of analysis on 5 disease free carcasses is depicted in Figure 1–3 (Widdowson, 1965). The data are presented as the mean with the range of values shown by the vertical bars. Water content was 60 percent with a range of 50 to 73 percent. Protein and fat were both nearly identical at 17 and 18 percent. Ash represented approximately 5 percent of total body weight (this represents the sum of the many macro and micro minerals, some of which are listed in Table 1–2). Such analysis is both cumbersome and difficult to perform, yet it provides a background of information which is essential for comparison with the indirect methods used in studies of living human subjects.

Indirect Methods

There are several methods used for assessing body composition. The indirect methods fall into several groups. The first are the simple rules which can be used to assess body weight and, by inference, body fatness. The second group are the anthropometric measurements

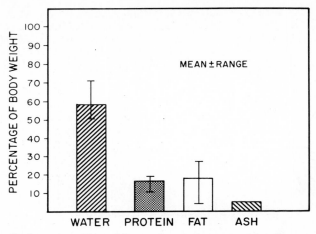

Figure 1–3. Body composition of five cadavers determined by direct analysis. The height of the individual bars indicates the mean for five patients and the vertical lines represent the range. Body components are plotted as a percentage of the total body weight. (Calculated from Widdowson, E. M. *In* Human Body Composition: Approaches and Applications, (J. Brozek, ed.), London, Pergamon Press, 1965.)

which rely on external body dimensions to estimate fatness. The third group uses measurements of density to divide the body weight into its fat and fat free body mass. The fourth group of methods are those involving dilutional techniques. They are more specialized and thus of more limited practical value.

SIMPLE RULES

There are several simple rules for testing body fatness. The following is one of the simplest. At a height of 60 inches (150 cm), 100 pounds (45 kg) is a desirable weight for a woman and 106 pounds (48 kg) for a man. For each extra inch (2.5 cm) above this height, 5 pounds is added to the woman's weight and 6 pounds to the man's weight. The Broca index which is also widely used estimates the appropriate weight in kilograms by subtracting 100 from the height in centimeters.* If body weight is greater than the height in centimeters −100, then you are "overweight" and in most instances "obese." This rule is applied to both males and females, although it lacks reliability due to the differences in fat content which occur between males and females.

Another rule of thumb is the so-called "magic 36." If the waist dimension in inches subtracted from the height in inches is less than 36, the individual is probably obese. On the other hand, if the waist circumference taken from the height in inches is more than 36, the

---

*To calculate height in centimeters from height in inches, one needs to multiply the height in inches by 2.54 (cm); and to convert weight in kilograms to weight in pounds, one needs to divide the weight in pounds by 2.2 (kg).

individual may be presumed to be of normal weight. The ruler test is a fourth simple test. With the subject supine a ruler is laid between the manubrium (lower end of the breast bone) and the pubic bone. If body fat content is normal the ruler should not touch the skin on the abdomen. Still another test is the belt test in which a belt is placed around the waist and then around the chest at the breast line. If the waist measurement is larger than the chest measurement, obesity is probably present.

Finally, one can use the "mirror test." This is the simplest and most commonly used method of self-assessment of obesity. It requires individual scrutiny before a mirror to determine whether or not one is "fat." These indirect measures are obviously limited in value since factors such as sex, age and physical conditioning, all of which play a role in determining the distribution of body weight between muscle and fat, have not been considered. Moreover, these methods do not quantify the deviation (if any) and are thus of value only to one's personal assessment. The exception is Broca's index which has been used to assess overweight in several studies.

ANTHROPOMETRIC MEASUREMENTS

Several techniques are available for measuring body size and fat. They include measurement of skinfold thickness, circumferences of arms, legs and chest, diameters of shoulders and hips, and measurement of fat thickness by soft x-ray and ultrasound.

HEIGHT AND WEIGHT. The measure of body weight has provided an enormous amount of information about relative degrees of overweight in many populations. In general, the appropriate or desirable weight for each height is determined by reference to some appropriate table of heights and weights. The most widely used reference table is one prepared by the Metropolitan Life Insurance Company based on the distribution of body weights at which minimal mortality rates were observed among insured policy holders. For children under 5 years of age the tables of Tanner and Whitehouse (1973) are most useful.

This table has the advantage of selecting ranges of appropriate body weights independent of measured values since it was based upon minimal rates of mortality. Weights are divided into three ranges based on body frame size. Unfortunately there are no criteria for determination of an appropriate "frame size." In the absence of such criteria, an adaptation of this table may be utilized in which the average weight for the middle frame is used as a reference point, with acceptable body weights ranging between the lowest level for the small frame and highest level for the large frame (Table 1–3). Individuals deviating above the upper limits of this top weight for height

TABLE 1-3. *Average Weight in Relation to Height**

HEIGHT		MEN				WOMEN			
		Pounds		Kilograms		Pounds		Kilograms	
Feet	Meters	Average	Range	Average	Range	Average	Range	Average	Range
4'10"	1.47	–	–	–	–	102	92-119	46.3	41.7-54.0
4'11"	1.50	–	–	–	–	104	94-122	47.1	42.6-55.3
5' 0"	1.52	–	–	–	–	107	96-125	48.5	43.5-56.7
5' 1"	1.55	–	–	–	–	110	99-128	50.0	44.9-58.1
5' 2"	1.58	123	112-141	55.8	50.8-63.9	113	102-131	51.3	46.3-59.4
5' 3"	1.60	127	115-144	57.6	52.2-65.3	116	105-134	52.6	47.6-60.8
5' 4"	1.63	130	118-148	58.9	53.5-67.1	120	108-138	54.4	49.0-62.6
5' 5"	1.65	133	121-152	60.3	54.9-68.9	123	111-142	55.8	50.3-64.4
5' 6"	1.68	136	124-156	61.7	56.2-70.8	128	114-146	58.1	51.7-66.2
5' 7"	1.70	140	128-161	63.5	58.1-73.0	132	118-150	59.9	53.5-68.0
5' 8"	1.73	145	132-166	65.8	59.9-75.3	136	122-154	61.7	55.3-69.9
5' 9"	1.75	149	136-170	67.6	61.7-77.1	140	126-158	63.5	57.2-71.7
5'10"	1.78	153	140-174	69.4	63.5-78.9	144	130-163	65.3	59.0-73.9
5'11"	1.80	158	144-179	71.7	65.3-81.2	148	134-168	67.1	60.8-70.2
6' 0"	1.83	162	148-184	73.5	67.1-83.5	152	138-173	68.9	62.6-78.5
6' 1"	1.85	166	152-189	75.3	68.9-85.7	–	–	–	–
6' 2"	1.88	171	156-194	77.6	70.8-88.0	–	–	–	–
6' 3"	1.91	176	160-199	79.8	72.6-90.3	–	–	–	–
6' 4"	1.93	181	164-204	82.1	74.4-92.5	–	–	–	–

*Adapted from the table of the Metropolitan Life Insurance Company.
It is recommended that height be taken while the subject is without shoes, and that weight be measured with the subject in light clothing or no clothing.

can be said to be overweight. These upper limits are approximately 15 percent above the median weight for the normal frame size. Body weight generally needs to deviate from the average figure shown in Table 1–3 by more than 30 percent to have medical significance. (The medical consequences are presented in Chapter 6.)

The chief advantage of utilizing height and weight tables to assess overweight is the simplicity with which these measurements can be made. Their limitations, however, are serious. First, insurance company figures are often based on patients' statements about their weight and height and may not reflect actual measurement (Keys, 1975). Second, weights were obtained in street clothing, adding a variable amount of weight ranging from 2 to nearly 10 pounds depending upon climate and time of year. Third, height was measured in shoes. The insurance company tables allow two inches for heels on women's shoes and one inch for heels on men's shoes. Since heel sizes vary from year to year, the recording of height, even when measured, is probably not a "true" height.

No matter how careful the procedure for measurements of height and weight, the weights provide only fair estimates of body fat (Keys et al., 1972; Benn, 1970, 1971; Florey, 1970; Kannel and Gordon, 1974). There are several ways in which height and weight can be related. Relative weight is the most common correlation. It expresses measured weight as a percentage of the appropriate weight according to height using a standard table. Three ratios are also in wide use. These are weight/height, weight/(height)^2 (the body mass index), and height/$^3\sqrt{\text{weight}}$, (the ponderal index).

In a study of the properties of these various relationships between weight and height Benn (1971) and Florey (1970) concluded that weight/height is the most appropriate index for women and weight/(height)^2 is most appropriate for men. Keys et al. (1972) have recently compared these three ratios with body fat measured by density and skinfolds. In general the ratios had correlations of $r = 0.7$ to $r = 0.8$ with the independent measures of body fat. Among these three ratios, the body mass index [weight/(height)^2] had the highest correlation in over half of the comparisons. In all comparisons of height and weight the ponderal index (height/$^3\sqrt{\text{weight}}$) was the least satisfactory. Therefore, for epidemiologic studies where only height and weight are available, it would appear to be most appropriate to use weight/height or weight/(height)^2 as the measures of choice. It would be far better, however, to incorporate an additional measure of fatness such as skinfold thickness or body circumferences (Seltzer et al. 1970).

Height and weight can also be used to estimate surface area. The most widely used equation is that of DuBois and DuBois (1916).

$$\text{Surface area (SA)} = 0.007184 \ (\text{ht})^{0.725} \ (\text{wt})^{0.425} \ ; \tag{1}$$
$$\text{ht in cm, wt in kg, SA in square meters.}$$

Van Graan and Wyndham (1964) have evaluated the DuBois formula against two independent methods. The surface area derived from measurement of surface radiation and from a "coating technique" agrees closely and are both 6.6 per cent higher than the DuBois formula.

SKINFOLD THICKNESS. Since the quantities of subcutaneous fat and the fat located within the body cavities are correlated (Alexander, 1964), the measurement of skinfold thickness can provide a potentially useful technique for evaluating total body fat. Because the thickness of the skin from site to site usually deviates between 0.8 and 1.1 mm, most of the distance between a fold of skin represents subcutaneous fat. By measuring this thickness one can estimate body fatness by referring to appropriate tables; Table 1–4 for children (Seltzer and Mayer, 1965) and Table 1–5 for adults (Durnin and Womersley, 1974).

The major problem with measurements of skinfold thickness is the selection of an appropriate site for measurement, obtaining an appropriate instrument, defining precisely the area to be measured, and having sufficient practice to obtain reproducible and reliable results. The two primary instruments in use for determining skinfold thickness are the Harpenden calipers and the Lange calipers (see Figure 1–4). They both apply a known pressure across the caliper tips whose distance can be read from a calibrated dial.

Variations in skinfold thickness are related to diverse factors, in-

TABLE 1–4. *Obesity Standards for Caucasian Americans**
(Miminum triceps skinfold thickness in millimeters indicating obesity.)†

AGE (YEARS)	SKINFOLD MEASUREMENTS	
	Males	Females
5	12	14
6	12	15
7	13	16
8	14	17
9	15	18
10	16	20
11	17	21
12	18	22
13	18	23
14	17	23
15	16	24
16	15	25
17	14	26
18	15	27
19	15	27

*Adapted from Seltzer, C. C. and Mayer, J.: A simple criterion of obesity. Postgrad. Med. 38:A101-107, 1965, copyright McGraw-Hill.

†Figures represent the logarithmic means of the frequency distributions plus one standard deviation.

TABLE 1–5. *The equivalent fat content, as a percentage of body weight, for a range of values for the sum of 4 skinfolds (biceps, triceps, subscapular and suprailiac) of males and females of different ages.* *

	PERCENTAGE FAT							
SKIN-FOLDS mm	Males 17 to 29	30 to 39 years	40 to 49	50+	Females 16 to 29	30 to 39 years	40 to 49	50+
15	4.8				10.5			
20	8.1	12.2	12.2	12.6	14.1	17.0	19.8	21.4
25	10.5	14.2	15.0	15.6	16.8	19.4	22.2	24.0
30	12.9	16.2	17.7	18.6	19.5	21.8	24.5	26.6
35	14.7	17.7	19.6	20.8	21.5	23.7	26.4	28.5
40	16.4	19.2	21.4	22.9	23.4	25.5	28.2	30.3
45	17.7	20.4	23.0	24.7	25.0	26.9	29.6	31.9
50	19.0	21.5	24.6	26.5	26.5	28.2	31.0	33.4
55	20.1	22.5	25.9	27.9	27.8	29.4	32.1	34.6
60	21.2	23.5	27.1	29.2	29.1	30.6	33.2	35.7
65	22.2	24.3	28.2	30.4	30.2	31.6	34.1	36.7
70	23.1	25.1	29.3	31.6	31.2	32.5	35.0	37.7
75	24.0	25.9	30.3	32.7	32.2	33.4	35.9	38.7
80	24.8	26.6	31.2	33.8	33.1	34.3	36.7	39.6
85	25.5	27.2	32.1	34.8	34.0	35.1	37.5	40.4
90	26.2	27.8	33.0	35.8	34.8	35.8	38.3	41.2
95	26.9	28.4	33.7	36.6	35.6	36.5	39.0	41.9
100	27.6	29.0	34.4	37.4	36.4	37.2	39.7	42.6
105	28.2	29.6	35.1	38.2	37.1	37.9	40.4	43.3
110	28.8	30.1	35.8	39.0	37.8	38.6	41.0	43.9
115	29.4	30.6	36.4	39.7	38.4	39.1	41.5	44.5
120	30.0	31.1	37.0	40.4	39.0	39.6	42.0	45.1
125	30.5	31.5	37.6	41.1	39.6	40.1	42.5	45.7
130	31.0	31.9	38.2	41.8	40.2	40.6	43.0	46.2
135	31.5	32.3	38.7	42.4	40.8	41.1	43.5	46.7
140	32.0	32.7	39.2	43.0	41.3	41.6	44.0	47.2
145	32.5	33.1	39.7	43.6	41.8	42.1	44.5	47.7
150	32.9	33.5	40.2	44.1	42.3	42.6	45.0	48.2
155	33.3	33.9	40.7	44.6	42.8	43.1	45.4	48.7
160	33.7	34.3	41.2	45.1	43.3	43.6	45.8	49.2
165	34.1	34.6	41.6	45.6	43.7	44.0	46.2	49.6
170	34.5	34.8	42.0	46.1	44.1	44.4	46.6	50.0
175	34.9					44.8	47.0	50.4
180	35.3					45.2	47.4	50.8
185	35.6					45.6	47.8	51.2
190	35.9					45.9	48.2	51.6
195						46.2	48.5	52.0
200						46.5	48.8	52.4
205							49.1	52.7
210							49.4	53.0

*Durnin, J. G. V. A., and J. Womersley, Brit. J. Nutr., 32:77-97, 1974.

cluding sex (Durnin and Womersley, 1974; Clemente et al., 1973; Edwards, 1951), ethnic origin (Robson, 1971; Young, 1965), and age (Durnin and Womersley, 1974). There is no single skinfold measure which is a reliable index of total body fat for both men and women.
Reliability also varies with the degree of experience of the indi-

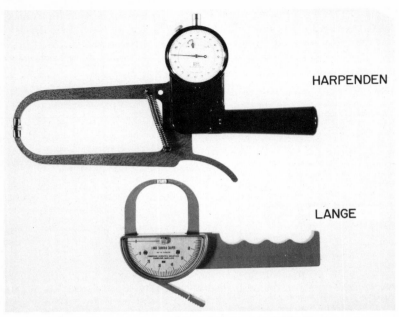

HARPENDEN

LANGE

Figure 1–4.   Harpenden and Lange skinfold calipers.

vidual using the calipers. In one study in which three observers measured skinfold thickness on 21 subjects on three occasions, the degree of variability depended upon whether the region to be measured was marked by the first observer. When site selection was not designated, differences in measurement averaged 2 mm higher for the two inexperienced observers than for the individual with experience in the use of calipers (Burkinshaw et al., 1973). The variability in skinfolds is particularly prominent over the triceps area (Ruiz, Colley and Hamilton, 1971). The skinfold 2.5 cm above the midpoint of the triceps has been found to be significantly thicker than that at the midpoint; whereas 2.5 cm below the midpoint it is significantly thinner. Deviations in caliper placement toward the medial or lateral side also produce significant deviations in the "recorded" measurement of triceps skinfold. Durnin, Armstrong, and Womersley (1973) have reported similar findings indicating the serious limitations in the use of skinfold calipers except by experienced observers.

Another problem with the use of skinfolds as a measure of body fatness is age (Durnin and Womersley, 1974). For a given skinfold measurement, body fat content increases with age. This may mean that the fat content in subcutaneous sites other than those being measured is rising with age, or that the deposition of body fat with age occurs at sites other than subcutaneous tissue. It would appear that with age proportionally less fat is deposited in commonly measured subcutaneous areas than in other depots. A final problem with skinfold calipers arises in measuring obese patients. Variability of measurements by five physicians working in an obesity clinic was smaller when measuring lean subjects. When more obese people were examined, the variability of measurements between different doctors rose. The fatter the patient the less reliable were the estimates of skinfold thickness. We have thus concluded that skinfold calipers are probably useful in large scale epidemiologic studies but that they have limited use in quantifying fat in obese patients.

Several investigators have developed equations correlating measurements of skinfolds at several sites on the body with measurements of circumferences or diameters in an effort to improve the estimation of body fat (Clemente et al., 1973; Garn, 1955; Hermansen and von Döbeln, 1971; Parizkova and Buzkova, 1971; Steinkamp et al., 1965). One group has even developed a nomogram for this purpose (Sloan and Weir, 1970). Steinkamp et al. have shown that correlations as high as $r = .98$ for measurements of skinfold thickness and circumferences with body fat can be obtained by using multiple measurements of body dimensions. The independent measurements of body fatness were obtained from measurements of density or dilution of radioactive water (see below).

The body measurements recommended by Steinkamp et al. are often used but, unfortunately, those which provide the most reliable estimate of body fat for white males aged 25 to 35 are not the same measurements which provide the best estimate of fat for older white males (ages 35 to 45), nor for black males of either age. Moreover, calculations of fatness for females require yet another set of measurements. Thus accurate assessment of body fat by measuring skinfolds requires appropriate indices for the subjects under question as well as skill and experience in their use.

Clemente et al. (1973) examined the correlation between body fat as assessed from measurements of cell mass (^{40}K), weight/(height)^2 (body mass index), and skinfolds. They found that, for females, body fat (^{40}K) had a correlation of $r = .909$ with weight/(height)^2, and was only improved to $r = .927$ by the addition of 4 skinfold measurements. For males weight/(height)^2 provided a reasonably adequate assessment of fatness with an $r = .827$, but the correlation was improved considerably by the inclusion of several skinfolds. The data of Crook et al. (1966) indicated that the subscapular skinfold was better than the triceps skinfold or the percent overweight in its correlation with body fat estimated by ^{40}K.

Similarly Montoye, Epstein, and Kjelsberg (1965) found that the subscapular skinfold reflected changes in body weight more accurately than the triceps skinfold. Hermansen and von Döbeln (1971) measured 11 separate skinfolds which were used singly and in various combinations to correlate with body density as an independent measure of body fat. They showed that in the 19 male and 19 female students the abdominal and suprapatellar skinfold gave the most accurate estimate of fat. The addition of any or all of the other 9 skinfolds did not significantly improve this relationship.

Seltzer and Mayer (1965) have proposed a criterion for obesity based on the measurement of the triceps skinfold (Table 1–4). This criterion was used alone in the Ten State Nutrition Survey (1972), and with other skinfolds and body weight measurements (Ruffer, 1970). Comparative studies point out the difficulties in measuring the triceps skinfold (Ruiz et al., 1971), and the relatively lower correlation it has with other measures of fatness (Parizkova and Buzkova, 1971; Montoye, Epstein and Kjelsberg, 1965; Seltzer and Mayer, 1967).

Parizkova and Buzkova measured 4 skinfolds in 101 males, using density as the independent measurement of body fat. Triceps skinfold had the poorest correlation with percentage of body fat at (r = .43); the subscapular skinfold correlation was r = .56; the suprailiac fold was r = .67; and the biceps was r = .59. These data would support the relative superiority of the subscapular fat fold for predicting body fat. When more than one skinfold is used, the correlation is generally improved (Table 1–5). With the current state of the art of measuring skinfold thickness, it would appear reasonable to encourage the measurement of skinfolds in at least two sites. Skinfold measurements, if carefully performed and referred to, are appropriate standards in population studies and serve as an important addition to the use of height/weight relationships in estimating obesity.

CIRCUMFERENCES AND DIAMETERS. Measurements of the distance around the neck, chest, waist, hips or thighs can be used for assessing body structure, as can the diameters or distances between the shoulders or hips (biacromal—distance between acromial joints; bideltoid—distance between deltoid muscles; biiliac—distance between iliac crests; bitrochanteric—distance between greater trochanters). Behnke and Wilmore (1974) (Wilmore and Behnke, 1968, 1970) have developed sophisticated formulas for estimating body fat from these data. Each individual measurement on a subject is compared with standards obtained from the dimensions of the "reference" male or female. The deviations of the actual measurements from the normal measurements are plotted on a somatogram. This allows a graphic representation of the deviations from normal of various parts of the body. During weight reduction, for example, the largest changes on the somatogram occur in the abdominal region. The complexity of preparing the somatograms makes the method interesting, but of less than practical value.

The studies of Steinkamp et al. (1965) showed the value of measuring the circumference of the chest, waist or hips. The circumference at the iliac crest, for example, had a correlation coefficient with body fat which ranged from r = 0.815 to r = 0.938. The circumference was almost as good. Although other circumferences or skin-folds were sometimes better in selected age groups, these two had the widest applicability.

Vague and his colleagues have also explored the use of circumferences to classify obesity (Vague et al., 1974). They compared a number of anthropometric methods for estimating fatness and concluded that the measurement of skinfold thickness at the proximal part of the upper arm and thigh, along with the circumference at the same point, was the most valuable. The ratio of the skinfold thickness divided by the circumference at each site is termed the adipomuscular ratio for the arm (BAMR) or for the leg (FAMR). For a normal weight male the BAMR is 0.21 and the FAMR 0.19, giving a B/F AMR of 1.10 for the male. In the female, however, there is more fat on the thighs. Thus the BAMR is 0.48, indicating a relatively thicker triceps fat fold than in the male. The FAMR, however, is 0.63, showing that the thigh is relatively fatter than the arm in women. The ratio of these two numbers for the normal female 25 to 30 years of age is 0.77 (compared to 1.10 in the male), indicating that the thigh has more fat than the arm.

In our experience the variability of measurements of circumferences between one subject and the next is smaller than for the measurements of skinfolds. More important, however, is that the variation in measuring the circumferences in obese patients is not less accurate than similar measurements in lean subjects. This implies that formulas involving circumferences should be more reliable and easier to use than those involving skinfolds.

SOMATOTYPING.   The concept of the "somatotype" is generally associated with Dr. Sheldon who has done the most to develop it (Sheldon, 1954). This technique involves the analysis of three photographs of each subject. One picture is from the front, one from the back, and one from the side. These are analyzed for the endomorphy, ectomorphy and mesomorphy, which are the three primary components of body structure (see Fig. 1–5). Each component is given a rating which ranges from 1 (minimum for the trait) to 7 (maximum for that trait). Endomorphy is the first component and refers to the roundness of the subject and to the fact that these individuals put on fat easily. The second component, referred to as mesomorphy, denotes the muscular structure. The third component, ectomorphy, refers to linearity or tallness. Seltzer and Mayer (1964) have utilized this technique to compare lean and obese teenagers. They clearly showed the preponderance of endomorphic traits in the obese girls and the low level of ectomorphy. Interestingly, the two groups of lean and obese girls had similar levels of mesomorphy. The concept of assigning a body type to an individual is attractive, but it requires considerable skill and training. For this reason it has not received wide use.

DENSITY.   The measurement of density is another approach to assessing body composition. Over 2000 years ago Archimedes intro-

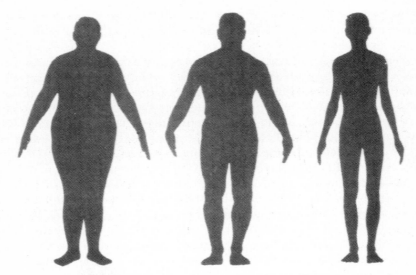

Endomorphic   Mesomorphic   Ectomorphic

Figure 1–5. Outlines of the three primary components of body structure. (Medcom-New York, 1973, p. 16. Obesity: Data and Directions for the 70's. Frederek Stare, Editor).

duced this technique. With it he determined the content of gold in a crown which the king thought might also contain lead. In the study of body fat this technique was first systematically applied by Behnke (1942; Behnke, Feen and Welham, 1942; Welham and Behnke, 1942; Keys and Brozek, 1953). The basic principle behind the measures of density is that any submerged object displaces its own weight in water. The density of a patient can thus be determined by weighing the individual before and after submersion in water, or by determining the volume of water which he displaces (Krzyswicki and Chinn, 1967; Pearson, Purchas and Reincke, 1968; Friis-Hansen, 1965; Parizkova, 1963; Wilmore and Behnke, 1968, 1970; Brozek et al., 1963).

The simplest technique involves placing the subject in an appropriate tank strapped to a chair or other supporting structure which is in turn attached to a sensitive scale. After the subject has maximally exhaled and the body is totally submerged, its weight is accurately recorded. A measurement of residual lung volume taken simultaneously is essential for the most accurate calculation of density from underwater weighing. Estimating residual volume increases the error slightly. From the measurements of density, the percentage of body fat can be calculated using one of several equations (see Pierson and Lin, 1972). The constants in these equations are based on the assumption of an average density for the fat and nonfat components. Brozek et al. (1963) found that at 36° the density of fat is 0.9007. Assuming the density for the nonfat body to be 1.10, then the average density of the reference body is 1.064. Figure 1–2 shows the fractionation of body

(Booth, Goddard and Paton, 1966; Strakova and Markova, 1971; Alsmeyer, Hiner and Thornton, 1963; Hawes et al., 1972). The technique consists of placing an ultrasound generator over the skin and measuring the reflection from various layers. The first reflection to be detected is from the fat and muscle interface. Thus the measurement obtained by ultrasound includes both skin and fat. Since skin thickness is fairly uniform, the differences are primarily a function of the fat layer.

Strakova and Markova found no significant differences between the thickness of subcutaneous fat as measured by skin fold calipers and ultrasound measurements over the biceps, triceps, chest or abdomen, but they did find significant differences in the measurement of fat thickness of the scapular and thigh regions. Booth et al. compared 26 males and 15 females whose fat thickness was measured by ultrasound, electrical conductivity and Harpenden skinfold calipers. Ultrasound proved the most reliable. Electrical conductivity was also accurate but was unpleasant. The skin calipers were the least reliable. The correlation coefficients between skin-fat thickness as estimated by ultrasound or electrical conductivity was $r = .98$. For the Harpenden calipers the correlations with conductivity and ultrasound were both $r = 0.81$, substantially lower than with ultrasound alone. Thus the ultrasound technique performed by a skilled technician provides the potential for quantifying fat thickness with high reliability.

FACTORS WHICH INFLUENCE BODY COMPOSITION

Body composition varies with sex, age, physical activity and dietary habits. Each of these variables is examined below.

Sex

Body fat content differs significantly between men and women (Ljunggren, 1965). Before puberty, however, there is little or no difference in the body composition of males and females (Anderson, 1963; Friis-Hansen, 1965; Forbes, 1972; Cheek, 1968; Flynn et al., 1972; Tanner, 1965). In a study of skinfold thicknesses measured at ten sites in newborn infants, Parizkova (1959) noted no significant differences in the group of 48 boys and 48 girls, though the sum of the skinfold thicknesses tended to be slightly larger for the girls. Skinfold thickness over the hips, however, was significantly greater in girls, and this difference persisted even during the period of weight loss between the second and fifth postnatal day. This has recently been confirmed by Huenemann (1974).

At the onset of puberty, the skinfold thicknesses of females become significantly higher than those in males. The increase in body

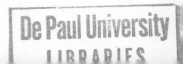

fat content during puberty is accompanied by a decrease in potassium content in females (Parizkova, 1963; Seltzer and Mayer, 1965; Anderson and Langum, 1959; Anderson, 1963; Forbes, 1968). At the end of puberty females have between 18 to 25 percent body fat, whereas males have only 12 to 18 percent (Friis-Hansen, 1965; Cheek et al., 1970). These changes in fat determined by measurements of density or by counting total body potassium are supported by the studies using soft x-ray.

Garn and Haskell (1959a, b) observed a statistically significant correlation between the thickness of subcutaneous fat over the lower thoracic vertebrae and the skeletal age of children. They also noted that the age of fusion of the tibial epiphysis and the age of menarche in girls could be predicted from this measurement. Between the ages of 12 and 17 this fat pad evinced no increase in boys but showed a progressive increase in girls, corresponding with the known rise in body fat and increased skinfold thickness in females during puberty. In summary, the development of secondary sexual characteristics at puberty is associated with significant alterations in body composition; there is an increase in the percentage of fat in females, and an increase in cell mass and a decrease in the percentage of body fat of males.

Age

Body fat content changes not only at the time of puberty but throughout adult life. These changes in body fat are accompanied by reciprocal changes in body water and cell mass (see Fig. 1–7). During the first trimester of pregnancy, body water accounts for 94 percent of the body weight of the fetus (Friis-Hansen, 1965; Fomon, 1967). This falls to 82 percent during the third trimester when fetal body fat content is rising from barely detectable levels to the 12 percent found at birth. By the end of the first month of life, body fat content has risen further to 16 percent and reaches a maximum of about 30 percent by the end of the first year of life. There is then a gradual decline of nearly one third in the percentage of body fat from age one through age 9. At the beginning of puberty, body fat content represents only 15 to 20 percent of total body weight. As previously noted, the body fat content of males and females diverges with the onset of puberty. Girls show a striking rise and males show both an absolute and relative decrease in total body fat during sexual maturation (Pierson and Lin, 1972).

Changes in body composition do not end with attainment of adult stature (Garn and Harper, 1955b; Lesser, Kumar and Steele, 1963). From the end of puberty onwards, there is a steady increase in the percentage of body fat and a small decline in lean body mass (Fig. 1–7). The data from several cross sectional studies of men and women have been summarized by Forbes and Reina (1970) (see also Behnke,

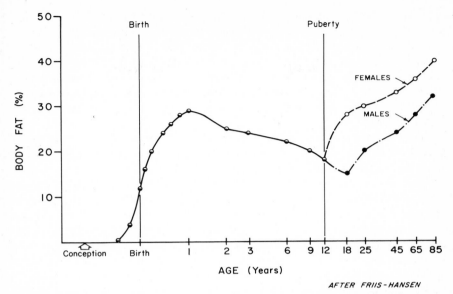

Figure 1–7. Changing body composition from gestation through adult life. (From Friis-Hansen: *In* Human Body Composition. (J. Brozek, ed.), Oxford, Pergamon Press, 1965, pp. 191–209.)

1963; Krzywicki and Chinn, 1967; Young et al., 1963; Norris, Lundy and Shock, 1963; Flynn et al., 1968). The cross sectional and longitudinal data both show a decline in lean body mass and an increase in the percentage of body fat in men and women from age 20 through the fifth or sixth decade. This rise in fat is concomitant with the decline in body water and the gradual decrease in body density, which falls from 1.072 to 1.041 g/cc in men and from 1.040 to 1.016 in women during adult life (Brozek, 1965).

Physical Activity

Physical activity can also alter body composition. This has been demonstrated clearly by Welham and Behnke (1942) using measurements of body density applied to overweight professional football players who were muscular (not fat) and who had a higher body density than normal subjects. The effects of physical training on body composition in children and adults have also been studied by Parizkova (1963, 1965), Björntorp et al. (1975) and by Keys and Brozek (1953). All of the studies performed on normal subjects during exercise show a decrease in total fat content and an increase in muscle mass with or without change in body weight.

For example, Behnke and Taylor (1959) found that body density of five athletes ranged from 1.069 to 1.094 gm/sq cm. This latter figure is just below the density assumed for lean body mass (e.g., 1.100) and indicates little fat and mainly muscle. The body composition of adult men can also be modified by long term continued exercise. The longitudal studies reported by Forbes and Reina (1970) and by Keys et al. (1973) showed that body composition could be maintained relatively constant over many years when the subjects undertook regular exercise. Thus the increasing fatness observed with age appears to result from decreased physical activity and can be prevented by regular exercise.

Parizkova (1963) showed that the increase in muscle mass and decrease in body fat associated with athletic training for the Olympic games or other athletic events is reversed in the post-training period. In subjects preparing for the Olympic games, body density in female athletes increased from 1.054 to 1.058 g/cc. Total skinfold thicknesses decreased from just over 100 mm to approximately 85 mm. Body weight, however, showed no significant change, remaining at 54 kg. At the end of the training period, the body density fell to less than 1.050. This indication of increasing body fatness was associated with an increase in skinfold thickness to a level higher than that recorded in the pre-training period. Body weight also increased, indicating that decrease in lean tissue was more than offset by a rise in the mass of adipose tissue.

Physical activity also has a significant effect on body composition of animals other than man. When male guinea pigs were maintained on a regimen of severe exercise, body weight was reduced 15 percent and body fat content was reduced by more than 20 percent when compared to sedentary animals (Pitts, 1956). There are also significant differences in the body fat content of animals living in their natural environment, as compared to those in captivity (Pitts and Bullard, 1968). The latter tend to be fatter than those living in the wild.

This investigation also noted a highly significant association between body fat content and body weight. In the small mouse, body fat content was 3.5 percent, while in the whale it was 35 percent of lean body weight. It is interesting to note that many adult human beings have a body fat content that is proportionally as high or higher than in the whale! An extreme example of the effect of inactivity is the gross obesity (Ingle, 1943) which develops when rodents are confined in small cages to restrict their activity but allowed free access to a nutritious and palatable diet. Under such circumstances body weight will increase to nearly twice that of animals of the same age and sex which are allowed adequate physical activity.

Miscellaneous Factors

A number of other factors, in addition to sex, age and physical activity, can also modify body composition. One of these is the frequency with which food is ingested. Cohn and his collaborators

(Cohn, 1963; Cohn and Joseph, 1959) showed that body fat content was increased when rats were given food by stomach tube twice daily in an amount equal to that eaten during the entire 24 hours by control rats. Although gross body weight did not differ, the fat content of the animals fed by stomach tube was often twice as high as in the animals allowed to eat their food ad libitum. The observation that decreasing the frequency of ingestion, but not the amount, can cause an increase in body fat content has been confirmed in many laboratories. Whether the effect applies to species other than the rat, however, is not yet settled. In an animal study, Reid et al. (1968) compared one group of sheep which was allowed to eat eight times per day with another group allowed to eat only once per day. They could find no difference in the quantity of body fat relative to lean body tissue in the sheep. Data on other species are needed to interpret this phenomenon as it relates to obesity.

Diabetes in the mother is another factor which influences body composition of newborn infants (Osler and Pedersen, 1960; Fee and Weil, 1963). These infants are considerably fatter than normal at birth. In the series published by Osler and Pedersen, the 122 diabetic infants weighed on the average 550 gm. more than the control infants. Body water and extracellular water were both decreased in the diabetic infants, but intracellular water was preserved, indicating maximal stores of glycogen.

Body fat was higher at all gestational ages and represented 20 percent of the body weight of full term infants of diabetic mothers, compared to 10 percent in infants of nondiabetic mothers (Fee and Weil, 1963). Although birth weights were heavier, skeletal growth as measured by ossification centers was not advanced and may even have been retarded in the diabetic infants. The presumptive explanation for this effect is the increased levels of insulin during prenatal life of children of diabetic mothers. This increase is a result of the high circulating levels of glucose in the mother and in the fetus. The high fat content at birth declines rapidly during the first weeks of life and these infants develop body fat contents comparable to those of other infants of the same age.

It is common knowledge that many cigarette smokers gain weight when they stop smoking, but evidence documenting this effect is contradictory. Khosla and Lowe (1972) reported on the body weight of 17,836 Welsh miners. Men over 40 years of age who had never smoked were, on the average, 12 pounds heavier than the smokers. This effect was observed in all social classes. In men who had previously smoked, body weight increased to approach that of the nonsmokers. However, Waller and Brooks (1972) failed to find any effect of smoking. They measured the height and weight of 2169 men. Although height decreased as age increased the older men were heavier than the younger men. There were no significant differences in weight between smokers and nonsmokers. The larger sample in the study by Khosla and Lowe, as well as the fact that their data is more consistent with the usual experience, leads the author to believe that smokers are probably significantly lighter than nonsmokers.

BODY COMPOSITION IN OBESITY

An increased content of body fat is the hallmark of obesity. Up to this point the normal limits of fat for the human body have not been defined because, at present, a precise definition is unattainable. Since sex, age, and physical activity all significantly modify the fraction of body weight which is fat, any definition or standard must consider these variables. As a working guideline, however, males with a body fat content in excess of 20 percent and females with an excess of 28 percent are probably obese.

Numerous studies have examined body fat content in obese patients. These have utilized two different approaches: static measurements of body fat content in normal and overweight individuals and examination of the changes in body fat content during weight gain or weight loss. In 1964 Forbes noted that one group of obese children had a higher content of body potassium than another group of obese children. He suggested that there might be two kinds of childhood obesity, one of which was associated with a greater lean body mass than the other. More recent studies on childhood obesity (Cheek et al., 1970; Mellits et al., 1970; Friis-Hansen, 1965; Flynn, 1968) have not supported this concept. It appears, rather, that changes in lean body tissue in relation to height are comparable in obese and lean individuals. What Forbes had observed was that many obese children show an earlier increase in height (see Chapter 5). When body composition is plotted against height, the major difference between lean and obese children is in the total body fat.

Differences in body composition of a 70 and 100 kg male are presented in Table 1–6 (Olesen, 1965). The increase of 30 kg was accounted for by a 51 percent increase in fat, a 26 percent increase in cell mass, and a 23 percent increase in extracellular water and other components. An increment of 30 kg in a 25 year old female was associated with a greater fractional deposition of fat. In this instance, the increased body fat content represented 63 percent of the total weight gain, whereas cell mass represented 18 percent, and the remainder only 19 percent.

Gundersen and Shen (1966) examined the relationships between body water and body weight in grossly obese individuals. They observed that as body weight increased, the fraction of body water decreased as a logarithmic function of the increasing body weight. In studies by Bray et al. (1970), a significant positive correlation was

TABLE 1–6. *Body Composition of a 70 kg and a 100 kg Man**

| COMPONENT | BODY WEIGHT | | | |
| | 70 kg Man | | 100 kg Man | |
	kg	percent	kg	percent
Fat	13.7	19.6	29.1	29.1
Extracellular water	17.2	24.6	21.8	21.8
Body cell mass	30.6	43.7	38.3	38.3
Remainder	8.5	12.1	10.8	10.8

*Adapted from Olesen: *In* Human Body Composition: Approaches and Applications. (J. Brozek, ed.), London, Pergamon Press, 1965, pp. 177–190.

found between body weight and body water as well as body weight and ^{42}K, indicating that with obesity there was an increase of lean body components as well as fat. This outcome was to be expected since the fraction of body weight as muscle needed to carry the extra fat must increase somewhat in order to accommodate the extra load of tissue.

A second approach to the study of body composition in obesity has been the examination of the tissue gained or lost during changes in body weight. When calories are consumed in excess of those needed for weight maintenance (Chapters 2–4), they are stored in various body compartments. In short term experiments Passmore and his colleagues concluded that essentially all of the weight gain due to overeating could be accounted for as triglyceride and protein which were stored within the already existing cellular structures (1955). Sims et al. (1968) observed that the weight gain was about 70 percent triglyceride with the remainder divided between cellular and extracellular components. This is somewhat higher than the estimates obtained by Oleson (1965).

Keys et al. (1955) and Brozek et al. (1963) concluded that the composition of the tissue added during weight gain was different from the composition lost during periods of weight loss. Fat represented 64 percent of the weight gained and of the tissue lost (Fig. 1–8). Cell residue, however, was 22 percent of the weight gain and 32 percent when weight was lost. The concept of adipose tissue differing in composition during weight gain and weight loss has been developed from the studies of Brozek (1963) and Keys et al. (1953) and has been supported by a large body of data, mostly derived from studies during weight reduction. With caloric deprivation, body weight declines. The initial composition differs from the composition of the weight loss observed later (see Chapter 8). Initially, the caloric value of the weight loss approximates 3000 kCal/kg. This rises to between 7000 and 8000 kCal/kg (Goldman, 1963; Passmore et al., 1958, 1959) as the weight loss shifts from a composition containing a large quantity of water to a predominantly fat one. A more detailed consideration of body fat and weight loss will follow in the discussion of diet.

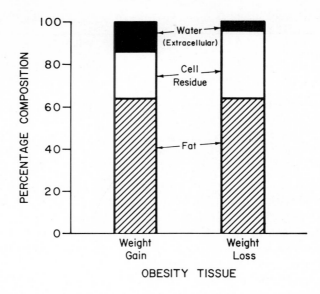

Figure 1–8. Composition of the tissue stored during weight gain and lost during weight reduction.

PREVALENCE OF OBESITY

Several kinds of studies have provided estimates on the prevalence of obesity. These include life insurance statistics (Build and Blood Pressure, 1959), national health surveys conducted in the United States (1964, 1967) and elsewhere, and investigations of the etiologic factors in cardiovascular disease and diabetes (Chapman et al., 1970; Kannel and Gordon, 1974; Keys, 1970). In each of these studies some criterion for the assessment of obesity has been employed. These have generally been of two types—relative weight or skinfold thickness. Although these criteria are arbitrary, they can nonetheless give some insight into the distribution of body weights and skinfold thickness in the population under study.

Analysis of the relationship between body weight and mortality rates among individuals insured by the large insurance companies in the United States has provided one of the largest bodies of data on this subject. The insurance companies have examined the relationships between mortality rates and deviations of body weight from the average weight for the insured group. On the basis of the lowest mortality rate in relation to body weight, the insurance industry has defined a table of "best weights" (Build and Blood Pressure Study, 1959; Metropolitan Life Insurance Company, 1960). Using this criterion, up to 60 percent of the American population aged 40 to 49 for men and 50 to 59 for women exceed their "best" weight by more than 10 percent (Table 1–7). It should be noted, however, that the data from which life

TABLE 1-7.   *Percentage of Persons Deviating from Best Weight**

AGE (YEARS)	MEN		WOMEN	
	10 to 19 percent above best weight	*20 percent or more above best weight*	*10 to 19 percent above best weight*	*20 percent or more above best weight*
20 to 29	19	12	11	12
30 to 39	28	25	16	25
40 to 49	28	32	19	40
50 to 59	29	34	21	46
60 to 69	28	29	23	45

*Adapted from Metropolitan Life Insurance Company; Frequency of overweight and underweight, Statistical Bulletin, *41*:4, 1960.

insurance tables are made does not represent the U.S. population. It is rather a selection of people who chose to buy life insurance and who have an above average life expectancy (see Chapter 6). Because of the large size of the sample on which life insurance data are based, this table of best weights has frequently been used in other studies on the prevalence of obesity (Table 1-3).

In cross sectional studies a general increase in the height of the population has been noted (Fig. 1-9). This figure shows the height of 10 year olds in the United States over the past century. There has been a steady rise, presumably reflecting improving standards of living. Taller 10 year olds become taller adults, a finding shown by the increasing height of cohorts of adults. Body weight has also increased in men. In a British study Montegriffo (1968, 1971) noted males were heavier and females lighter than their counterparts of the same height measured 25 years earlier in a study by Kemsley. For similar heights, Montegriffo found that both British females and males were lighter than Americans. Defining overweight as a weight greater than the midpoint for the large frame size in the Metropolitan table, Montegriffo observed a frequency of overweight of 59 percent for males aged 40 to 49, and 64.4 percent for women aged 50 to 59.

The National Health Surveys conducted by the United States Public Health Service (1964, 1967, 1970) have estimated the frequency of deviations from best weight for men and women as a function of age, as summarized in Table 1-7. It can be seen that the percentage of men 10 to 19 percent above their best weight increased from 19 percent of the group aged 20 to 29 to nearly 30 percent of the group aged 30 to 39. A more consistent rise was noted in the percent deviating 20 percent or more from their "best" weight. This figure ranged from 12 percent for men aged 20 to 29 to 46 percent in the group aged 50 to 59.

More severe deviations also have been examined. For women, 97

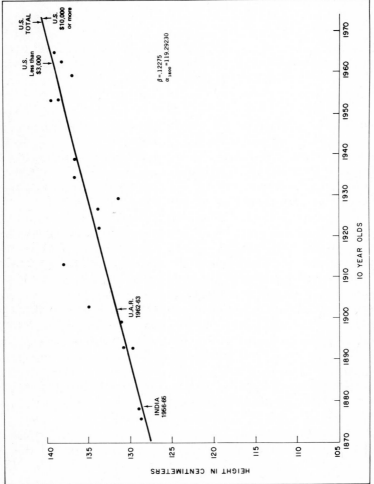

Figure 1–9. Regression line shows the growth of U.S. 10 year old children during the last century according to income groups. (National Health Survey Series 11, No. 119, 1972)

to 99 percent weighed between 93 and 236 pounds (42 to 107 kg) (National Health Survey, 1964). Thus less than 0.1 percent weigh in excess of 250 pounds (113 kg) and less than 0.1 percent weigh over 300 pounds (136 kg) (Karpinos, 1958).

The most recent examination of the nutritional status of the American population was conducted by the United States Public Health Service in a Ten State Nutrition Survey conducted between 1968 and 1970 (Ten State Nutrition Survey, 1972). In the ten states sampled, 62,532 individuals were examined for many factors including body weight, height, and thickness of the triceps skinfold. For these studies the prevalence of obesity in adolescents was defined by the thickness of triceps fatfold using the criteria of Seltzer and Mayer (1965). For adults a triceps skinfold greater than the 85th percentile was used to designate "obesity." In males the upper limit was 18.6 mm and in females 25.1 mm. By these criteria the percentage of obese adolescents varied with age from 11 to 39 percent for white males and from 9 to 19 percent for white females. In general white male adolescents had a higher percentage of obesity than black males of comparable age (Table 1–8). The prevalence of obesity in adult black males ranged from 5 to 33 percent, whereas in black females the range was 6 to 32 percent. For the adolescent groups little consistent relationship between obesity and the level of income was evident.

Ethnic differences in the frequency of obesity were clearly present among adults as measured by skinfold thickness. Obesity was consistently more common in white than in black males. This finding was reversed for women. Black women showed a consistently higher prevalence of obesity at all ages than did white females. In contrast to the findings in adolescents, income level was a significant factor in the appearance of obesity in adults. For both black and white males, the lower income levels were associated with a lower prevalence of obesity.

TABLE 1–8. *Frequency of Obesity in American Males and Females of Various Ages**

| AGE | MALES | | FEMALES | |
| | Black | White | Black | White |
	percent		percent	
21	8.3	15.1	18.1	16.6
30	12.0	21.0	36.4	25.9
40	16.4	23.1	46.1	36.5
50	13.2	23.9	52.7	41.9
60	19.1	18.6	46.7	37.8
70	8.8	14.8	32.6	30.9
80	10.0	13.7	28.1	26.7

*Adapted from the Ten State Nutrition Survey p-III-85.
Obesity = triceps skinfold > 18.6 mm for males; 25.1 mm for females.
Age is the midpoint of group in years.

The results were more complex for women. Lower income ranges were associated with a lower prevalence of obesity in older women of both ethnic groups. For younger women obesity was sometimes more prevalent in the lower socioeconomic groups. Among adult males the prevalence of obesity varied between 5 and 25 percent. Among adult women who were frequently more obese than males, the prevalence ranged from 10 to 55 percent. In general, middle-aged men and women had the highest prevalence of obesity.

The impact of social factors on the prevalence of overweight had originally been pointed out by Moore, Stunkard and Srole (1962) and was expanded by the work of Goldblatt, Moore and Stunkard (1965), Silverstone, Gordon and Stunkard (1969) and Stunkard et al. (1972). In the study by Moore et al. obesity was defined as greater than 15 percent overweight derived from verbal replies to questionnaires. Actual weights were not measured. Women of lower socioeconomic groups had an incidence of overweight of 30 percent versus 4 percent for women in the highest socioeconomic status.

In general social factors were more prominently related to overweight in women than in men. This is shown in Fig. 1–10. Whether the social status was based on the respondent's own socioeconomic status or the socioeconomic background from which they came, 30 percent of the lower income women were overweight, compared to 5 percent for the women with high socioeconomic status. Additional factors of social importance were ethnic origin, social mobility and number of generations in the United States. Women who were recent immigrants tended to have a higher prevalence of obesity (24 percent) than fourth generation Americans (5 percent) of the same ethnic background and the same socioeconomic status. Moreover, 41 percent

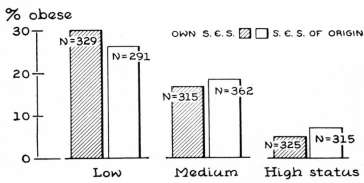

Figure 1–10. Decreasing prevalence of obesity with increasing socioeconomic status. The ordinate is the percentage of obese among each group. The cross-hatched bars show the socioeconomic status (SES) of the subject and the open bars show the socioeconomic status of the family from which the subject came. Data exclude one female about whom no information on the socioeconomic status of origin was available. (From Goldblatt et al.: J.A.M.A., *192*:1039–1044, 1965.)

of women of Czechoslovakian ancestry were overweight, as compared with 27 percent Italian and 10 percent of women of British ancestry. Finally, the prevalence of overweight decreased with upward social mobility.

In a study of 563 patients, Silverstone et al. (1969) defined obesity as weight greater than 20 percent above the figures for body weight provided by the Build and Blood Pressure Study of 1959. For the entire sample, 37 percent of the males and 49 percent of the females were overweight. In their study the incidence of obesity in the lower socioeconomic group of females was 72 percent, compared to 39 percent in the highest socioeconomic group. For males the relationship between social class and overweight was less striking. Among the three variables of age, social class and sex, social class proved to have the most significant correlation with obesity.

Socioeconomic factors could be traced into the childhood years. Overweight children from the lower socioeconomic groups could be identified by age 6 (Fig. 1–11). Among the upper socioeconomic

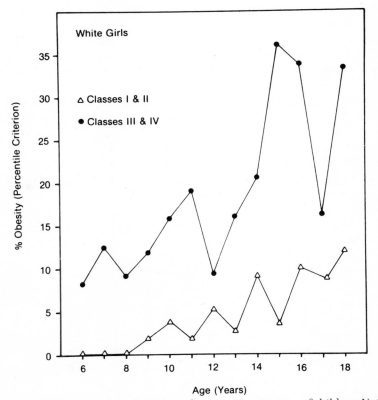

Figure 1–11.   The correlation of weight and socioeconomic status of children. Note that overweight was lower in the children from the higher socioeconomic groups at all ages. (From Stunkard et al.: J.A.M.A., *221*:579–584, 1972.)

group, overweight was of lower frequency at all ages in childhood and could not be identified before age 8. However, Huenemann (1974) has not found this early difference in overweight to be related to social class.

Another perspective on the factors relating to overweight is provided by a longitudinal study conducted in Framingham, Massachusetts (Kannel and Gordon, 1974). Over 5000 individuals were examined between 1948 and 1950 and were followed up with periodic examinations thereafter. The last available data are for the examination conducted between 1968 and 1970. Examination of cross sectional and cohort data revealed a number of interesting facts. Over 15 percent of the men and 20 percent of the women in this population had a relative body weight which was more than 30 percent above those specified in the tables of desirable weight.

Even more striking was the evidence that body weight of more than 50 percent above desirable weight was observed in 3 percent of the men and 9 percent of the women. Men born later in the twentieth century were shown to have a higher relative body weight than those born in earlier years. Each cohort of men in Framingham (i.e., men born in the same year) is heavier at corresponding ages than their earlier cohorts, although within each cohort weight increased with age (Fig. 1–12). This finding has also been observed by Montoye, Epstein and Kjelsberg (1965), as well as in studies of the weights of inductees into the military service (Karpinos, 1945).

The contrary finding is true for women. That is, women born more recently, i.e., the younger cohorts, are lighter at corresponding ages than women born earlier in the century (Fig. 1–12). The influence of life style on the weight of men and women suggests that body weight can be influenced significantly by environmental factors. The effect of fashion, i.e., shorter skirts and the exposure of larger portions of the body, may be an important factor in the declining relative weight for comparable ages of women. However, within any given cohort, both men and women become heavier with age up to age 45 to 49 years of age. After attaining that age both sexes tend to level off or to lose weight.

The epidemiologic study of coronary heart disease by Keys et al. (1970, 1975) provided data on the prevalence of overweight and obesity in different geographic regions. The criteria used were relative weight and skinfold measurements. American males proved to be among the fattest in the world when either skinfold or relative weight criteria were used. Among the European males, those from Scandinavia and the Netherlands had a lower prevalence of obesity and overweight than men from Southern Europe. These data again emphasize the importance of ethnic and geographic influences on body weight.

The frequency of overweight in East Germany has been studied

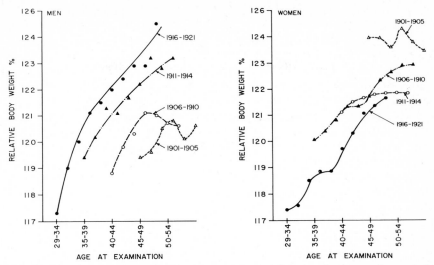

Figure 1–12. Body weight of cohorts in the Framingham Study during the periods 1948 to 1950 and 1968 to 1970. (Data of Kannel and Gordon: *In* Obesity. W. L. Burland, J. Yudkin and P. Samuel, eds., Edinburgh, Churchill Livingstone Publishers, 1974.)

by Muller, Paul and Brasch (1970). Overweight was designated as a deviation of more than 20 percent over the Broca index. This occurred in 19.2 percent of males and 42.2 percent of females. Body weights more than 50 percent above the Broca index occurred in 8 percent of the group aged 19 to 29 years and in more than 20 percent of those 50 to 69 years of age. Finally, overweight in rural areas of East Germany averaged 37.8 percent as compared to 24.5 percent in the larger cities.

Studies of black and oriental populations have also shown marked differences in the prevalence of overweight in males and females. Johnson (1970) studied Nigerians using standard weights of the Metropolitan Life Insurance Company as well as the triceps skinfold thickness. Subjects were overweight if their body weight deviated by 10 percent from the standard weight and were considered "obese" if their body weight deviated by more than 20 percent. Using these criteria, a maximum of 7.2 percent of the males aged 35 to 44 and 29 per cent of the females aged 55 to 64 were categorized as "obese." Using the 10 percent overweight criterion 41.9 percent of the women and 9.6 percent of the men were overweight. These data in Africa confirm the evidence from other parts of the world that overweight and obesity have a significantly higher prevalence in females than in males. A study by Slome et al. (1960) in South Africa found that the weights of 5.7 percent of the males and 37.9 percent of the females deviated by more than 25 percent from the life insurance actuarial tables published in 1913.

Studies on populations living in the Pacific area have been performed by Morioka and Brown (1970) on Hawaiians and by Prior and Davidson on the inhabitants of the Polynesian islands (1966). The study in Hawaii compared body weights and skinfold thicknesses of policemen and firemen in Honolulu. Policemen were found to have a higher incidence of overweight or obesity than firemen. The percentage of men categorized as overweight (i.e., above desirable weight) was 70.5 percent for the policemen and 65.3 percent for the firemen. Using Seltzer and Mayer's criteria for obesity, 18.7 percent of the policemen and 5 percent of the firemen were categorized as obese. The frequency of obesity and overweight was higher in Hawaiian descendants than in Caucasian descendants. Orientals living in Hawaii had the lowest incidence of obesity and overweight.

Prior and Davidson (1966) compared the body weight of Caucasians and Polynesians living in New Zealand and in the Polynesian islands to standard tables of body weights published in 1913. According to these criteria body weights greater than 40 percent above standard weight were found in more females than males. In the Maori group living in rural New Zealand 21 percent of the females were overweight, compared with 19 percent of those living in urban communities. Among the Caucasians, on the other hand, only 3 percent of females were 40 percent above average weight. The frequency of overweight was lower for males in all populations studied. Similar conclusions have been reached from study of the skinfolds of adults and children in New Guinea (Jansen, 1963).

Comparative studies on the prevalence of obesity between countries are infrequent, making a recent study by Keys and his collaborators all the more significant (Keys et al., 1970). In this study in seven countries similar techniques were used to measure height and weight and to obtain the thickness of triceps and subscapular skinfolds

TABLE 1–9. *Prevalence of Overweight and Obesity in Groups of Men from Seven Countries**

COUNTRY	OVERWEIGHT†	OBESE‡
	Percent of Sample	
Japan	2	2
Greece	11	11
Finland	15	14
Yugoslavia	19	29
Italy	33	28
Netherlands	13	32
United States	32	63

*Adapted from Keys et al.: American Heart Association Monograph #29, April 1970.
†Overweight = men 10 percent or more over standard weight.
‡Obesity = men with sum of triceps and subscapular skinfold > 28 mm.

on more than 12,000 men aged 40 to 59. The percentage of men who were more than 10 percent over the standard weight from the Metropolitan table has been summarized in Table 1–9. The highest number of overweight men were found in the United States, where 60 percent of the railway men included in this study were 10 percent or more overweight. The high prevalence of obesity as defined by skinfold thicknesses is also apparent and has an international distribution similar to that of overweight. From this comparative data we can conclude that obesity is indeed a major public health dilemma in many countries.

In summary, obesity is a significant problem both in affluent nations and in many developing countries as well. Both overweight and obesity are more prevalent in females than in males and its frequency is influenced by ethnic, social, and economic factors. A more detailed discussion of prevalence data can be found in a review by Christakis (1975).

REFERENCES

Alexander, M. K.: The postmortem estimation of total body fat, muscle and bone. Clin. Sci., 26:193–202, 1964.

Alsmeyer, R. H., Hiner, R. L. and Thornton, J. W.: Ultrasonic measurements of fat and muscle thickness of cattle and swine. Ann. N.Y. Acad. Sci., 110:23–30, 1963.

Anderson, E. C.: Three compartment body composition analysis based on potassium and water determinations. Ann. N.Y. Acad. Sci., 110:189–210, 1963.

Anderson, E. C. and Langham, W. H.: Average potassium concentration of the human body as a function of age. Science, 130:713–714, 1959.

Behnke, A. R.: Anthropometric evaluation of body composition throughout life. Ann. N.Y. Acad. Sci., 110:450–464, 1963.

Behnke, A. R., Jr.: Physiologic studies pertaining to deep sea diving and aviation, especially in relation to the fat content and composition of the human body. Harvey Lect. 37:198–226, 1942.

Behnke, A. R., Jr., Feen, B. G. and Welham, W. C.: The specific gravity of healthy men: body weight ÷ volume as an index of obesity. J.A.M.A., 118:495–498, 1942.

Behnke, A. R. and Taylor W. A.: U.S. Naval Radiology Defense Lab Rept. No. USNRDL-TR 339, 1959.

Behnke, A. R. and Wilmore, J. H.: Evaluation and regulation of body build and composition. Englewood Cliffs, Prentice-Hall, 1974.

Benn, R. T.: Indices of height and weight as measures of obesity. Brit. J. Prev. Soc. Med., 24:64, 1970.

Benn, R. T.: Some mathematical properties of weight-for-height indices used as measures of adiposity. Brit. J. Prev. Soc. Med., 25:42–50, 1971.

Bjorntorp, P.: Effects of physical conditioning in obesity. In: Obesity in Perspective. (G. A. Bray, ed.), Fogarty International Center Series on Preventive Medicine, Vol. II, Part 2, U.S. Government Printing Office, 1976.

Booth, R. A. D., Goddard, B. A. and Paton, A.: Measurement of fat thickness in man: a comparison of ultrasound, Harpenden calipers and electrical conductivity. Brit. J. Nutr., 20:719–725, 1966.

Bowmer, E. J.: Daniel Lambert, the great. J.A.M.A., 210:906, 1969.

Bray, G. A., Schwartz, M., Rozin, R. R. and Lister, J.: Some relationships between oxygen consumption and body composition of obese patients. Metabolism, 19:418–429, 1970.

Brooke, C. G. D.: Determinations of body composition of children from skinfold measurement. Arch. Dis. Child., 46:182–184, 1971.

Brozek, J.: Research on body composition and its relevance for human biology. *In*: Human Body Composition: Approaches and Applications. (J. Brozek, ed.) Symposia of the Society for the Study of Human Biology, Vol. 7, London, Pergamon Press, pp. 85–119, 1965.

Brozek, J., Grande, F., Anderson, J. T. and Keys, A.: Densitometric analysis of body composition: Revision of some quantitative assumptions. Ann. N.Y. Acad. Sci., 110:113–140, 1963 a.

Brozek, J., Kohlberg, J. K., Taylor, H. L. and Keys, A.: Skinfold distributions in middle-aged American men: A contribution to norms of leanness-fatness. Ann. N.Y. Acad. Sci., 110:492–502, 1963 b.

Build and Blood Pressure Study, Society of Actuaries, Chicago, 1959.

Burkinshaw, L., Jones, P. R. and Krupowicz, D. W.: Observer error in skinfold thickness measurements. Hum. Biol., 45:273–279, 1973.

Chapman, J. M., Coulson, A. H., Clark, V. A. and Boruh, E. R.: The differential effect of serum cholesterol blood pressure and weight on the incidence of myocardial infarction and angina pectoris. J. Chronic. Dis., 23:631–647, 1971.

Cheek, D. B., Schultz, R. B., Parra, A. and Reba, R. C.: Overgrowth of lean and adipose tissues in adolescent obesity. Pediatr. Res., 4:268–279, 1970.

Cheek, D. B.: Human growth. Philadelphia, Lea and Febiger, 1968.

Christakis, G.: The prevalence of adult obesity. *In*: Obesity in Perspective. (G. A. Bray, ed.), Fogarty International Series on Preventive Medicine, Vol. II, Part 1 and Part 2, U.S. Government Printing Office, 1975.

Clemente, G. A., Gerro-Luzzi, A., Mariani, G., Santaroni, G. B. and Tranquilli, F.: Evaluation of analytical models based on anthropometry and age for the prediction of body fat. Nutr. Rep. Intern., 7:157–168, 1973.

Cohn, C.: Feeding frequency and body composition. Ann. N.Y. Acad. Sci., 110:395–409, 1963.

Cohn, S. H. and Dombrowski, C. S.: Absolute measurement of whole-body potassium by gamma-ray spectrometry. J. Nucl. Med., 11:239–246, 1970.

Cohn, C. and Joseph, D.: Changes in body composition attendant on force feeding. Am. J. Physiol., 196:965–968, 1959.

Consolazio, C. F., Johnson, R. E. and Pecora, L. J.: Physiological measurements of metabolic functions in man. McGraw-Hill Co., New York, 1963.

Corsa, L., Jr., Olney, L. M., Steenburg, R. W., Ball, M. R. and Moore, F. D.: The measurement of exchangeable potassium in man by isotope dilution. J. Clin. Invest., 29:1280–1295, 1950.

Crook, G. H., Bennett, C. A., Norwood, W. D. and Mahaffey, J. A.: Evaluation of skinfold measurements and weight chart to measure body fat. J.A.M.A., 198:39–44, 1966.

DuBois, D. and DuBois, E. F.: A formula to estimate the approximate surface area if height and weight be known. Arch. Int. Med., 17:863–871, 1916.

Durnin, J. V. G. A., Armstrong, W. H. and Womersley, J.: An experimental study on the variability of measurement of skinfold thickness by three observers on 23 young women and 27 young men. Hum. Biol., 45:281–292, 1973.

Durnin, J. V. G. A. and Womersley, J.: Body fat assessed from total body density and its estimation from skinfold thickness: Measurements on 481 men and women aged from 16 to 72 years. Brit. J. Nutr., 32:77–97, 1974.

Edwards, D. A. W.: Observations on the distribution of subcutaneous fat. Clin. Sci., 9:259–270, 1950.

Fee, B. A. and Weil, W. B., Jr.: Body composition of infants of diabetic mothers by direct analysis. Ann. N.Y. Acad. Sci., 110:869–897, 1963.

Florey, C. V.: The use and interpretation of ponderal index and other weight-height ratios in epidemiological studies. J. Chron. Dis., 23:93–103, 1970.

Flynn, M. A., Hanna, F., Long, C. H., Asfour, R. Y., Lutz, R. N. and Zobrisky, S. E.: Deuterium-Oxide dilution as a predictor of body composition in children and pigs. *In*: Body Composition in Animals and Man. Proc. of a Symposium May 4–6, 1967 at Univ. of Missouri, Publ. #1598, Natl. Acad. Sci., Washington, D.C. 1968, pp. 480–491.

Flynn, M. A., Woodruff, C., Clark, J. and Chase, G.: Total body potassium in normal children. Pediatr. Res., 6:239–245, 1972.

Fomon, S. J.: Body composition of the male reference infant during the first year of life. Pediatrics, 40:863–870, 1967.

Fomon, S. J., Jensen, R. L. and Owen, G. M.: Determination of body volume of infants by a method of helium displacement. Ann. N.Y. Acad. Sci., 110:80–90, 1963.

Forbes, G. B.: Changes in body water and electrolyte during growth and development. In: Body Composition in Animals and Man. Proc. of a Symposium May 4–6, 1967 at Univ. of Missouri, Publ. #1598, Natl. Acad. Sci., Washington D.C. 1968, pp. 80–86.

Forbes, G. B.: Lean body mass and fat in obese children. Pediatrics., 34:308–314, 1964.

Forbes, G. B.: Relation of lean body mass to height in children and adolescents. Pediatr. Res., 6:32–37, 1972.

Forbes, G. B. and Hursh, J. B.: Age and sex trends in lean body mass calculated from [40]K measurements: with a note on the theoretical basis for the procedure. Ann. N.Y. Acad. Sci., 110:255–263, 1963.

Forbes, G. B. and Lewis, A. M.: Total sodium, potassium and chloride in adult man. J. Clin. Invest., 35:596–600, 1956.

Forbes, G. B. and Reina, J. C.: Adult lean body mass declines with age: some longitudinal observations. Metabolism, 19:653–663, 1970.

Forbes, R. M., Cooper, A. R. and Mitchell, H. H.: The composition of the adult human body as determined by chemical analysis. J. Biol. Chem., 203:359–366, 1953.

Forbes, R. M., Mitchell, H. H. and Cooper, A. R.: Further studies on the gross composition and mineral elements of the adult human body. J. Biol. Chem., 223:969–975, 1956.

Friis-Hansen, B.: Hydrometry of growth and aging. In: Human Body Composition. (J. Brozek, ed.). Oxford, Pergamon Press, 1965, pp. 191–209.

Garn, S. M.: Relative fat patterning: an individual characteristic. Hum. Biol., 27:75–89, 1955 a.

Garn, S. M. and Harper, R. V.: Fat accumulation and weight gain in the adult male. Hum. Biol., 27:39–40, 1955 b.

Garn, S. M.: Comparison of pinch-caliper and x-ray measurements of skin plus subcutaneous fat. Science, 124:178–179, 1956.

Garn, S. M. and Haskell, J. A.: Fat and growth during childhood. Science, 130:1711–1712, 1959 a.

Garn, S. M. and Haskell, J. A.: Fat changes during adolescence. Science, 129:1615–1616, 1959 b.

Goldblatt: P. E., Moore, M. E. and Stunkard, A. J.: Social factors in obesity. J.A.M.A. 192:1039–1044, 1965.

Goldbourt, U. and Medalie, J. H.: Weight-height indices: Choice of the most suitable index and its association with selected variables among 10,000 adult males of heterogenous origin. Br. J. Prev. Soc. Med., 28:116–126, 1974.

Goldman, R. F., Bullen, B. and Seltzer, C.: Changes in specific gravity and body fat in overweight female adolescents as a result of weight reduction. Ann. N.Y. Acad. Sci., 110:913–917, 1963.

Guinness Book of World Records (McWhirter, N. D. and McWhirter, A. R., eds.) 1974.

Gundersen, K. and Shen, G.: Total body water in obesity. Am. J. Clin. Nutr., 19:77–83, 1966.

Gurney, J. M. and Jelliffe, D. B.: Arm anthropometry in nutritional assessment: Nomogram for rapid calculation of muscle circumference and cross-sectional muscle and fat areas. Am. J. Clin. Nutr., 26:912–915, 1973.

Hawes, S. F., Albert, A., Healy, M. J. R. and Garrow, J. S.: A comparison of soft-tissue radiography, reflected ultrasound, skinfold calipers and thigh circumference for estimating the thickness of fat overlying the iliac crest and greater trochanter. Proc. Nutr. Soc., 31:91A, 1972.

Hermansen, L. and Döbeln, W. V.: Body fat and skinfold measurements. Scand. J. Clin. Lab. Invest., 27:315–319, 1971.

Huenemann, R. L.: 1. Obesity in six-month-old children. Environmental factors associated with preschool obesity. J. Am. Diet. Assoc., 64:480–487, 1974.

Hytten, F. E., Taylor, K. and Taggart, N.: Measurement of total body fat in man by absorption of [85]Kr. Clin. Sci., 31:111–119, 1966.

Ingle, D. J.: A simple means of producing obesity in the rat. Proc. Soc. Exp. Biol. Med., 72:604–605, 1949.

Jansen, A. A.: Skinfold measurements from early childhood to adulthood in Papuans from Western New Guinea. Ann. N.Y. Acad. Sci., 110:515–531, 1963.

Jasani, B. M. and Edmonds, C. J.: Kinetics of potassium distribution in man using isotope dilution and whole-body counting. Metabolism, 20:1099–1106, 1971.

Johnson, T. O.: Prevalence of overweight and obesity among adult subjects of an urban African population sample. Brit. J. Prev. Soc. Med., 24:105–109, 1970.

Johnston, L. C. and Bernstein, L. M.: Body composition and oxygen consumption of overweight, normal and underweight women. J. Lab. Clin. Med., 45:109–118, 1955.

Johny, K. V. Worthley, B. W., Lawrence, J. R. and O'Halloran, M. W.: A whole body counter for serial studies of total body potassium. Clin. Sci., 39:319–326, 1970.

Kannel, W. B. and Gordon, T.: Obesity and cardiovascular disease. The Framingham Study. Symposium. In: Obesity. Proceedings of a Servier Research Institute on Obesity. Servier Inst. Monograph. Burland, W. L., Yudkin, J. and Samuel, P. eds., Edinburgh, Churchill Livingstone Publishers, 1974.

Karpinos, B. D.: Height and weight of selective service registrants processed for military service during World War II. Hum. Biol., 30:292–321, 1958.

Keys, A. (ed.): Coronary heart disease in seven countries. American Heart Assn. Monograph #29, April, 1970.

Keys, A., Anderson, J. T. and Brozek, J.: Weight gain from simple overeating. I. Character of the tissue gained. Metabolism, 4:427–432, 1955.

Keys, A., Fidanza, F., Karvonen, M. J., Kimura, N. and Taylor, H. L.: Indices of relative weight and obesity. J. Chron. Dis., 25:329–343, 1972.

Keys, A., Taylor, H. L. and Grande, F.: Basal metabolism and age of adult man. Metabolism, 22:579–587, 1973.

Keys, A. and Brozek, J.: Body fat in adult man. Physiol. Rev., 33:245–325, 1953.

Keys, A.: Overweight and the risk of heart attack and sudden death. In: Obesity in Perspective. (Bray, G. A., ed.) Fogarty International Series on Preventive Medicine, Vol. II, Part 2, Washington, D.C., U.S. Government Printing Office, 1976.

Khosla, T. and Lowe, C. R.: Obesity and smoking habits by social class. Brit. J. Prev. Soc. Med., 26:249–256, 1972.

Kreisberg, R. A., Bowdoin, B. and Meador, C. K.: Measurement of muscle mass in humans by isotopic dilution of creatine ^{14}C. J. Appl. Physiol., 28:264–267, 1970.

Krzywicki, H. J. and Chinn, K. S. K.: Human body density and fat of an adult male population as measured by water displacement. Am. J. Clin. Nutr., 20:305–310, 1967.

Lesser, G. T., Deutsch, S. and Markofsky, J.: Use of independent measurement of body fat to evaluate overweight and underweight. Metabolism, 20:792–804, 1971.

Lesser, G. T., Kumar, I. and Steele, J. M.: Changes in body composition with age. Ann. N.Y. Acad. Sci., 110:578–588, 1963.

Lim, T. P. K.: Critical evaluation of the pneumatic method for determining body volume: Its history and technique. Ann. N.Y. Acad. Sci., 110:72–74, 1963.

Ljunggren, H.: Sex difference in body composition. In: Human body composition: Approaches and Applications, Symposia of the Society for the Study of Human Biol. Vol. 7 (Brozek, J., ed.), London, Pergamon Press, 1965, pp. 129–138.

McCance, R. A. and Widdowson, E. M.: A method of breaking down the body weights of living persons into terms of extracellular fluid, cell mass and fat, and some applications of it to physiology and medicine. Proc. Roy. Soc. B., 138:115–130, 1951.

Mellits, E. D. and Cheek, D. B.: The assessment of body water and fatness from infancy to adulthood. Monographs Soc. Res. Child Develop., 35:12–26, 1970.

Meneely, G. R., Heyssel, R. M., Ball, C. O. T., Weiland, R. L., Lorimer, A. R., Constantinides, C. and Meneely, E. U.: Analysis of factors affecting body composition determined from potassium content in 915 normal subjects. Ann. N.Y. Acad. Sci., 110:271–281, 1963.

Metropolitan Life Insurance Company: Frequency of overweight and underweight. Statistical Bulletin, 41:4, 1960.

Mitchell, H. H., Hamilton, T. S., Steggerda, F. R. and Bean, H. W.: The chemical composition of the adult human body and its bearing on the biochemistry of growth. J. Biol. Chem., 158:625–637, 1945.

Montegriffo, V. M. E.: A survey of the incidence of obesity in the United Kingdom. Postgrad. Med. J., 47:(Suppl June) 418–422, 1971.

Montegriffo, V. M. E.: Height and weight of a United Kingdom adult population. Ann. Hum. Genet., 31:389–399, 1968.

Montoye, H. J., Epstein, F. H. and Kjelsberg, M. O.: The measurement of body fatness: a study in a total community. Am. J. Clin. Nutr., 16:417–427, 1965.

Moore, F. D., Olesen, K. H., McMurrey, J. D., Parker, H. V., Ball, M. B. and Boyden, C. M.: The Body Cell Mass and Its Supporting Environment. Philadelphia, W. B. Saunders Co., 1963, p. 484.

Moore, M. E., Stunkard, A. and Srole, L.: Obesity, social class, and mental illness. J.A.M.A., 181:962–966, 1962.

Morioka, H. M. and Brown, M. L.: Incidence of obesity and overweight among Honolulu policemen and firemen. Public Health Reports, 85:5, 433–439, 1970.

Muller, F., Paul, I. and Brasch, C.: The incidence of obesity in the German Democratic Republic. Z. Gesamte Inn. Med., 25:1001–1009, 1970.

National Academy of Sciences. Body composition in animals and man. Washington, D.C. National Academy of Sciences, 1968.

National Health Survey (National Center for Health Statistics): Changes in cigarette smoking habits between 1955–1966. PHS No. 1000, Series 10, No. 59, 1970.

National Health Survey (National Center for Health Statistics): Blood pressure of adults by age and sex, United States 1960–1962. PHS. No. 1000, Series 11, No. 4, 1964.

National Health Survey (National Center for Health Statistics) Serum cholesterol levels of adults, United States 1960–1962. PHS No. 1000, Series 11, No. 22, 1967.

Norris, A. H., Lundy, T. and Shock, N. W.: Trends in selected indices of body composition in men between the ages 30 and 80 years. Ann. N.Y. Acad. Sci., 110:623–639, 1963.

Olesen, K. H.: Body composition in normal adults. In: Human Body Composition: Approaches and Applications, Symposia of the Society for the Study of Human Biology Vol. 7, (Brozek, J., ed.) London, Pergamon Press, 1965, pp. 177–190.

Olsson, K. E.: Determination of total body water and its turnover rate. Acta Chir. Scand., 136:647–656, 1970.

Osler, M. and Pedersen, J.: Body composition of newborn infants of diabetic mothers. Pediatrics., 26:985–992, 1960.

Pace, N. and Rathbun, E. N.: Studies on body composition: body water and chemically combined nitrogen content in relation to fat content. J. Biol. Chem., 158:685–691, 1945.

Panaretto, B. A.: Estimation of body composition by the dilution of hydrogen isotopes. In: Body Composition in Animals and Man. Proc. of a Symposium May 4–6, 1967 at Univ. of Missouri, Publ. #1598, Natl. Acad. Sci., Washington, D.C., 1968, pp. 153–169.

Parizkova, J.: The development of subcutaneous fat in adolescents and the effect of physical training and sport. Physiol. Bohemoslov. 8:112–117, 1959.

Parizkova, J.: Impact of age, diet, and exercise on man's body composition. Ann. N.Y. Acad. Sci., 110:661–674, 1963.

Parizkova, J.: Physical activity and body composition. In: Human Body Composition: Approaches and Applications. Symposia of the Society for the Study of Human Biology Vol. 7 (Brozek, J., ed.) London, Pergamon Press, 1965, pp. 161–176.

Parizkova, J. and Buzkova, P.: Relationship between skinfold thickness measured by Harpenden caliper and densitometric analysis of total body fat in men. Hum. Biol., 43:16–21, 1971.

Passmore, T., Meiklejohn, A. B., Dewar, A. D. and Thow, R. K.: The analysis of the gain in weight of overfed thin young men. Brit. J. Nutr., 9:27–37, 1955.

Passmore, R., Strong, J. A. and Ritchie, F. J.: The chemical composition of the tissue lost by obese patients on a reducing regimen. Brit. J. Nutr., 12:113–122, 1958.

Passmore, R., Strong, J. A., and Ritchie, F. J.: Water and electrolyte analysis of obese patients on a reducing regimen. Brit. J. Nutr., 13:17–25, 1959.

Pearson, A. M., Purchas, R. W. and Reineke, E. P.: Theory and potential usefulness of body density as a predictor of body composition. In: Body Composition in Animals and Man. Proc. of a Symposium May 4–6, 1967 at Univ. of Missouri, Publ. #1598, Natl. Acad. Sci., Washington, D.C., 1968, pp. 153–169.

Pierson, R. N., Jr. and Lin, D. H.: Measurement of body compartments in children: whole body counting and other methods. Semin. Nucl. Med., 2:373–382, 1972.

Pitts, G. C.: Body fat accumulation in the guinea pig. Am. J. Physiol., 185:41–48, 1956.

Pitts, G. C. and Bullard, T. R.: Some interspecific aspects of body composition in mammals. In: Body Composition in Animals and Man. Proc. of a Symposium May 4–6, 1967 at Univ. of Missouri. Publ. #1598, Natl. Acad. Sci., Washington, D.C. 1968, pp. 45–70.

Prior, I. A. M. and Davidson, F.: The epidemiology of diabetes in Polynesians and Europeans in New Zealand and the Pacific. N.Z. Med. J., 65:375–383, 1966.

Reid, J. T., Bensadown, A., Bull, L. S., Burton, J. H., Gleeson, P. A., Han, I. K., Joo, Y. D., Johnson, D. E., McManus, W. R., Paladines, O. L., Stroud, J. W., Tyrrell, H. F., Van Niekerk, B. D. H. and Wellington, G. W.: Some Peculiarities in the Body Composition of Animals. In: Body Composition in Animals and Man. Proc. of a Symposium May 4–6, 1967 at Univ. of Missouri, Publ. #1598, Natl. Acad. Sci., Washington, D.C., 1968, pp. 19–44.

Robson, J. R.: Ethnic differences in skinfold thickness. Am. J. Clin. Nutr., 24:864–868, 1971.

Roessler, G. S. and Dunavant, B. G.: Comparative evaluation of a whole-body potassium counter 40 method for measuring lean body mass. Am. J. Clin. Nutr., 20:1171–1178, 1967.

Ruffer, W. A.: Two simple indexes for identifying obesity compared. J. Am. Diet Assoc., 57:326–330, 1970.

Ruiz, L., Colley, J. R. T. and Hamilton, P. J. S.: Measurement of triceps skinfold thickness. An investigation of sources of variation. Brit. J. Prev. Soc. Med., 25:165–167, 1971.

Salans, L. B., Cushman, S. W. and Weismann, R. E.: Studies of human adipose tissue. Adipose cell size and number in nonobese and obese patients. J. Clin. Invest., 52:929–941, 1973.

Seltzer, C. C., Stoudt, H. W., Jr., Bell, B. and Mayer, J.: Reliability of relative body weight as a criterion of obesity. Am. J. Epidemiol., 92:339–350, 1970.

Seltzer, C. C. and Mayer, J.: A simple criterion of obesity. Postgrad. Med., 38A:101–107, 1965.

Seltzer, C. C. and Mayer J.: Body build and obesity—who are the obese? J.A.M.A., 189:677–684, 1964.

Seltzer, C. C. and Mayer, J.: Greater reliability of the tricep skinfold over the subscapular skinfold as an index of obesity. Am. J. Clin. Nutr., 20:950–953, 1967.

Sheldon, W. H.: Atlas of men. New York, Harper and Bros., 1954.

Silverstone, J. T., Gordon, R. P. and Stunkard, A. J.: Social factors in obesity in London. Practitioner, 202:682–688, 1969.

Sims, E. A. H., Goldman, R. F., Gluck, C. M., Horton, E. S., Kelleher, P. C. and Rowe, D. W.: Experimental obesity in man. Trans. Assoc. Am. Physicians, 81:153–170, 1968.

Sloan, A. W. and Weir, J. B.: Nomograms for predictions of body density and total body fat from skinfold measurements. J. Appl. Physiol., 28:221–222, 1970.

Slome, C., Gampel, B., Abramson, J. H. and Scotch, N.: Weight, height and skinfold thickness of Zulu adults in Durban. S. Afr. Med. J., 34:505–509, 1960.

Steinkamp, R. C., Cohen, N. L., Siri, W. E., Sargent, T. W. and Walsh, H. E.: Measures of body fat and related factors in normal adults, I, J. Chron. Dis., 18:1279–1289, 1965.

Steinkamp, R. C. et al.: Measures of body fat and related factors in normal adults, II. A simple clinical method to measure body fat and lean body mass. J. Chron. Dis., 18:1291–1307, 1965.

Strakova, M. and Markova, J.: Ultrasound used for measuring subcutaneous fat. Rev. Czech. Med., 17:66–73, 1971.

Stunkard, A., D'Aquili, E., Fox, S. and Filion, R. D. L.: Influence of social class on obesity and thinness in children. J.A.M.A., 221:579–584, 1972.

Tanner, J. M.: Radiographic studies of body composition in children and adults. In: Human Body Composition, (Brozek, J., ed.) Oxford, Pergamon Press, 1965, pp. 211–236.

Tanner, J. M. and Whitehouse, R. H.: Height and weight charts from birth to five years allowing for length of gestation for use in infant welfare clinics. Arch. Dis. Child., 48:786–789, 1973.

Ten State Nutrition Survey, 1968-1970. U.S. Dept. of HEW, Publ. (HSM) 72-8131, 1972.

Tyson, I., Genna, S., Jones, R. L.: Studies of potassium depletion using a direct measurement of total body potassium. J. Nucl. Med., 11:426–434, 1970.

Vague, J., Rubin, P., Jubelin, J. and Vague, P.: The various forms of obesity. In: Triangle. Sandoz, J. Med. Sci., 13:41–50, 1974.

Van Graan, C. H. and Wyndham, C. H.: Body surface area in human beings. Nature, (Lond.) 204:998, 1964.

Waller, R. E. and Brooks, A. G. F.: Heights and weights of men visiting a public health exhibition. Brit. J. Prev. Soc. Med., 26:180–185, 1972.

Walsh, G. C., Carruthers, B. M., Seraglia, M. and Olson, M.: Determination of total body water by deuterium oxide dilution and cryoscopy. J. Lab. Clin. Med., 72:836–841, 1968.

Welham, W. C. and Behnke, A. R.: Specific gravity of healthy men: body weight divided by volume and other physical characteristics of exceptional athletes and of naval personnel. J.A.M.A., 118:498–501, 1942.

Widdowson, E. M., McCance, R. A. and Spray, C. M.: The chemical composition of the human body. Clin. Sci., 10:113–125, 1951.

Widdowson, E. M.: Chemical analysis of the body. In: Human Body Composition: Approaches and Applications, Symposia for the Society for the Study of Human Biology, Vol. 7 (Brozek, J., ed.), Oxford, Pergamon Press, 1965, pp. 31–55.

Willoughby, D. P.: Extraordinary case of obesity and review of some lesser cases. Hum. Biol., 14:166–177, 1942.

Wilmore, J. H. and Behnke, A. R.: an anthropometric estimation of body density and lean body weight in young women. Am. J. Clin. Nutr., 23:267–274, 1970.

Wilmore, J. H. and Behnke, A. R.: Predictability of lean body weight through anthropometric assessment in college men. J. Appl. Physiol., 25:349–355, 1968.

Womersley, J. K., Boddy, P. C., King, J. V. and Durnin, G. A.: A comparison of the fat-free mass of young adults estimated by anthropometry, body density and total body potassium content. Clin. Sci., 43:469–475, 1972.

Young, C. M., Blondin, J., Tensuan, R. and Fryer, J. H.: Body composition studies of "older" women, thirty to seventy years of age. Ann. N.Y. Acad. Sci., 110:589–607, 1963.

Young, H. B.: Body composition, culture, and sex: Two comments. In: Human Body Composition: Approaches and Applications. Symposia of the Society for the Study of Human Biology Vol. 7, (Brozek, J., ed.) London, Pergamon Press, 1965, pp. 139–159.

157

CHAPTER 2

PATHOGENESIS OF OBESITY: FOOD INTAKE

The problem of obesity is essentially a problem of *energy balance*. Excess caloric intake, relative to caloric expenditure, leads at various rates to storage of extra fat. To explore more fully the implications of this proposition, "energy" should be examined from a biological standpoint. Energy, defined as the capacity to do work, has several forms and can be measured in a number of ways. In biological systems energy is usually expressed in terms of heat and is measured as calories or joules. A calorie is defined as the quantity of heat needed to raise the temperature of 1 gram of water from 15 to 16° C at normal atmospheric pressure.

To illustrate the problem of maintaining energy balance, it is useful to examine the caloric requirements for one year's normal activity for a man. The caloric needs of a normal 22 year old American male have been set at 3000 kCal/day, and 2100 kCal/day maintain the needs of an average woman of the same age (Table 2–1). Hence an average young male will ingest just over one million kilocalories during a twelve month period (3000 × 365). Of these million kilocalories, nearly all will be metabolized, and only a small percentage stored. Differences between intake and storage are reflected in gains or losses in stored energy as evidenced by changes in body weight.

Careful studies on the caloric value of adipose tissue show that it contains approximately 3500 calories per pound (454 g) (Lusk, 1928). If an individual ingests and stores 100 kCal more than is required for all needs, then 36,500 excess calories will be accumulated during the course of a year. The net storage of 36,500 calories will result in a ten pound (4.59 kg) weight gain in one year. If this rate is continued,

44

weight would increase 100 pounds (45.4 kg) in 10 years. A consistent weight gain of this sort fortunately occurs only in very rare instances.

There are three possible explanations for an increase in caloric storage: (1) caloric intake could be increased in the face of normal levels of caloric expenditure; (2) caloric intake could be unchanged but caloric expenditure could be reduced; or (3) caloric storage could result from a combination of increased caloric intake and decreased caloric expenditure. A careful analysis of the factors which relate food intake and energy expenditure is essential for understanding the nature of the problem of caloric storage.

STABILITY OF BODY WEIGHT

A pattern of slow changes in body weight over many years has been demonstrated in several studies, supporting the hypothesis that body weight is regulated. However, this conclusion is not shared by all (Garrow, 1974; Polin and Wolford, 1973). Both longitudinal and cross sectional studies show that there is only a small change in average body weight during adult life. The Ten State Nutrition Survey (1972) documents this very clearly in cross sectional studies. Among white males from the high income group, body weight increased from 72.9 kg at age 21 to 77.2 kg in men aged 30, but remained almost constant from age 30 to age 60. Among white males from lower income groups, weight at age 21 was slightly lower at 68.5 kg, and rose to 75 kg in men aged 30; thereafter it remained within 2 kg of the weight at age 30 until after age 60.

In the groups of white females, there was a rise in weight from 59.6 kg at age 21 to 63.1 kg in women of age 30, and a further small rise to 66.2 kg in women who were 40 years old. Thereafter weight remained constant through age 70. A similar stability of weight over the middle years of life also occurs among black males and females. It should be noted that stability of weight does not necessarily imply a stability of body composition. The fraction of body weight which is fat increases, while the percentage which is lean tissue declines during the adult years (Fig. 2–1). In summary, weight itself shows an increase between ages 21 and 30, with only small changes thereafter (Forbes and Reina, 1970).

Variations in short term body weight have been investigated by Adams et al. (1961). They found that among 64 young soldiers who were weighed daily for up to 7 weeks body weight changed by 0.5 kg from day to day in over 30 percent of the weighings. However, there was no relationship between these changes and daily intake or caloric expenditure.

In the prospective study conducted at Framingham, Massachusetts, Kannell et al. (Gordon and Kannell, 1973; Kannell and Gordon,

TABLE 2–1. *National Research Council Recommended Daily Dietary Allowances (1974)*

	Age (years)	Weight (kg)	Weight (lbs)	Height (cm)	Height (in)	Energy (kcal)*	Protein (g)	FAT-SOLUBLE VITAMINS Vitamin A activity (RE)†	(IU)	Vitamin D (IU)	Vitamin E activity§ (IU)
Infants	0.0–0.5	6	14	60	24	kg×117	kg×2.2	420‡	1,400	400	4
	0.5–1.0	9	20	71	28	kg×108	kg×2.0	400	2,000	400	5
Children	1–3	13	28	86	34	1,300	23	400	2,000	400	7
	4–6	20	44	110	44	1,800	30	500	2,500	400	9
	7–10	30	66	135	54	2,400	36	700	3,300	400	10
Males	11–14	44	97	158	63	2,800	44	1,000	5,000	400	12
	15–18	61	134	172	69	3,000	54	1,000	5,000	400	15
	19–22	67	147	172	69	3,000	54	1,000	5,000	400	15
	23–50	70	154	172	69	2,700	56	1,000	5,000		15
	51+	70	154	172	69	2,400	56	1,000	5,000		15
Females	11–14	44	97	155	62	2,400	44	800	4,000	400	12
	15–18	54	119	162	65	2,100	48	800	4,000	400	12
	19–22	58	128	162	65	2,100	46	800	4,000	400	12
	23–50	58	128	162	65	2,000	46	800	4,000		12
	51+	58	128	162	65	1,800	46	800	4,000		12
Pregnant						+300	+30	1,000	5,000	400	15
Lactating						+500	+20	1,200	6,000	400	15

*Kilojoules (KJ) = 4.2 × kcal.

†Retinol equivalents.

‡Assumed to be all as retinol in milk during the first six months of life. All subsequent intakes are assumed to be half as retinol and half as β-carotene when calculated from international units. As retinol equivalents, three fourths are as retinol and one fourth as β-carotene.

§Total vitamin E activity, estimated to be 80 percent as α-tocopherol and 20 percent other tocopherols. See text for variation in allowances.

**The folacin allowances refer to dietary sources as determined by *Lactobacillus casei* assay. Pure forms of folacin may be effective in doses less than one fourth of the recommended dietary allowance.

††Although allowances are expressed as niacin, it is recognized that on the average 1 mg of niacin is derived from each 60 mg of dietary tryptophan.

‡‡This increased requirement cannot be met by ordinary diets; therefore, the use of supplement iron is recommended.

1974) noted a correlation coefficient of r = 0.75 for the weight at entry into the study and the body weights determined 18 years later. Over the 18 years spanned by the Framingham Study the average difference between highest and lowest weights for men and women was 21.2 ± 7.0 lb. This reflects primarily short term variation with persistent changes occurring very slowly.

Abraham, Collins and Nordsieck (1971) studied the stability of body weight in 1087 of the 1963 white males who had entered the school system in Hagerstown, Maryland between 1923-1928, and who were reweighed 33 to 40 years later. Only 4 percent of the males who were below average weight in childhood had become markedly overweight as adults, and only 17 percent reached weights above average. On the other hand, none of the markedly overweight children were below average weight as adults and only 16 percent were average weight. Of the subjects who were below average as children, 50 percent remained in the same group as adults. Sixty-three percent of the

TABLE 2-1. *National Research Council Recommended*
Daily Dietary Allowances (continued)

Ascorbic acid (mg)	Folacin** (μg)	Niacin†† (mg)	Riboflavin (mg)	Thiamin (mg)	Vitamin B₆ (mg)	Vitamin B₁₂ (μg)	Calcium (mg)	Phosphorus (mg)	Iodine (μg)	Iron (mg)	Magnesium (mg)	Zinc (mg)
35	50	5	0.4	0.3	0.3	0.3	360	240	35	10	60	3
35	50	8	0.6	0.5	0.4	0.3	540	400	45	15	70	5
40	100	9	0.8	0.7	0.6	1.0	800	800	60	15	150	10
40	200	12	1.1	0.9	0.9	1.5	800	800	80	10	200	10
40	300	16	1.2	1.2	1.2	2.0	800	800	110	10	250	10
45	400	18	1.5	1.4	1.6	3.0	1,200	1,200	130	18	350	15
45	400	20	1.8	1.5	2.0	3.0	1,200	1,200	150	18	400	15
45	400	20	1.8	1.5	2.0	3.0	800	800	140	10	350	15
45	400	18	1.6	1.4	2.0	3.0	800	800	130	10	350	15
45	400	16	1.5	1.2	2.0	3.0	800	800	110	10	350	15
45	400	16	1.3	1.2	1.6	3.0	1,200	1,200	115	18	300	15
45	400	14	1.4	1.1	2.0	3.0	1,200	1,200	115	18	300	15
45	400	14	1.4	1.1	2.0	3.0	800	800	100	18	300	15
45	400	13	1.2	1.0	2.0	3.0	800	800	100	18	300	15
45	400	12	1.1	1.0	2.0	3.0	800	800	80	10	300	15
60	800	+2	+0.3	+0.3	2.5	4.0	1,200	1,200	125	18†‡	450	20
80	600	+4	+0.5	+0.3	2.5	4.0	1,200	1,200	150	18	450	25

markedly overweight boys were markedly overweight as adults. The findings of Sohar et al. (1973) also demonstrate the constancy of relative body weight in growing children. Among 404 school children, weights at ages 6 and 7 correlated with weights at ages 13 and 14 with a coefficient of r = 0.81. In only 6 percent of the children did relative weight change by 20 percent or more.

Two other studies in adults also lend support to the concept that body weight is regulated. Comstock and Stone (1972) found that over 5 years weight gain was only 1.1 to 1.5 pounds in men whose smoking status did not change. Chinn et al. (see Garrow 1974) examined body weight in Welsh populations over a period of years. Although there were some with a significant change in weight between the two weighings, most were close to their initial weight. In summary, the data which we have reviewed indicate that body weight can change but that long term changes occur slowly and are relatively small.

Several groups of investigators have proposed the concept that total energy reserves are regulated (Baile and Forbes, 1972; Baile, 1968, 1971; Bray and Campfield, 1975, Cioffi and Speranza, 1972; Hirsch, 1972; Hamilton, 1973; Lepkovsky, 1973a, b). The diagram in Figure 2-2 shows one way of approaching the problem of controlling body fat by using concepts of feedback control. It is analogous to the regulation of temperature in a house. The thermostat in the house measures the temperature; when it rises too high, the furnace is shut off. Conversely, when the temperature in the house falls below the level set on the thermostat, the reverse occurs and heat increases. For

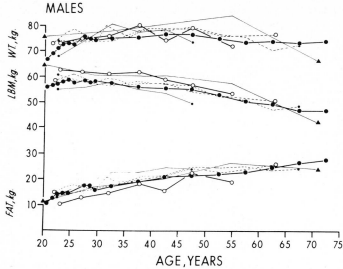

Figure 2–1. Changes in body composition with age in males. These data are a composite of several studies in which cross sectional measurements were made. Note the relative stability of body weight compared with the rise in the percentage of body fat and the fall in the percentage of lean tissue. (Forbes and Reina: Metabolism, *19*:653–663, 1970, with permission.)

the living animal, the regulation of total energy is controlled by varying caloric intake and caloric expenditure in response to some as yet unknown factor(s) related to caloric stores (Bray and Campfield, 1975).

Experimental evidence from four kinds of experiments favors the concept of a regulatory mechanism which controls body weight. The first shows that when mature animals are underfed to reduce weight (McCance, 1962) or force-fed to gain weight (Cohn and Joseph, 1962), they spontaneously readjust their food intake when allowed to. When the caloric restriction is stopped or the forced feeding terminated, the animal modifies its food intake to return to a body weight which is at or near the expected level. The starved animal will eat an excess amount of food until the body weight returns to its original level (McCance, 1962). Conversely, animals which are force-fed will decrease their food intake and will return to the normal weight (Cohn and Joseph, 1962).

Environmental temperature is a factor in the weight loss. At temperatures of 20° C (68° F) the force-fed animals sometimes remained significantly fatter than the controls (Cohn and Joseph, 1962). A similar experiment with overfeeding has been performed with human subjects who voluntarily overate (Mann et al., 1955; Sims et al., 1968, 1973). In these studies of self-induced gorging, body weight increased during the period of overeating. When the experiment ended, however, the subjects voluntarily restricted food intake until body weight

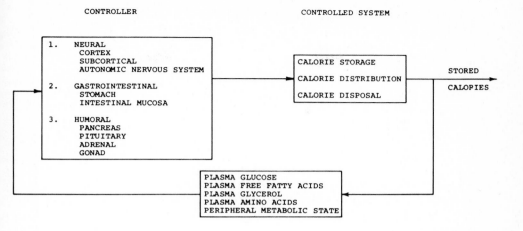

CONTROLLER

CONTROLLED SYSTEM

1. NEURAL
   CORTEX
   SUBCORTICAL
   AUTONOMIC NERVOUS SYSTEM

2. GASTROINTESTINAL
   STOMACH
   INTESTINAL MUCOSA

3. HUMORAL
   PANCREAS
   PITUITARY
   ADRENAL
   GONAD

CALORIE STORAGE

CALORIE DISTRIBUTION

CALORIE DISPOSAL

STORED

CALORIES

PLASMA GLUCOSE
PLASMA FREE FATTY ACIDS
PLASMA GLYCEROL
PLASMA AMINO ACIDS
PERIPHERAL METABOLIC STATE

FEEDBACK ELEMENTS

Figure 2–2.   Diagram for the control of stored energy. The controlled system stores and releases the energy from foods. These processes are regulated by the many switches which respond to various feedback elements (the "controllers"). (Bray and Campfield: Metabolism, 24:98–117, 1975, with permission.)

returned to its original level. This readjustment usually took only a few weeks.

Experiments with the transplantation of adipose tissue are a second experimental approach indicating internal regulation of body fat. Liebelt et al. (1965) transplanted fat from one mouse to a second mouse from which variable amounts of fat had been surgically excised before the transplantation. They found that the percentage of successful intra-abdominal transplants of adipose tissue between mice rose from about 10 percent when no fat was removed from the recipient to more than 80 percent when both gonadal fat organs had been removed prior to the implantation of fat.

In a second study these authors examined the relation between total body fat and its distribution in individual fat organs in animals treated with gold thioglucose. In the mouse the gonadal fat organ contains approximately 25 percent of the total body fat, and removal of this organ thus reduces body fat by nearly one fourth. Treatment with gold thioglucose damages the ventromedial region of the hypothalamus and obesity develops (see below). When animals with intact or removed gonadal fat organs were treated with gold thioglucose, they both became obese and the final quantity of body fat was the same. In the obese animals with intact gonadal fat organs, final body lipid was 12.1 g. In the animals without gonadal fat organs, it was 13.8 g, indicating that the remaining fat deposits had accumulated more fat. The inguinal fat organ, for example, had doubled in weight.

In similar experiments Chlouverakis and Hojnicki (1974) have examined the effect of removing intra-abdominal fat from mice which had one form of a genetically transmitted obesity (ob/ob—see Chapter 5). After the operation the body weights increased, and total body fat was the same in operated subjects and in the unoperated controls. This group of experiments suggests that the total body fat is integrated into a single functional component (compartment) with compensatory changes occurring in each fat depot. However, the way in which all of the deposits of adipose tissue are integrated into the total body economy is as yet unknown.

Studies with parabiosed* animals provide a third line of evidence supporting the regulation of total stored calories. When one animal of such a pair becomes obese following destructive lesions in the ventromedial nucleus, the unlesioned parabiotic animal becomes thin by loss of body fat. The body fat of the hyperphagic-parabiotic animal will rise to 30 to 40 percent and the fat content of the lean animal will fall to 1 to 2 percent, compared to a normal value of 8 to 10 percent body fat for rats (Hervey, 1959). Fleming (1969) repeated these experiments and found a small but statistically significant reduction in food intake in the lean rat parabiosed to a hyperphagic lesioned animal ($r =$ .789, $p < .02$). Coleman and Hummel (1969) obtained similar results after parabiosis of genetically diabetic mice (genotype db/db) to lean littermates. This group of experiments suggests that the lean animal is detecting some signal from the fat animal which indicates an increased store of calories. To compensate, the lean animal reduces its food intake and its caloric stores of fat decrease.

The final kind of evidence supporting the regulation of caloric stores comes from studies with hypothalamic injury. After effective hypothalamic injury, there is an initial rapid rate of weight gain with marked hyperphagia. This is followed by a new stability of body weight in which food intake returns to nearly normal levels (Brobeck, 1946; Brooks, Marine and Lambert, 1946; Hetherington and Ranson, 1942b; Stevenson, 1969). Disturbance of this higher but plateaued weight by starvation is followed by increased caloric intake until weight is restored to the plateau from which it started.

The data reviewed above imply the existence of some kind of controlling mechanisms for body weight and body fat. Unfortunately, stability of weight and fat is not always maintained. Meal eating is a periodic phenomenon. A meal starts, lasts for a period of time, and then ends. This process is repeated one or more times a day. Yet the body's need for energy is not periodic. Basal energy requirements are continuous and demands for activity are superimposed. The body is

---

*Parabiosis involves attaching two animals side to side with the skin and peritoneal surfaces of one attached to the other.

thus faced with continuing demand for energy (calories) and periodic or intermittent supplies of food. Le Magnen has examined the relation between the size of individual meals and the interval between meals (Le Magnen, 1967; Le Magnen et al., 1973). This data suggests that a large meal is followed by a longer intermeal period than is a short meal. He thus suggests that meal eating is in part "anticipatory," but not all workers can confirm this (Revusky, 1970).

Several factors must be examined in an effort to understand the way in which the control goes awry in obesity: the factors regulating food ingestion, the factors involved in the distribution and storage of calories, and the control of energy expenditure. These subjects will be examined in this and the next two chapters.

REGULATION OF FOOD INTAKE

Neuroanatomical Basis

Studies using the experimental animal have increased our understanding of the anatomical basis for the regulation of food intake. The principal neural components which integrate this system are located in the hypothalamus and are shown schematically in Figure 2–3.

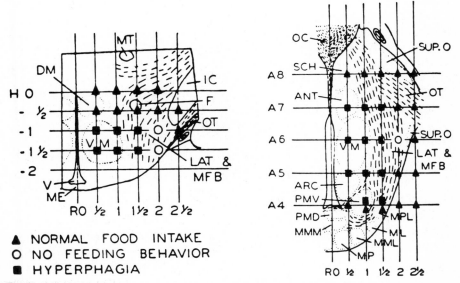

▲ NORMAL FOOD INTAKE
O NO FEEDING BEHAVIOR
■ HYPERPHAGIA

Figure 2–3. Hypothalamic structures involved in feeding. This diagram shows transverse (left) and longitudinal (right) views of a rat brain. The lines represent a 1 mm grid. The effects of lesions at various areas are shown. The open circles (o) are those areas which abolished feeding. The solid squares (□) are the areas where lesions produced hyperphagia. Note that the area producing hyperphagia is larger than the VM nucleus. (From Stevenson, J. A. F. *In*: The hypothalamus, 1969. Courtesy of Charles C Thomas, publisher, Springfield, Illinois.)

Anatomically the third ventricle divides the hypothalamus into two lateral halves. Adjacent to the third ventricle are several midline nuclei which can be subdivided into anterior, medial and posterior groups. The ventromedial nucleus occupies a prominent position in the middle hypothalamus. Bilateral destructive lesions in this area have consistently produced obesity in all species studied.

Careful mapping of these regions of the hypothalamus has determined a clear anatomic location for the important structures. These structures include: (1) the larger part of the anterior ventromedial nucleus along with some of the tissue lateral to it; (2) the caudal end of the ventromedial nucleus involving the premamillary area and some of the adjacent lateral hypothalamus; and (3) the area dorsal and lateral to the mamillary body. In contrast, lesions in the anterior hypothalamus, fornix, most of the mamillary body, ventral septal system, olfactory tubercle, and in the midline near the floor of the third ventricle produced no similar effect (Hetherington, 1944; Hetherington and Ranson, 1942a). Effective lesions involve the ventromedial nuclei and extend laterally to involve fiber tracts which course anteriorly. Anand and Brobeck (1951) have prepared a neurological map of these critical areas (adapted as shown in Figure 2–3).

The lateral hypothalamus is also involved in the control of energy balance. In contrast to the medial region, the nuclear structures in the lateral hypothalamus are less clearly defined. The importance of this area for regulation of food intake has been well established by studies which demonstrate that destructive lesions produce profound aphagia and death (Anand, 1962; Anand and Brobeck, 1951; Cheng et al., 1971; Teitelbaum et al., 1969a, b). Aphagia or hypophagia has been observed in rats (Hetherington and Ranson, 1942b), cats (Clark et al., 1939) and monkeys (Ingram et al., 1936). The syndrome of aphagia and adipsia occurs with injury to the far lateral hypothalamus. Current evidence thus suggests that the lateral and far lateral hypothalamus play a critical role in the initiation of food seeking behavior.

It has been difficult to demonstrate that fiber tracts run from the ventromedial to the lateral hypothalamic regions, although two studies have strongly suggested that such connections do exist. In the first case, knife cuts between the ventromedial hypothalamus were found to produce hyperphagia similar to that resulting from destruction of the ventromedial hypothalamus (Jansen and Hutchinson, 1969; Albert et al., 1971; Grossman and Grossman, 1971; Gold, 1973a, b). Secondly, Arees and Mayer (1967) (see also Mayer and Arees, 1968) have followed the degeneration of fibers in the ventromedial nucleus after treatment with gold thioglucose. Fibers leaving the ventromedial area appear to travel in the bundle of Schutz to the head of the vagal nerve and to the lateral hypothalamus.

Alterations in food intake with damage to other parts of the brain have been reported on many occasions (for a review see Stevenson,

1969; Grossman, 1972). Three principal techniques of investigation have been used in these studies: electrical stimulation, electrical lesions and chemical stimulation by microinjection of norepinephrine into the brain. Table 2–2 summarizes some of this data. Consistent effects have been observed in studies of the amygdaloid complex and of the globus pallidus. Morgane and Kosman (1959, 1960) observed that food intake was increased in cats after aspiration of the amygdala. This effect was not dependent on simultaneous injury to the ventromedial hypothalamus. Indeed destruction of the ventromedial hypothalamus enhanced the effects of lesions of the amygdala.

Additional evidence indicating an important function of the amygdala has come from experiments using electrical stimulation. When the basolateral part of the amygdaloid complex is stimulated, food intake is inhibited in cats (Fonberg and Delgado, 1961). Reciprocal effects of destruction increasing and stimulation decreasing food intake suggest an important role for the amygdaloid complex in the control of energy balance (Fonberg, 1975).

Anatomical connections between the amygdala and the ventromedial nucleus consist of two groups of fibers which run in the fornix (Sutin, 1975). This close anatomic connection provides a basis for the functional relationship noted above.

In addition to the hypothalamus and amygdala, food intake can be modified by stimulating or destroying the septal region, the globus pallidus, the caudate nucleus, the cingulate gyrus and the frontal lobe. In general, stimulation and destruction have reciprocal effects (for review see Grossman, 1972; Stevenson, 1969).

TABLE 2–2. *Effect of Experimental Manipulation of Various Regions of the Brain on Food Intake**

REGION OF BRAIN	CHANGE IN FOOD INTAKE AFTER		
	Destructive Lesion	*Electrical Stimulation*	*Chemical Stimulation With Norepinephrine*
Hypothalamus			
Medial	↑	–	↑
Lateral	↓	↑	↑
Septal Area	–	↑	No effect
Thalamus	?	↑	↑
Globus Pallidus	↓	–	↑
Caudate Nucleus	↓	↓	–
Tegmentum	↓	↑	
Amygdaloid Complex	↑	Variable	No effect
Frontal Lobotomy	↑	–	–
Cingulate Gyrus	–	↑ or variable	↑

*Adapted from Grossman: Adv. Psychosom. Med., 7:49–72, 1972.

Physiological Factors

Several different techniques have been used to investigate the functional relationships within the hypothalamus. These are summarized in Table 2–3 (for review see Hoebel, 1971; and Mogenson, 1975). From examination of this table it is obvious that the medial and lateral regions of the hypothalamus have reciprocal responses to most of the experimental manipulations listed. The reciprocal function of these two areas led Anand and Brobeck (1951) to propose the "dual center" hypothesis for the control of food intake. In this hypothesis the ventromedial nucleus serves as a "satiety center" and acts as an inhibitor of a "feeding center" located in the lateral hypothalamus. The "dual center" hypothesis has provided a fruitful and stimulating basis for the study of hypothalamic control of food intake. It has received support from a number of experimental observations including the various reciprocal functions listed in Table 2–3.

From the standpoint of electrophysiology it has received support from the work of Anand et al. (1964) and Oomura et al. (1967, 1975). The former study shows that the electrical firing rate of neural units in the ventromedial hypothalamus of starved animals is slower than that of neural units in the lateral hypothalamus. Glucose given intravenously decreases the unit electrical activity of the lateral feeding area and increases the firing activity of the ventromedial area. Oomura et al. (1967) expanded upon these findings to show that there is reciprocal electrical activity in the ventromedial and lateral hypothalamic area of cats. The correlation between the firing rate of the ventromedial and lateral area was $r = 0.78$ ($y = -1.1 \times +18$).

In all species thus far studied, hyperphagia is produced by injury to the ventromedial hypothalamus (VMH), suggesting that this region plays an important role in regulation of caloric balance in most, if not all, higher animals (Hetherington and Ranson, 1942b; Brobeck et al., 1943; Anand and Brobeck, 1951; Montemurro, 1971; Hamilton and

TABLE 2–3. *Experimental Manipulations Which Support the Dual Center Hypothesis*

| | CHANGE IN FOOD INTAKE | |
EXPERIMENTAL MANIPULATION	VENTRAL MEDIAL AREA	LATERAL AREA
Lesion	↑	↓
Electrical stimulation	—	↑
Procaine	↑	↓
Hypertonic NaCl	↓	↑
Glucose	↑ (long latency)	— (insulin induced feeding)
Norepinephrine	↑	↑
Isoproterenol	—	↓

Brobeck, 1964; Hamilton et al., 1972; Lepkovsky, 1973a, b; Knobil et al., 1974, personal communication).

Figure 2–4 shows a characteristic response to bilateral hypothalamic injury by electric current in the rat (Brooks, 1946). After an effective injury there is a decrease in running activity, a rise in food intake, and a disturbance to the reproductive cycle (Brooks, 1946; Brobeck, 1946; Bernardis, 1972). The normal diurnal rhythm of greater food intake at night is lost (Kakolewski et al., 1971). The electrolytic lesion also changes the pattern of hormonal activity. Growth hormone is released over the first minutes after electrolytic lesioning, but then falls to low levels (Frohman and Bernardis, 1968; Frohman et al., 1969; Bernardis and Frohman, 1971b). VMH lesions in weaning rats are associated with stunting (Bernardis, 1966; Bernardis and Skelton, 1965, 1966; Han et al., 1965, 1968; Han and Liu, 1966). Conversely, insulin concentrations are increased (Hales and Kennedy, 1964; Han, 1967; Frohman et al., 1969; Bernardis and Frohman, 1970, 1971a; Hustfelt and Lovo, 1972). These two hormonal changes may play an important pathogenetic role in this syndrome (see Chapters 5 and 7).

Several other techniques in addition to electrolytic destruction have been used to study the response of the ventromedial hypothalamus. Pfaff (1969) showed that the nucleoli in the ventromedial nucleus were smaller in fasted rats than in fed ones. Epstein (1960) used injections of procaine, a local anesthetic, or of hypertonic saline into the hypothalamus to study its function. When the medial hypothalamus was anesthetized with procaine, food intake increased. Local anesthesia in the lateral hypothalamus, on the other hand, depressed food intake. The increase in food intake in sheep (Baile and Mayer, 1966) and in chickens (Shapiro et al., 1973) after injecting

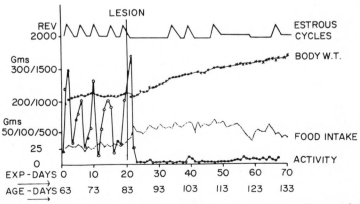

Figure 2–4.   The effects of hypothalamic injury in the rat. Following the introduction of bilateral hypothalamic lesions, there was an increase in food intake, a decrease in activity and a gradual rise in body weight. (Brooks: Am. J. Physiol., *147*:708–716, 1946.)

pentobarbital into the third ventricle may be due to anesthetizing the ventromedial hypothalamus. Injections of hypertonic saline into the hypothalamus depressed food intake when applied locally to the ventromedial hypothalamus, and stimulated feeding when applied laterally (Table 2–3).

Several chemicals in addition to procaine have been used to investigate hypothalamic control of food intake, most notable of which are the catecholamines (see below), gold thioglucose (Brecher and Waxler, 1949), monosodium glutamate (Olney, 1969), 4-nitroquinoline-1-oxide (Yamamoto et al., 1970), and bipiperidyl mustard (Rutman et al., 1967). Gold thioglucose produces particularly interesting results. It enters many regions of the brain but damages primarily the ventromedial hypothalamus (Brecher and Waxler, 1949; Debons et al., 1968; Marshall, Barnett and Mayer, 1955). More recent data (Brecher et al., 1965) have indicated that the ventromedial nucleus is not the central focus of the lesion produced by this drug. Although anatomic lesions were present in over 90 percent of the animals to which the drug was administered, only the 30 percent with large lesions involving part of the ventromedial nucleus developed obesity.

Microsurgical knife cuts have been used to interrupt various fiber tracts in order to explore hypothalamic function (Gold et al., 1973b; Albert et al., 1971; Grossman and Grossman, 1971; Jansen and Hutchisen, 1969). Knife cuts which isolate the entire hypothalamus produce obesity in monkeys (Knobil et al., 1974) as do knife cuts lateral to the ventromedial nucleus which produce a syndrome essentially identical with that produced by electrolytic destruction of the ventromedial nucleus; however, weight gain is somewhat less (Albert et al., 1971). Knife cuts anterior to the ventromedial nucleus enhance food intake slightly in female rats but have no effect in males. Posterior knife cuts do not modify food intake. Knife cuts in the lateral hypothalamus result in inhibited food intake, as do electrolytic lesions (Sclafani, 1971; Sclafani et al., 1973b).

Recent data have suggested that the ventral noradrenergic bundle, rather than the ventromedial nucleus itself, is the critical structure in the hypothalamus for control and regulation of body weight (Gold, 1973a; Ungerstedt, 1971; Mogenson, 1975). This bundle ascends from the midbrain and has terminals near the ventromedial region of the hypothalamus and fibers placed more anteriorly (Fig. 2–5). Destruction of this pathway or interruption of the pathways between the ventromedial and lateral hypothalamus is followed by hyperphagia and obesity.

Kapatos and Gold (1973) made cuts between the ventromedial and lateral hypothalamus on one side of the brain. They found that subsequent damage to the ventral noradrenergic bundle anywhere between the midbrain and the mamillary body on the opposite side was effective in producing hyperphagia. Ahlskog and Hoebel (1973)

Noradrenergic   Dopaminergic

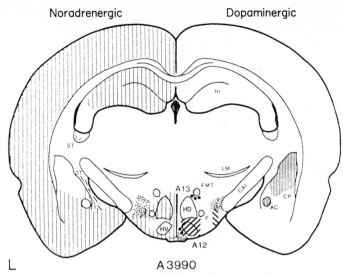

L   A 3990

Figure 2–5. Distribution of norepinephrine and dopamine in the rat brain. The drawing is based on the stereotaxic atlas of König and Klippel and on Craigie's Neuroanatomy. This section is 3990 micra (μ) anterior to the zero plane. HI = hippocampus; LM = medial lemniscus; CAI = internal capsule; AC = central amygdaloid nucleus; CP = caudate putamen; FMT = mamillothalamic tract; HD = dorsomedial nucleus; HV = ventromedial hypothalamic nucleus; F = fornix; ST = stria terminalis. The regions of the ventral hypothalamus in which destructive lesions produce hyperphagia (ventromedial = HV) or aphagia (lateral) have been superimposed as cross hatched areas. (From Ungerstedt: Acta Physiol. Scand., Suppl. 367:1–122, 1971.)

came to a similar conclusion using 6-hydroxydopamine, a chemical which selectively destroys noradrenergic nerve fibers. When this compound was injected into the ventral noradrenergic bundle, it produced hyperphagia in rats. These two observations suggest that the ventromedial nucleus is a convenient landmark and possibly a point of interaction with messages ascending in the brain over the noradrenergic bundle. The noradrenergic bundle, however, appears to have the central role in controlling food intake.

Stimulation by electrical or chemical means has also been used to explore the relation between the medial and lateral hypothalamus. Hess (1951) was the first to show that stimulation just above the mamillothalamic tract of the hypothalamus of the cat induces feeding. Delgado and Anand (1953) performed similar experiments in cats in which the electrodes were chronically implanted. Various parts of the brain were stimulated and it was found that electrical stimulation of the lateral hypothalamus for one hour per day significantly increased food intake. Electrical stimulation of the hypothalamus results in increased food intake in goats (Larsson, 1954), rabbits (Traczyk, 1962), and rats (Smith et al., 1961; Coons et al., 1965).

Morgane (1961) noted that stimulation of the far lateral hypothalamic area could increase both the basic drive to eat and the intake of food provided as a reward for the pressing of a lever (so-called motivated feeding). With stimulation of the more medial portion of the lateral perifornical area in the hypothalamus, basic feeding, but not motivated feeding, increased. Steinbaum and Miller (1965) showed that regular stimulation of the lateral hypothalamus in the presence of food was followed by the development of obesity. If food were absent during these periods of stimulation, there was no increase in body weight. The rise in body weight by stimulating the lateral hypothalamus 3 times daily is shown in Fig. 2–6 (Steffens, 1975). Body weight continued to increase as long as the stimulation was continued.

The effect of electrical stimulation on food intake was further studied by Wendt and Olds (1957). They found that there is a similarity in the regions of the hypothalamus in which food intake can be stimulated and those areas of the brain which rats will self-stimulate* to produce intrahypothalamic current. As noted above, stimulation of electrodes in the lateral hypothalamus elicits feeding in the satiated rat. When these electrodes are left in place for two weeks after implantation and then tested, rats will press a bar to receive an electrical stimulus through the same electrodes that elicit food intake (Margules and Olds, 1962). Electrolytic lesions made by passing a higher current through these electrodes will cause aphagia and abolish self-stimulatory behavior.

After stimulation of the ventromedial hypothalamus (VMH), both feeding and bar-pressing for self-stimulation decreased (Hoebel and Teitelbaum, 1962). Thus rats ceased pressing the lever when each press stimulated both the medial and lateral hypothalamus. Medial stimulation alone, however, did not cause cessation of bar-pressing for self-stimulation in the lateral hypothalamus. Finally, if the VMH is ablated or anesthetized with procaine, lateral hypothalamic self-stimulation increases (Hoebel, 1965). The introduction of food into the stomach or the ingestion of a meal also decreases the rate of self-stimulation through electrodes in the lateral hypothalamus. Similarly gastric distention with a rubber balloon reduces the rate of self-stimulation (Hoebel and Thompson, 1969). Anesthesia to or destruction of the ventromedial hypothalamus restores the rate of self-stimulation of the fed animal to its previous level.

The relation of lesions in the ventromedial hypothalamus to self-stimulation through electrodes in the lateral hypothalamus has been re-examined by Ferguson and Keesey (1971). They observed a positive correlation between the weight gain of the animal and the rate of self-stimulation on the day of the ventromedial hypothalamic lesion, but a significant negative correlation between weight gain and the rate

---

*Self-stimulation is the act of pressing a bar to introduce an electrical current into the brain.

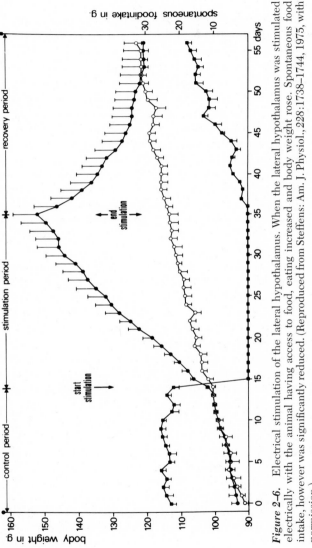

Figure 2-6. Electrical stimulation of the lateral hypothalamus. When the lateral hypothalamus was stimulated electrically with the animal having access to food, eating increased and body weight rose. Spontaneous food intake, however was significantly reduced. (Reproduced from Steffens: Am. J. Physiol., 228:1738–1744, 1975, with permission.)

of self-stimulation on the postoperative days. This suggests that the increased food intake of the lesioned hyperphagic rat substitutes nutrient stimulation or reward to the hypothalamus for the reward of self-stimulation, which increases following the introduction of the VMH lesion and accounts for the rise in self-stimulation on the first postoperative day.

The role of the lateral hypothalamus in relation to food intake has been extensively explored using destructive lesions (Anand and Brobeck, 1951; Teitelbaum et al., 1969b). Bilateral destructive lesions in the lateral hypothalamus abolish feeding behavior with eventual death unless animals are carefully nursed and tubefed during the early postoperative days. With time and good nursing care there is a gradual recovery, and animals will eventually eat enough spontaneously to maintain body weight.

The sequence of events from aphagia through recovery has been subdivided into several stages. This sequence of recovery affects both food and water intake and is similar to the normal sequence of events during maturation of the hypothalamus in the first few weeks after birth. During early recovery, the injection of norepinephrine into the lateral ventricle increases food intake, but this does not happen immediately after the lesion (Berger et al., 1971). Injections of nerve growth factor also facilitate recovery from lateral injury (Berger et al., 1973). Rats which have recovered from lateral lesions will maintain body weight and will eat more in the cold, as well as adjust the bulk of food eaten to maintain a constant caloric intake. Rats which have recovered from lateral lesions will, however, not eat extra food after injections of insulin, although such injections in normal rats elicit food intake (Epstein and Teitelbaum, 1967).

The lateral hypothalamic syndrome is associated with injury to the dopaminergic pathways (Fig. 2–5). These pathways ascend from the striatum and terminate in subcortical areas. An analog of dopamine which destroys the dopamine-containing neurons (either injections of 6-hydroxydopamine or knife cuts which interrupt these pathways and reduce dopamine) produce this syndrome (Grossman, 1975; Stricker and Zigmond, 1975). Animals with injury to these pathways are somnolent but, when aroused by vigorous stimulation, they may eat (Wolgin et al., 1975), suggesting that part of the lateral hypothalamic syndrome represents loss of mechanisms for arousal.

Powley and Keesey (1970) have recently suggested that the lateral region of the hypothalamus may play an important role in "setting" one limit of the desired level of body weight. Animals which had been deprived of food and lost weight prior to a lateral hypothalamic lesion resumed eating much earlier than those of normal weight at the time of the lesion. Powley and Keesey interpreted this to mean that injury to the lateral hypothalamic area lowers the limits on weight. By analogy the ventromedial injury would set a higher limit. Injury to the lateral hypothalamus would destroy fibers and make the remaining neurons "think" the body was "heavier" than normal and thus inhibit food intake. Conversely, injury to the ventromedial area would make the animal think it is lighter than it should be and the animal would eat more. Animals will maintain the lower or higher weight after hypothalamic injury (Keesey, 1975).

Nerve endings which release norepinephrine may be involved in the transmission of neurochemical information within the hypothalamus. The injection of norepinephrine into the ventromedial nucleus of the satiated rat stimulates food intake (see Table 2–3) (Grossman, 1960, 1972; Leibowitz, 1970a, b, 1975; Margules and Dragovich, 1973). This effect of norepinephrine can be blocked with phentolamine, an alpha-adrenergic blocking drug, but cannot be blocked by propranolol which is a beta blocking drug. This suggests that norepinephrine inhibits the ventromedial nucleus by interacting with receptors on the surface of these neurons and releasing the lateral hypothalamus to initiate food seeking. The ventromedial nucleus thus has an alpha-adrenergic hunger system. Injection of a beta-adrenergic drug such as isoproterenol into the lateral hypothalamus of a hungry rat will inhibit food intake. This effect is blocked by propranolol, a beta-adrenergic blocking drug, but not by phentolamine. This suggests the possibility of a beta satiety system in the lateral hypothalamus. The hypothesis of an alpha-receptor-mediated hunger and beta-receptor-mediated satiety area provides many challenging possibilities for further research.

The calcium ion may be another component of the intercellular system for transmission of neurochemical information. Myers et al. (1972) increased the calcium concentration in the lateral cerebral ventricles from 2.5 to 151.2 mM and noted that satiated rats started eating. Injecting magnesium or sodium ions had no effect. The stimulatory effect of calcium was slightly augmented by propranolol and partially attenuated by phentolamine in some, but not all, of the animals. These findings suggest that catecholamines may modify feeding behavior by regulating transmembrane ionic concentrations of calcium (Panksepp, 1974).

Additional Factors

CALORIES VERSUS TASTE

The normal rat will eat for calories. This has been clearly shown in two kinds of experiments (Adolph, 1947; Strominger and Brobeck, 1953; Carlisle and Stellar, 1969; Mayer and Thomas, 1967). When the caloric density (i.e., calories per gram) of a stock diet for rats is decreased by adding a bland, but indigestible, substance like cellulose or kaolin, the animals will promptly increase the volume of food which they ingest in order to maintain a constant intake of calories. The time required for this adjustment is less than 24 hours.

Eating for calories has been observed in rats which have been fitted with intragastric tubes through which food is injected when the rat presses a lever (Epstein, 1967). The total daily intake, the size of individual meals, and their number each day vary within narrow limits. When the caloric density of the intragastric formula is decreased by diluting it with water, the animal adjusts the volume pumped into the stomach to maintain a constant caloric intake. This adjustment is usually completed during the first night. These two kinds of studies show that caloric regulation in rodents is accurate, adjusts rapidly to changes in the caloric density of the diet, and does not require oropharyngeal contact to make the adjustment.

Under many circumstances, however, the regulation is not so precise and the taste of the diet becomes as important as the calorie value. This is particularly true in the hungry or deprived animal, or when the caloric density of the diet is very high. The relation of caloric density and taste of the diet has been succinctly stated by Jacobs as follows: ". . . an animal eats for calories when he does not need them and eats for taste when he needs calories," (Jacobs and Sharma, 1969). Soulairac, observed as early as 1944, that hungry rats would drink more of a 10 percent saccharine solution than would normal rats. The effect of a sweet taste on the quantity of indigestible cellulose eaten by rats is shown in Figure 2–7. After 22 hours without food the animals were allowed a two hour feeding period. Less than 1 gram of dry cellulose was ingested. When the cellulose was moistened with water, nearly two grams were eaten. When 0.75 percent saccharine and 0.9 percent Tween-80 (polysorbate 80) were mixed with the cellulose, the rats ate over 6 grams of food in two hours.

Greasiness is another component of taste or palatability. In 1955 Mickelsen et al. reported that rats fed a 60 percent fat diet became grossly obese (see also Chapter 5). In these animals eating for "calories" was overcome by the palatability of a high fat diet (Schemmel et al., 1970). When Carlisle and Stellar (1969) examined the relationship between "greasiness" and caloric density of diets fed to normal rats and to rats with lesions in the ventromedial hypothalamus, they found that both groups prefer the greasy diets over pellets regardless of the caloric density. When the greasy texture was held constant, calorically dense rations were preferred over the more dilute ones. Thus both greasy and sweet tastes have for the animal rewards of their own which are independent of caloric value.

The rat with a ventromedial hypothalamic lesion is alleged to react differently to the sensory qualities of its food than does the lean rat (Teitelbaum, 1955; Corbit and Stellar, 1964; Khairy et al., 1963; Lipton, 1969). Miller, Bailey, and Stevenson (1950) noted for example

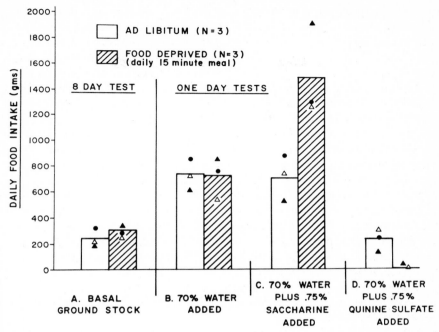

Figure 2-7. Taste versus calories. Rats were given various diets after being fed ad libitum or after being deprived of food. The rats ate more moist food than dry food. The rats deprived of food ate more when saccharine was present and less when quinine was present. (Reproduced from Jacobs and Sharma: Ann. N. Y. Acad. Sci., *157*:1084–1125, 1969, with permission.)

that the VMH-lesioned, obese rat has an increased food intake but a decreased desire to strive to obtain food. Thus VMH-lesioned rats would not cross an electric field as readily as lean ones when food was the reward, nor would they work as hard to lift a lid on a jar of food. Quinine adulteration of the food reduced food intake of VMH rats more than that of normal rats. This phenomenon does not occur in genetically obese rats but was observed in VMH-lesioned obese rats of the same strain (Bray and York, 1972). These studies appear to indicate that laziness and finickiness are part of the syndrome which follows ablation of the VMH area.

This conclusion has come into question because studies have been conducted which have compared food intake of lesioned and control rats at different levels of body weight. If rats which have VMH lesions are maintained at their preoperative weight, they will work as hard or harder for food than the lean control animals (Marks and Remley, 1972; Porter and Allen, 1972; Beatty, 1973; Kent and Peters, 1973; Sclafani, 1975). Beatty has summarized this situation as follows, "It is . . . clear that body weight level, deprivation conditions, session length, preoperative training conditions, the response requirements of the behavioral task, the method by which lesions are produced, and the ambient temperature during the test are also important variables" in comparing lean animals to those with VMH lesions.

The effects of preoperative training have been explored by Singh (1973). He compared rats which had been trained in the bar-pressing techniques before VMH injury with rats which had not. Rats which had been trained before the lesions were unchanged in their postoperative performance. The animals which were not trained before surgery had lower responses and less "motivation" after surgery. Thus the finickiness which is attributed to VMH rats may be a function of the experimental procedures rather than a changed physiology.

Levison et al. (1973) showed that "palatability" of the diet can be more readily modified in the VMH rat than in normal rats. When the caloric density of the diet was reduced 20 percent by adding kaolin, food intake fell in the VMH rats. When the diet was sweetened with saccharine or confectioners' sugar, the sweetening produced a greater food intake in the VMH-lesioned rats than in the lean animals. Sclafani and Grossman (1971) suggest that the concept of decreased appetitive drive to hunger as proposed by Miller et al. (1950) may not be an adequate explanation for the differential reactivity in VMH-lesioned rats to quinine and electric shock.

Bait-shyness is a third component of taste which plays a role in food intake (Garcia and Koelling, 1971). If a rodent ingests something and shortly afterward becomes sick, the animal will henceforth avoid ingesting this substance. Exposure to x-irradiation, for example, will make rats ill. When rats are exposed to a dose of irradiation which does not produce overt illness at the same time that they are drinking saccharine-flavored water, they will subsequently display an aversion to saccharine-flavored water which may persist for many weeks. Several aspects of this phenomenon are now well established. The stronger the flavor, the greater the aversion induced by simultaneous illness. When the flavor is held constant, the aversion is greater with a more severe illness. Finally, given a constant flavor and constant illness, the strength of the aversion falls off with increasing duration between time of illness and time of consumption of the flavor.

GASTROINTESTINAL FACTORS

Although eating for calories is well regulated, this precision breaks down when both oral and intragastric loads are given at the same time. In dogs the oral intake of food was only partially suppressed when the animal received 50 to 100 percent of its total daily intake directly into the stomach and was allowed to have food orally. Only when the stomach load was 175 percent of total daily intake was oral ingestion completely eliminated. Acute preloading of the stomach in dogs twenty minutes before eating does, however, decrease food intake by an equivalent amount (Janowitz and Grossman, 1949a, b). An inert material which distends the stomach also has some effect. However, the distention must occur immediately before eating to be effective (Share, Martyniuk, and Grossman, 1952). In esophagostomized dogs (i.e., dogs whose esophagus exits through the neck and does not enter the stomach) sham feeding greatly exceeds the deficit in calories. Preloading the stomach of these animals does not inhibit oral ingestion, but the introduction of food into the stomach during the act of feeding partially reduces oral food ingestion. These studies in dogs indicate that gastric distention plays a role in terminating food intake and that both oral and gastric factors are involved in its precise regulation.

The effects of intragastric loads on the oral feeding of rats have also been studied (Berkun et al., 1952). When solutions of sodium chloride were placed in the stomach, rats drank 19.7 ml of milk. When allowed to drink the first 10 ml by mouth, the animals drank significantly less (7.1 ml) than when the 10 ml of milk had been placed directly into the stomach. These experiments in rats and dogs indicate that an intragastric load of calories does not reduce oral intake by an equivalent amount.

Most animals have selective sensitivity for food nutrients. Richter (1943) showed that growing animals with access to a "cafeteria" of basic foods would select a reasonably balanced diet for growth. Deficiency of essential components from the choices can be detected and will result in a decreased total intake. Distortion of the amino acid content of the diet can depress food intake. This effect is most clearly observed when one of the essential amino acids is deleted (Peng et al., 1972; Harper, 1975). The neuroanatomic basis for the inhibition of food intake by deletion of an amino acid from the diet has not been clearly established but the nervous system plays an important role in this response. Injection of the deficient amino acid into the carotid artery stimulates food intake, whereas the same quantity of the amino acid injected into the jugular vein does not. The ventromedial region of the hypothalamus has been largely excluded from monitoring the deficiency of amino acids, as shown by the reduced food intake of rats with ventromedial lesions when amino acids are omitted from the diet. The response to injections of amino acids is blunted but not abolished by lesions in the hippocampus. Further work is needed to establish the basis for the effect.

The ingestion of food may serve to inhibit food intake in one of three ways: (1) distention of the gastrointestinal tract during the ingestion of food may activate neural pathways to the nervous system; (2) ingestion of food may trigger the release of hormones from the gastrointestinal tract; and (3) early absorption of nutrients may signal an end to eating. The possibility that food in the G.I. tract could serve to modify the awareness of gastric contractions has been tested repeatedly since its original proposal by Carlson and by Cannon and Washburn in 1912. Gastric distention will diminish food intake and esophageal or gastric fistulas will prevent satiety. Distention of the stomach increases the firing rate of the vagus and this may be the mechanism by which these effects are relayed to the central nervous system (Paintal, 1954). Following vagotomy in rats, the size of individual meals is reduced by 25 to 50 percent and the frequency of eating increases; however, caloric intake is maintained constant (Snowden, 1970). On the other hand, stimulation of vagal afferents or gastric distention increases the unit activity in the VMH (Sharma et al., 1961). Ablation of the VMH prevents the inhibition of gastric contractions which usually follow the injection of glucagon (Sudsaneh and Mayer, 1959).

Finally, stimulation of the feeding area in the lateral hypothalamus inhibited gastric motility if the stomach were active. If the stomach were quiescent, however, stimulation of the lateral hypothalamus increased gastric activity (Glacheva et al., 1972). These findings taken together suggest that gastric distention may stimulate the vagus and serve as one factor in regulating meal size. Booth (1975) and Davis, Collins and Levine (1975) have recently proposed that the absorption of nutrients across the intestinal tract may serve as a major indicator of energy balance.

Humoral or hormonal mechanisms are a second way in which food in the gastrointestinal tract might provide signals to stop eating. When 50 percent of the blood from satiated rats was cross transfused into hungry rats, food intake was depressed for up to three hours (Davis et al., 1969, 1971). Fleming (1969) explored this problem using parabiotic rats. He showed that when one rat of a parabiotic pair ate one hour before the other, the food intake of the second rat was suppressed. No difference was noted if the animals were fed simultaneously. This implies that some circulating factor was transferred from one rat to the other.

Gibbs, Young and Smith (1973a, b) have recently suggested that the gastrointestinal hormone cholecystokinin-pancreozymin (CCK-PZ) may be one of these humoral factors. Rats with gastric fistulas were adapted to eating a liquid formula diet. If the gastric cannula were opened, the orally ingested liquid diet drained out and the animals ate large quantities of food with no inhibition of eating. However, when the gastric cannula was closed, feeding behavior was similar to normal. Injection of small doses of cholecystokinin (CCK-PZ) into animals with open gastric fistulas inhibited food intake as would closing of the gastric cannula (Fig. 2–8). The doses of cholecystokinin were within the physiologic range for producing contraction of the gall bladder. These data provide evidence for one humoral mechanism which inhibits food intake in experimental animals.

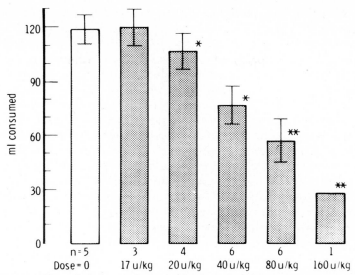

Figure 2–8. Effect of cholecystokinin on food intake of rats. Increasing amounts of cholecystokinin was injected into rats with open gastric fistulas. There was a dose-related reduction in food intake with doses above 20 u/kg. (From Gibbs, Young and Smith, copyright 1973 by the American Psychological Association. Reprinted with permission.)

The absorption of nutrients themselves may also influence dietary intake. After digestion, the macronutrients and micronutrients are absorbed across the gastrointestinal tract and enter the portal circulation. Glucose might influence subsequent food intake in two ways: first, by changing the blood concentration or the rate of glucose utilization, which might be detected by centers in the hypothalamus and inhibit food intake; and second, by activating neural inputs into the hypothalamus.

These possibilities have been assessed by using glucose itself and 2-deoxyglucose, an analog of glucose which can enter the cell and be phosphorylated, but cannot be further metabolized by the enzymes of the Embden-Mayerhof (the pentose phosphate pathway). Injection of 2-deoxyglucose into monkeys or rats increases food intake (Smith and Epstein, 1969) with a latency or lag time which is shorter than the increase in eating which follows the injection of insulin. Although 2-deoxyglucose enhances short term food intake, this effect is most marked during the daytime hours, and in long term studies the drug does not alter total daily food intake or body weight (Naito et al., 1973).

Recently Novin et al. (1973) found that the injection of 2-deoxyglucose into the portal vein of rabbits produced the onset of feeding more rapidly than if injected into a peripheral vein. This effect was delayed if the rabbits' vagus nerve were cut. These findings suggest that gluco-receptors in the liver may transmit messages related to acute changes in nutritional status to the central nervous system via the vagus nerve. Niijima (1969) showed that the firing rate of nerves from the liver of guinea pigs was reduced as the concentration of glucose perfusing the liver through the portal circulation was increased. These findings, along with those of Russek (1963, 1975), suggest that some of the gluco-receptors to which the brain responds may be in the liver and not in the central nervous system.

In addition to the hepatic gluco-receptors there appear to be gluco-receptors in the duodenum and hypothalamus. The increased firing of hypothalamic gluco-receptors has been clearly shown by putting glucose directly onto hypothalamic neurons (Oomura, 1975), as well as by giving glucose into the carotid artery (Marrazzi, 1975). The analysis which Oomura has done shows the presence of glucose-sensitive neurons in the lateral hypothalamus, and insulin-sensitive ones in the medial hypothalamus.

Duodenal gluco-receptors are also present. Novin (1975) infused glucose into the duodenum or portal vein of rabbits and found that the intraduodenal infusion suppressed food intake more than glucose given into the portal vein. The suppression of food intake by glucose in the duodenum was abolished by vagotomy. Mogenson (1975) has integrated these gluco-receptors as shown in Figure 2–9. The duodenal and hepatic gluco-receptors which are present both require an intact vagus nerve over which messages are transmitted. Although clearly present, the question of whether the hypothalamus gluco-receptors are directly involved in the modulation of food intake or only act through messages sent from peripheral gluco-receptors is presently unsettled.

HORMONAL FACTORS

Hormonal factors may also play a role in modifying food intake. Insulin, for example, acutely increases food intake. The possible role of insulin in the control of food intake has been reviewed by Woods

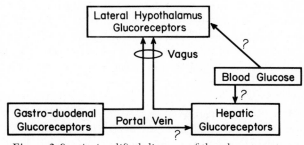

Figure 2–9.   A simplified diagram of the glucoreceptors.

(1974). Steffens (1969) has shown that insulin concentrations decline just before food ingestion begins. In addition, if rats are regularly injected with insulin, food intake increases and body weight rises (MacKay et al., 1940; Hoebel and Teitelbaum, 1966). This effect of insulin could result from peripheral hypoglycemia or from a direct action of insulin on the central nervous system. If small amounts of glucose are given into the lateral hypothalamus (Booth, 1968), the increased feeding behavior following the injection of insulin is inhibited, which suggests an indirect role for insulin. Animals which have recovered from the aphagia and hypophagia produced by lateral hypothalamic lesions will also not increase food intake following the injection of insulin although peripheral hypoglycemia and death results in 80 to 100 percent of the animals (Epstein and Teitelbaum, 1967). These two observations suggest that there is an area in the lateral hypothalamus which can respond to low levels of blood sugar by increasing food intake.

Evidence for a direct effect of insulin on the hypothalamus is less convincing. Injections of gold thioglucose destroy the ventromedial area of the hypothalamus, and this is followed by hyperphagia and obesity. If gold thioglucose is given to diabetic animals, there is no injury to the VMH nucleus until the diabetes is brought under control with insulin (Debons et al., 1968, 1969, 1970). Direct injection of large doses of insulin into the ventromedial hypothalamus of diabetic rats also restores the uptake of gold thioglucose. This suggests that insulin-sensitive receptors may reside in the VMH.

The electrophysiological studies of Oomura (1975) indeed show that insulin together with glucose alters the electrical properties of neurons in the ventromedial hypothalamus. The data of Panksepp (1974) do not support this, however. He found that glucose given into the VMH, but not into the lateral hypothalamus, depressed the 24 hour intake of food. Glucose and insulin together were no more effective than glucose alone. A study of Szabo and Szabo (1972) showed that injection of insulin into the carotid artery depressed glucose concentration with a latency of 10 minutes. This occurred when anti-insulin serum was given to prevent peripheral effects of insulin. The location in the brain of possible receptors for insulin has only recently been found (Oomura, 1975), suggesting that insulin may have an important role in altering function in the central nervous system and indirectly modulating peripheral metabolism.

The role of estrogens in the control of food intake has been investigated in the experimental animal (Wade, 1972). The rat normally has four to five days between estrus cycles. On the day of estrus there is an increase in running, a decrease in food intake, and a decrease in body weight. In the nonestrus phase of the cycle, food intake and body weight rise (ter Haar, 1972). This cyclic pattern of food intake and body weight in the female rat can be abolished by castration. When this is done, there is a gain in weight and an increase in body fat in the female rat. A pattern of cyclic depression of food intake can be produced by administration of estradiol every fourth or fifth day (Tartellin and Gorski, 1971). Finally, there is a depression of food intake with administration of estrogen and estrogen-like compounds (Sullivan and Smith, 1957). The action of estrogen is, in part, on the ventromedial hypothalamus but may also be elsewhere in the hypothalamus or in the periphery. Implantation of estradiol in the ventromedial nucleus of female rats will significantly depress food intake (Wade and Zucker, 1970). However, rats with ventromedial injury and hyperphagia show suppression of food intake after parenteral administration of estrogen. In the male there is very little cyclic variation in food intake. These studies suggest that estrogen acts both on the ventromedial nucleus and probably on the anterior and lateral hypothalamus as well, since male and female rodents respond differently.

Growth hormone is the third hormone which may be involved with regulation of food intake. Following hypophysectomy, food intake falls and growth ceases (Kennedy and Parrott, 1958) and obesity may develop in man (Tanner and Whitehouse, 1967) and chickens (Gibson and Nalbandov, 1966). Injection of growth hormone is accompanied by an increase in food intake and the longitudinal growth of both humans and experimental animals. The mechanism for decrease of food intake in the absence of growth hormone is at present unknown. However, growth hormone is not essential for the appearance of obesity although treatment with growth hormone may modify the magnitude of the obesity. Rats without pituitaries will become obese after injury to the VMH (Hetherington and Ranson, 1942a; Kennedy and Parrott, 1958; York and Bray, 1972; Bray, 1974; Valenstein et al., 1969).

HYPOTHESES FOR PERIPHERAL SIGNALS

A number of hypotheses have been advanced to account for the control of body calories. These include the glucostatic hypothesis, the aminostatic hypothesis, the lipostatic hypothesis and the thermostatic hypothesis. These are depicted schematically in Figure 2–9 (from Mogenson, 1975).

THE GLUCOSTATIC HYPOTHESIS.   Formulation of the glucostatic hypothesis is attributed to Mayer (1953, 1970). He postulated that the ventromedial nucleus of the hypothalamus might respond to changes in the rate of glucose utilization and thus modify food intake. The glucostatic hypothesis was based on several observations: first, the central nervous system (CNS) is known to depend largely on glucose for its metabolic needs, yet the CNS has little capacity to store glucose and is thus dependent on a continuing supply from the blood; second, the proportional change in glucose stored as glycogen between meals is much greater than for other substrates; third, the concentration of blood glucose is controlled by several endocrine mechanisms; and fourth, glucose oxidation regulates the oxidation and synthesis of fat.

The glucostatic hypothesis has been supported by several observations. When gold thioglucose is injected, the gold is localized in the highest concentration in the ventromedial hypothalamus (Debons et al., 1962). Both injected glucose and diabetes with hyperglycemia will reduce the deposition of gold thioglucose in the VMH. Moreover, when other gold-containing compounds such as gold thiomalate are injected, there is no accumulation of gold in the ventromedial hypothalamus. These observations suggest that the gold is accumulated by cells in the ventromedial hypothalamus which can transport glucose.

Measurement of glucose utilization by the VMH is not generally practical. However, injection of phloridzin, a drug which blocks glucose uptake by cells, into the ventricular system of the brain increases food intake (Glick and Mayer, 1968). Most other tests of the glucostatic hypothesis have, therefore, resorted to indirect measures, such as gastric contractions or the rates of peripheral glucose metabolism, and correlated them with food intake. There is a modest correlation between capillary-venous glucose concentrations (used to measure glucose metabolism) and reports or feelings of hunger (Quaade, 1962). Moreover, infusions of glucose into hungry individuals reduced the feelings of hunger as well as gastric contractions (Stunkard and Wolff, 1956).

Additional support for the glucostatic hypothesis was provided by the demonstration of the reciprocal electrical activity in the ventromedial and lateral hypothalamus (Anand et al., 1964; Oomuro et al., 1967). During periods of hunger and food seeking, the ventromedial nucleus was electrically inactive and the lateral area showed increased activity. With satiety which was associated with high glucose utilization, the ventromedial hypothalamus was active and the activity of the lateral hypothalamus was decreased.

This hypothesis has also been supported by studies using glucagon. Stunkard et al. (1955) noted in 16 studies that glucagon decreases hunger and gastric contractions within two minutes. Blood glucose also rises and glucose utilization probably increases. In animals with VMH lesions, however, glucagon does not effectively suppress the gastric contractions (Mayer and Sudsaneh, 1959).

Other lines of evidence also support this hypothesis. In a careful study of the relation between glucose and insulin concentrations and feeding behavior, Steffens (1969) found that insulin concentrations dropped to low levels just before the onset of a meal. A dropping concentration of insulin would be associated with reduced glucose utilization which according to the glucostatic hypothesis should initiate eating. Panksepp (1973, 1974) has examined the relationship of the ventromedial hypothalamus to the long term regulation of caloric stores and has suggested that this may be in part a glucostatic mechanism.

A major limitation of the glucostatic hypothesis is the evidence that the injection of glucose into the ventromedial hypothalamus does not promptly depress food intake (Epstein, 1960; Grossman, 1969; Wagner and DeGroot, 1963). However, if the intake of food was measured over a 24 hour period after injecting glucose there were reliable reductions in food intake. In addition, Panksepp (1972) has observed that radioactive glucose is accumulated in greater quantities in the ventromedial hypothalamus than in the lateral hypothalamus 6 hours after giving the glucose by stomach tube.

In summary, the hypothalamus contains cells which accumulate glucose readily and may be sensitive to insulin. These may function in the control of stored calories in the body. The peripheral gluco-receptors discussed earlier may be as important or more important than the central gluco-receptors.

THE LIPOSTATIC HYPOTHESIS.   The lipostatic hypothesis was proposed by Kennedy (1950, 1953, 1966, 1972) on the basis of studies in rats with injury to the VMH. He argued that body fat content was regulated in these animals. When overfed to increase weight or starved to reduce body weight, the rats would return to their original weight when allowed to eat spontaneously. The suggestion was that some metabolite from fat was produced which could accomplish this regulation. The principal metabolites released from adipose tissue are free fatty acids and glycerol, with prostaglandins representing a minor product. The rapid changes in the circulating concentrations of free fatty acids during the day, and their response to variations in metabolic state, make them an unlikely metabolic product for a control signal.

On the other hand, glycerol is a very reasonable candidate. It is released during the hydrolysis of triglycerides in adipose tissue (see Chapter 3). This glycerol cannot be revised by the adipose tissue because a key enzyme, glycerol kinase, is either absent or in very low concentration in this tissue. For that reason, the glycerol is released into the circulation in proportion to the rate of hydrolysis of tri-glycerides. The glycerol in the circulation is transported to the liver where it can be readily converted into glucose. Such glucose might in turn provide a signal to the hepatic gluco-receptors and thence to the brain.

Goodner et al. (1973) have found that the hypothalamus metabolizes glycerol more rapidly than does the cortex of brain, albeit at a slow rate compared with the liver or kidney. The hypothalamus did not display any special permeability of the blood-brain barrier for entry of glycerol. Thus glycerol remains a possible messenger, either indirectly through glucose formation in the liver or directly through specific glycerol receptors in the hypothalamus. Prostaglandins, which are derivatives of arachidic acid, are released during lipolysis in adipose tissue. One of the numerous prostaglandins might serve as a messenger, as evidenced by the observation of Martin and Baile (1973) that prostaglandin PGE will increase food intake if injected into the hypothalamus of sheep. Had PGE depressed food intake, it would be more consistent with the hypothesis.

A novel approach to the message or signal for the lipostatic hypothesis was first articulated by Hervey (1969, 1971, 1973). This proposal suggests that there is a mechanism for sensing the storage of energy and that total stored energy is mainly regulated through changes in food intake. Some "regulatory substance" produced by, or dissolved in, the fat must be "sensed" by the central nervous system. If the regulatory molecule were produced at a constant rate, the concentration in the blood would be inversely related to the quantity of fat. As the amount of fat increased, the quantity of this "regulatory substance" would decline as more entered the fat stores. A fall in concentration would signal the hypothalamus to reduce its food intake until the concentration of this "substance" in the circulation had risen to some threshold level. Steroids are one possible group of "regulatory substances." Progesterone is a steroid which will increase body fat. Since it has a central place in steroid metabolism, it is an attractive molecule to consider. This intriguing hypothesis awaits further testing.

THE THERMOSTATIC HYPOTHESIS. Heat production, reflected in changes of body temperature, was proposed by Brobeck (1948, 1960) as a regulator of food intake. This concept is supported by the observation that homeothermic animals eat more in cold than in hot environments. This adaptation is regulated in the preoptic region of the anterior hypothalamus. When this area of the hypothalamus is destroyed, control of body temperature is impaired. In such animals food intake does not show the appropriate responses to temperature; rather, the animals overeat in the heat and eat too little in the cold (Hamilton and Brobeck, 1966). Finally, when this area of the hypothalamus in rats was artificially heated, the intake of food increased. Conversely, cooling this area depressed feeding in rats (Spector et al., 1968). This effect in rats is unexpected and unexplained, and is contrary to the findings in goats where local cooling of the anterior hypothalamus produced feeding, whereas warming of this area inhibited eating even in the hungry goat (Andersson and Larsson, 1961; Andersson et al., 1962). Thus environmental temperature is an important modulator of feeding behavior that is integrated into the overall control process.

THE AMINOSTATIC HYPOTHESIS. Mellinkoff et al. (1956) observed an inverse relationship between the levels of amino acids and food intake and suggested that these nutrients might be important in regulating appetite. Experimental animals will reduce food intake if their diet is low in or devoid of a single amino acid, or if there is an excess of one amino acid (Harper, 1975). Adjustments in intake in a distorted diet are rapid. When isoleucine was omitted, for example, the food intake fell 75 percent in the first day. The plasma amino acid levels rose, except for the deficient amino acid, which fell (Peng et al., 1972).

The receptor system for detecting the deficiency of the amino acid appears to be in the brain. If a small quantity of the deficient amino acid is injected into the carotid artery, food intake is not depressed. The same quantity of amino acid injected into the jugular vein does not prevent the drop in food intake (Rogers and Leung, 1973). These receptors do not appear to be in the ventromedial hypothalamus. The depression of food intake when the diet is deficient in one amino acid returns toward normal when animals are exposed to cold. Under these conditions the animal increases its total diet and metabolizes the excess amino acid to provide heat (Beaton, 1967).

CONTROL OF FOOD INTAKE IN LEAN AND OBESE SUBJECTS

Internal Factors

The control of body weight and the regulation of caloric stores have been documented for humans as well as for experimental animals (Hamilton, 1972). Detailed studies on this process in man are, however, few in number compared with those already reviewed for experimental animals. The neuroanatomical structures involved in the control of body weight appear to be the same in man (Bray and Gallagher, 1975) and in monkeys (Hamilton et al., 1972) as in the other animals (see above).

The studies of Erdheim in 1904 demonstrated that the obesity associated with hypothalamic injury was probably the result of changes in the hypothalamus and not due to changes in the pituitary as had been argued by Fröhlich (1901). Confirmation of this proposition has been provided in animal studies and can also be seen in the careful anatomical study of a patient with a hypothalamic tumor for whom obesity was a major part of the clinical picture, as reported by Reeves and Plum (1969). Autopsy revealed that the tumor in this patient was limited almost entirely to the ventromedial hypothalamus. A more detailed discussion of hypothalamic obesity in man is presented in Chapter 5.

Two general techniques have been used to obtain information about the intake of calories in man. The first of these uses retrospec-

TABLE 2–4.   *The Caloric Intake of Overweight and*
Normal Weight Subjects*

Method	Number of Overweight	Calories/Day	Number of Normal Weight	Calories/Day
One day dietary record	59	1964	58	2198
Three day food record	12	1591	12	2196
Clinic diet history	30	2524	–	–
Research diet history	33	2829	20	2201

*From Beaudoin and Mayer: J. Am. Diet. Assoc., 29:29–33, 1953.

tive nutritional histories and records of foods eaten by the patient (Marr 1971). For adults the estimates of accuracy for the collection of data from nutritional histories are about ± 10 percent for both calories and protein (Reed and Burke, 1954). With children the accuracy is reduced to about 80 percent of actual intake in fourth graders and about 60 percent of actual intake in first graders (Emmons and Hayes, 1973). Van den Berg and Mayer (1954) noted that the one day dietary record errs on the low side due primarily to underreporting of certain foods and inadequate description of portion size of other foods. The latter is especially true of those foods with high caloric density.

The dietary history has been used to estimate caloric intake in normal and overweight individuals. The data of Beaudoin and Mayer are summarized in Table 2–4. The similarities among several methods for estimating the caloric intake of normal weight subjects are apparent in this table. Equally obvious is the discrepancy between estimates for the overweight group. These data suggest that estimation of the energy intake for overweight individuals has at least a moderate degree of uncertainty and may be very unreliable.

The recently conducted Canadian Nutrition Survey (1973) compiled data on caloric intake in Canadians. The respondents were divided into two groups based on ponderal index (see Chapter 1). The caloric intake of those with high ponderal index (i.e., the lean subjects) was the same as those with the lower ponderal index (the overweight) for all ages and both sexes. Thomson et al. (1961) have also provided data to show that, in population surveys from several authors, caloric intake does not rise with body weight (Fig. 2–10). When body weights were 45 to 49 kg for women and 55 to 64 kg for men the observed and desired values were similar. Above these levels food intake showed little increase as body weight rose. These data suggest that there is, on the average, no difference in caloric intake between the overweight and the normal weight group. However, the uncertainty of the methods leaves these data open to some question.

A second approach to the study of food intake in man has been developed in the laboratory. Under controlled conditions, it has been possible to manipulate both the internal and external environment

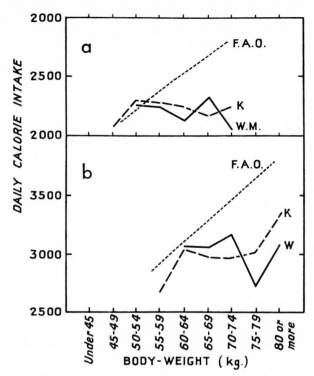

Figure 2–10. Food intake and body weight. Average food intake according to body weight for men (a) and women (b). The dotted line shows the calorie intake calculated from the FAO formula (1957). (Reproduced from Thomson, Billewicz and Passmore: Lancet, *1*:1027–1028, 1961, with permission.)

and to quantify the intake of food in normal weight and overweight subjects. Figure 2–11 shows the food intake at lunch time in one normal weight subject over 4 days (Jordan, 1973a, b). Lunch each day was obtained by pressing a lever which delivered a liquid diet into the mouth from a reservoir which was out of sight. The rate at which the liquid diet was injected into the mouth was most rapid at the beginning of the lunch period and slowed down over the ensuing 20 minutes. The daily intake for this subject was fairly constant from day to day. The influence of oral factors was assessed by having volunteers inject the food through a nasogastric tube directly into the stomach. Like the experimental animals discussed above, normal weight humans show reproducible daily intake when food was fed intragastrically (thus bypassing oral sensation). Man, like animals, will eat for calories when the environment is not disturbed, and when he is not "hungry" (Jordan, 1969, 1973b).

Human subjects will adjust their intake of food to changes in caloric density, but there is a difference of opinion about the rate of this adaptation. Campbell, Hashim and Van Itallie (1971) found that

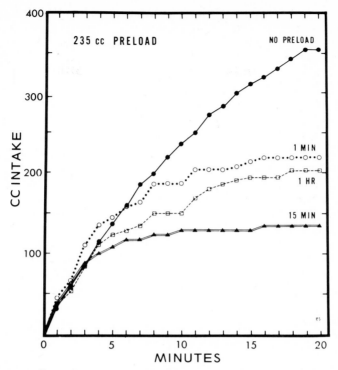

Figure 2–11. Effect of various preloads on the ingestion of a liquid formula diet. Liquid formula intake was measured over 20 minutes when no preload was given, and when a preload of 235 ml was given 1, 15, or 60 minutes earlier. The preload suppressed food intake but total ingestion (preload plus liquid diet) did not completely compensate. (Reproduced from Jordan: Obesity and Baria. Med., 2:42–48, 1973b, with permission.)

five lean subjects who were fed from a "feeding machine" adjusted the intake of liquid formula diet so that caloric intake was maintained constant (Hashim and Van Itallie, 1965). Obese subjects, however, took in too few calories to maintain weight under the same circumstances and did not adjust well to changes in the caloric density of the diet.

Spiegel (1973) noted that compensation for changes in the caloric density of the diet was slow, beginning only after two to five days and that some subjects did not adapt completely, even after several days. Indeed, the mean compensation was only 87 percent and the weight loss averaged 1 to 3 percent of body weight. Wooley et al. (1972) also noted the slow adaptation to changes in caloric density of the diet. The caloric value of a formula diet was adjusted up or down by a factor of two and taste was maintained constant. This showed that the *belief* held by the subject about the caloric content of the formula was more important in determining the volume which was ingested than the actual level of calories.

Ashworth et al. (1962) used a different design to evaluate this question. They provided five medical students with a dummy meal or with 1000 or 2000 calories at night and measured the food intake during the next day, as well as the weight gain throughout the study. With a supplement of 1000 calories at night for 20 days, there was no suppression of food intake on the following day and the subjects gained weight. With the 2000 calorie supplement, only one subject showed a significant reduction in voluntary daily intake of food. Pre-loading, however, does depress oral food intake when given one to 120 minutes before a meal (Walike, Jordan and Stellar, 1969). The adaptation to acute changes, like long term adaptation, was incomplete and the subjects overate. The conclusion which can be drawn from these studies is that humans, like animals, eat in part for calories but that adaptation to changes in caloric density of food is slow and may be inadequate in some people. It is obvious that this sluggish adaptive mechanism may be important in the development of obesity.

The role of taste and the response to gastric contractions have also been studied in man. Cabanac et al. (1971) have argued that humans show an alteration in taste sensitivity after weight loss (deprivation). The sensitivity of taste to varying solutions of sugar was decreased after ingesting glucose in normal individuals. After weight loss, however, the depression in pleasant ratings for sucrose solutions was not reduced. Canabac and Duclaux (1970) showed that obese subjects have higher ratings for pleasantness than lean subjects, and that this is unchanged by ingesting glucose.

Other investigators have obtained different results. Grinker (1975) compared taste preferences of normal and obese subjects using pairs of sucrose solutions varying from 1.95 to 19.5 percent. The obese subjects rated the higher concentrations as less pleasant and chose them less frequently (Underwood et al., 1973). This was in contrast to the increased preference of lean subjects for the sweeter solutions. Moreover, the ratings and the quantity of solution which the subjects drank were highly correlated for both obese and lean subjects. Of particular note is the fact that the aversion to sweet tasting solutions did not change after weight loss. We have also found an aversion to very sweet solutions by obese subjects (Bray et al., 1975).

The role of the gastrointestinal tract in signaling hunger or satiation in man has been the subject of considerable investigation. In a study of the sensations of hunger and satiety among 603 children and adults, Monello and Mayer (1967) found that numerous patterns are reported but that specific gastric sensations were usually part of this pattern of hunger. The physical sensations were more specific in males than in females. Satiation, on the other hand, tended to have fewer physical correlates. Satiety was most frequently described in terms of relaxation and calmness, and with sensations of gastric bulk (Linton et al., 1972).

The relationship of gastric contractions to the sensations of hunger has been reviewed by Stunkard and Fox (1971). Three experiments were performed to critically assess this relationship. Reports of hunger and recordings of gastric contractions were obtained over a 24 hour period in three women (Bloom et al., 1970). Reports of hunger began to increase shortly after the end of the meal and continued to increase until the onset of the next meal. Hunger increased whether gastric contractions were present or not. In a second experiment gastric contractions and reports of hunger were similar in normal weight and in obese individuals. Training the obese subjects to be aware of their gastric contractions did not alter their intake of food (Stunkard and Fox, 1971).

External Factors

In addition to modification of the internal environment which so clearly alters subsequent dietary behavior, there are a number of external factors which can also modify food intake.

Attention is focused on this possibility by the work of Schachter and his colleagues (1968, 1971, 1974). They have demonstrated that food deprivation influences neither self report of hunger nor actual eating for many overweight individuals. These investigators were aware of the reported relative insensitivity of obese patients to feelings of hunger during contractions of the gastrointestinal tracts, and postulated that obese people might be less sensitive to internally derived messages than are lean individuals.

One corollary of diminished internal awareness might be heightened sensitivity to external cues which could signal or inhibit eating. This hypothesis was tested in a number of different ways and it was concluded that obese people are not only more sensitive to external factors, but are less sensitive to internal (physiological) cues to eat than are lean subjects. This heightened sensitivity to external events occurs in other areas of life for the obese individual who seems to be generally more aware of his surroundings than the lean individual (Rodin, 1975).

Among the early experiments, Schachter, Goldman, and Gordon (1968) examined the effects of eating sandwiches on the subsequent ingestion of crackers by lean college students and by students who were 15 percent or more overweight. In this experiment subjects were instructed to come to the laboratory in the afternoon. Some were then invited to eat lunch while others were not. They were all subsequently given crackers whose taste they were to judge. When food had been ingested prior to coming to the laboratory, the lean subjects ate substantially fewer crackers than when they were hungry or had not eaten food. The overweight subjects, however, ate essentially the same number of crackers whether or not they had eaten food before coming into the laboratory. This same experiment examined the effects of food intake in situations of high or low emotion. When the level of fear was low, the normal weight subjects ate more than the overweight ones. However, when fear was introduced, the food intake of lean subjects dropped sharply, but the intake in the overweight individuals actually showed a small rise.

In a similar fashion these investigators have examined the effects of external variables such as time on the clock (Schachter and Gross, 1968), the intensity of the lighting, the ease with which food is available (Nisbett, 1968a), and the palatability of food items. When fasting on Yom Kippur was used as an index of internal deprivation, 83.1 percent of the obese Jews, but only 68.8 percent of the normal weight Jewish students, fasted. This suggests that the overweight individuals got "less hungry" during the fasting period (Schachter, 1968; Goldman et al., 1968).

When asked to taste ice cream containing various amounts of quinine, obese subjects ingested much less ice cream than did lean subjects (Nisbett, 1968b). That is, when there was little or no quinine in the ice cream, the obese subjects ate more than the normal or underweight groups, but when quinine was added, the overweight ate less than did the lean college students (shown in Fig. 2–12). Nisbett's

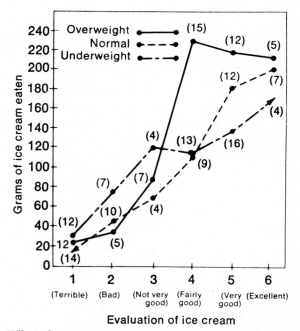

Figure 2–12. Effect of quinine on the ingestion of ice cream. Overweight subjects ate more ice cream with low amounts of quinine and less of the adulterated ice cream than lean or underweight subjects. (From Nisbett, copyright 1968 by the American Psychological Association. Reprinted with permission.)

original interpretation of this experiment was that overweight subjects are more sensitive to taste and eat larger portions of good tasting foods than do lean subjects.

In another experiment, Nisbett (1968a) tested the availability of food and the quantity that was eaten. The experimental subjects were instructed to skip lunch and arrive at the laboratory in the afternoon. While the students were filling out a questionnaire, a lunch of one or three sandwiches was available on the table, and a refrigerator full of sandwiches was across the room. Under these circumstances the lean subjects ate essentially the same number of sandwiches whether there was one or three sandwiches available on the table (1.96 vs 1.88). The overweight subjects, however, ate fewer sandwiches (1.48) when only one was available than when 3 were available (2.32). Thus those who were overweight ate more food if it was readily available than when they were obliged to walk across the room to acquire it. In summary, these studies and others reviewed by Schachter (1971), Schachter and Rodin (1974), and Rodin (1975) demonstrate that peripheral physiological correlates of food deprivation have less influence on the eating behavior of the overweight college student than they do on normal weight students. Eating thus appears to be determined more by external factors in the overweight and this concept has formed the basis for the development of behavior modification.

If the obese are more responsive to external cues or stimuli as signals to eat, they should eat more or less continuously since cues for available food are almost universally present. However, as noted above (Beaudoin and Mayer, 1953) and by others (Johnson, Burke, and Mayer, 1956; Ross, Pliner, Nisbett and Schachter, 1971) the obese tend to eat fewer meals. To reconcile these apparent discrepancies, Schachter and Rodin (1974) have suggested that the overweight eat only when the cues are highly potent, and when these are weak or absent, overweight individuals eat less.

This hypothesis is supported by observed eating behavior on weekdays as contrasted to weekends. During the week, almost all lean and overweight students ate lunch, but on weekends when food cues might be less acute, 89 percent of the lean and only 46 percent of the overweight subjects ate lunch (Ross, Pliner, Nisbett and Schachter, 1971). The prominence of food cues was also tested by varying the intensity of lighting (Ross et al., 1971). A variety of objects including chessmen, candlesticks, marbles, a toy car and cashew nuts illuminated by a 40 or 7½ watt bulb were situated in front of lean and overweight subjects. The overweight subjects ate twice as many nuts when brightly lit as when dimly lit, but the lean subjects showed no differences.

The tendency of overweight subjects to respond to manipulation of stimuli in the environment in ways different from lean subjects might be restricted to food cues or might be more generalized. Rodin

(1975) has investigated this possibility and finds that the obese have enhanced sensitivity to external objects. From a slide containing 13 items which was shown for five seconds, overweight subjects recalled 6.52 items as against 5.76 items for the lean (p < .002). Overweight subjects were found to be distracted more easily from tasks requiring concentration. Under conditions of "high" distraction, such as when listening to emotionally charged tape recordings, overweight subjects learned fewer incidental details than lean subjects, whereas they had previously learned more when there was no distraction. Overweight subjects were far more affected by external cues relating to time than were normal weight subjects. Lean and overweight subjects were asked to estimate the duration of a "boring" and an interesting tape recording whose actual lengths were 15 minutes. The estimates were just under 16 minutes for each tape for normal subjects. The overweight group estimated the boring tape to be 21 minutes long and the interesting one at just under 15 minutes in length.

Almost all of these studies have been conducted using normal and slightly overweight college students. Recently Rodin (1975) has compared the response of subjects who were more than 50 percent overweight with slightly overweight and normal subjects. Under these experimental conditions, the very obese do *not* behave like the moderately overweight, but in fact behave more like the normal weight subjects (Rodin, 1975). This variation in sensitivity to external factors may account for the variability in data being reported from different laboratories.

Whether the heightened sensitivity to environmental factors in overweight subjects is a cause for obesity or a consequence of obesity is not clearly established. In an analysis of this question, Nisbett (1972) has suggested that it may be a consequence. He compared the effects of semistarvation on behavior patterns of lean subjects studied in the 1940's by Keys et al. (1950) with the responsiveness of the overweight college student. Semistarvation with weight loss in the lean volunteers was accompanied by three changes in behavior: (1) the semistarved men became less interested in sexual relationships and in any interpersonal relationships with members of the opposite sex; (2) they became very irritable and were unable to carry on group discussions which had been conducted prior to the initiation of the experiment in semistarvation; and (3) their focus was almost entirely on food. Nisbett notes that some of these features are similar to those observed in the overweight college students. He suggests that the sensitivity of the overweight college student to food cues in the external environment may be a reflection of "semistarvation," in comparison with what the central weight regulating mechanisms would have him maintain.

The social pressure to be "thin" may keep the overweight student from eating as much as his internal drives might dictate. If this is so, then an overweight subject is below the weight he would achieve if he ate all of the food he wanted. Under these conditions of internal deprivation, external factors in food might become more important (see the discussion of calories and taste in the experimental animal).

REFERENCES

Abraham, S., Collins, G. and Nordsieck, M.: Relationship of childhood weight status to morbidity in adults. H.S.M.H.A. Health Reports, 86:273–284, 1971.

Adam, J. M., Best, T. W. and Edholm, O. G.: Weight changes in young men. J. Physiol. (London), 156:38P, 1961.

Adolph, E. F.: Urges to eat and drink in rats. Am. J. Physiol., 151:110–125, 1947.

Ahlskog, J. E. and Hoebel, B. G.: Overeating and obesity from damage to a noradrenergic system in the brain. Science, 182:166–169, 1973.

Albert, D. J., Storlien, L. H., Albert, J. G. and Mah, C. J.: Obesity following disturbance of the ventromedial hypothalamus: A comparison of lesions, lateral cuts and anterior cuts. Physiol. Behav., 7:135–141, 1971.

Anand, B. K.: Nervous regulation of food intake. Physiol. Rev., 41:677–708, 1962.

Anand, B. K. and Brobeck, J. R.: Hypothalamic control of food intake in rats and cats. Yale J. Biol. Med., 24:123–140, 1951.

Anand, B. K., Chhina, G. S., Sharma, K. N., Dua, S. and Singh, B.: Activity of single neurons in the hypothalamic feeding centers: effect of glucose. Am. J. Physiol., 207:1146–1154, 1964.

Andersson, B. and Larsson, B.: Influence of local temperature changes in the preoptic area and rostral hypothalamus on the regulation of food and water intake. Acta Physiol. Scand., 52:75–89, 1961.

Andersson, B., Gale, C. C. and Sundsten, J. W.: Effects of chronic central cooling on alimentation and thermoregulation. Acta Physiol. Scand., 55:177–188, 1962.

Arees, E. A. and Mayer, J.: Anatomical connections between the medial and lateral regions of the hypothalamus concerned with food intake. Science, 157:1574–1575, 1967.

Ashworth, N., Creedy, S., Hunt, J. N., Mahon, S. and Newland, P.: Effect of nightly food supplements on food intake in man. Lancet, 2:685–687, 1962.

Baile, C. A.: Regulation of feed intake in ruminants. Fed. Proc., 27:1361–1366, 1968.

Baile, C. A.: Control of feed intake and the fat depots. J. Dairy Sci., 54:564–582, 1971.

Baile, C. A. and Forbes, G. B.: Control of food intake and regulation of energy balance in ruminants. Physiol. Rev., 54:160–214, 1972.

Baile, C. A. and Mayer, J.: Hyperphagia in ruminants induced by a depressant. Science, 151:458–459, 1966.

Beaton, J. R.: Effect of increased metabolism and of hyperphagia on dietary amino acid imbalance in the rat. Canad. J. Physiol. Pharmacol., 45:1011–1019, 1967.

Beatty, W. W.: Influence of type of reinforcement on operant responding by rats with ventromedial lesions. Physiol. Behav., 10:841–846, 1973.

Beaudoin, R. and Mayer, J.: Food intakes of obese and non-obese women. J. Am. Diet Assoc., 29:29–33, 1953.

Berger, B. D., Wise, C. D. and Stein, L.: Norepinephrine: reversal of anorexia in rats with lateral hypothalamic damage. Science, 172:281–284, 1971.

Berger, B. D., Wise, D. and Stein, L.: Nerve growth factor: enhanced recovery of feeding after hypothalamic damage. Science, 180:506–508, 1973.

Berkun, M. M., Kessen, M. L. and Miller, N. E.: Hunger reducing effects of food by stomach fistula versus food by mouth measured by a consummatory response. J. Comp. Physiol. Psychol., 45:550–554, 1952.

Bernardis, L. L.: Development of hyperphagia in male rats following placement of ventromedial hypothalamic lesions at four divisions at four different ages. Experientia, 22:671, 1966.

Bernardis, L. L.: Hypoactivity as a possible contributing cause of obesity in the weanling rat ventromedial syndrome. Canad. J. Physiol. Pharmacol., 50:370–372, 1972.

Bernardis, L. L. and Frohman, L. A.: Effect of lesion size in the ventromedial hypothalamus on growth hormone and insulin levels in weanling rats. Neuroendocrinol., 6:319–328, 1970.

Bernardis, L. L. and Frohman, L.A.: Effects of hypothalamic lesions at different loci on development of hyperinsulinemia and obesity in the weanling rat. J. Comp. Neurol., 141:107–116, 1971a.

Bernardis, L. L. and Frohman, L. A.: Plasma growth hormone responses to electrical stimulation of the hypothalamus in the rat. Neuroendocrinol., 7:193–201, 1971b.

Bernardis, L. L. and Skelton, F. R.: Growth and obesity following ventromedial hypothalamic lesions placed in female rats at four different ages. Neuroendocrinol., 1:265–275, 1965/66.

Bloom, P. B., Filion, R. D. L., Stunkard, A. J., Fox, S. and Stellar, E.: Gastric and duodenal motility, food intake and hunger measured in man during a 24-hour period. Am. J. Dig. Dis., 15:719–725, 1970.

Booth, D. A.: Effects of intrahypothalamic glucose injection on eating and drinking elicited by insulin. J. Comp. Physiol. Psychol., 65:13–16, 1968.

Booth, D. A.: Normal metabolic control of hunger. In: Hunger: Basic Mechanisms and Clinical Implications. (Novin, D., Wyrwicka, W. and Bray, G. A., eds.) New York, Raven Press, 1975.

Bray, G. A.: Endocrine factors in the control of food intake. Fed. Proc., 33:1140–1145, 1974.

Bray, G. A. and Campfield, A.: Metabolic factors in the regulation of calorie stores. Metabolism, 24:99–117, 1975.

Bray, G. A. and Gallagher, T. F., Jr.: Manifestations of hypothalamic obesity in man: A comprehensive investigation of eight patients and a review of the literature. Medicine, 54:301–330, 1975.

Bray, G. A., Barry, R. E., Benfield, J., Castelnuovo-Tedesco, P. and Rodin, J.: Food intake and taste preferences for glucose and sucrose decrease after intestinal bypass surgery. In: Hunger: Basic Mechanisms and Clinical Implications. (Novin, D., Wyrwicka, W. and Bray, G. A., eds.) New York, Raven Press, 1975.

Bray, G. A. and York, D. A.: Studies on food intake of genetically obese rats. Am. J. Physiol., 233:176–179, 1972.

Brecher, G., Laqueur, G. L., Cronkite, E. P., Edelman, P. M. and Schwartz, I. L.: The brain lesion of gold thioglucose obesity. J. Exptl. Med., 121:395–401, 1965.

Brecher, G. and Waxler, S. H.: Obesity in albino mice due to single injections of gold thioglucose. Proc. Soc. Exptl. Biol. Med., 70:498–501, 1949.

Brobeck, J. R.: Food intake as a mechanism of temperature regulation. Yale J. Biol. Med., 20:545–552, 1948.

Brobeck, J. R.: Food and temperature. Recent Progr. Horm. Res., 16:439–459, 1960.

Brobeck, J. R.: Mechanism of the development of obesity in animals with hypothalamic lesions. Physiol. Rev., 26:541–559, 1946.

Brobeck, J. R., Tepperman, J. and Long, C. N. H.: Experimental hypothalamic hyperphagia in albino rat. Yale J. Biol. Med., 15:893–904, 1943.

Brooks, C. M.: The relative importance of changes in activity in the development of experimentally produced obesity in the rat. Am. J. Physiol., 147:708–716, 1946.

Brooks, C. M., Marine, D. N. and Lambert, E. F.: A study of the food-feces ratios and the oxygen consumption of albino rats during various phases of experimentally produced obesity. Am. J. Physiol., 147:717–726, 1946.

Cabanac, M. and Duclaux, R.: Obesity: Absence of satiety aversion to sucrose. Science, 168:496–497, 1970.

Cabanac, M., Duclaux, R. and Spector, N. H.: Sensory feedback in regulation of body weight: Is there a ponderostat? Nature, 229:125–127, 1971.

Campbell, R. G., Hashim, S. A. and Van Itallie, T. B.: Studies of food-intake regulation in man: Responses to variations in nutritive density in lean and obese subjects. New Engl. J. Med., 285:1402–1406, 1971.

Cannon, W. B and Washburn, A. L.: An explanation of hunger. Am. J. Physiol., 29:441–454, 1912.

Carlisle, H. J. and Stellar, E.: Caloric regulation and food preference in normal, hyperphagic and aphagic rats. J. Comp. Physiol. Psychol., 69:107–114, 1969.

Carlson, A. J.: The Control of Hunger in Health and Disease. Chicago, University of Chicago Press, 1912.

Cheng, M. F., Rozin, P. and Teitelbaum, P.: Starvation retards development of food and water regulations. J. Comp. Physiol. Psychol., 76:206–218, 1971.

Chlouverakis, C. and Hojnicki, D.: Lipectomy in obese hyperglycemic mice (ob/ob). Metabolism, 23:133–137, 1974.

Cioffi, L. A. and Speranza, A. : Physiological and psychological components of the body weight control system in the obese. Biblioteca Nutritio et Dieta, 17:154–176, 1972.

Clark, G., Magoun, H. W. and Ranson, S. W.: Hypothalamic regulation of body temperature. J. Neurophysiol., 2:61–80, 1939.

Cohn, C. and Joseph, D.: Influence of body weight and body fat on appetite of "normal" lean and obese rats. Yale J. Biol. Med., 34:598–607, 1962.

Coleman, D. L. and Hummel, K. P.: Effects of parabiosis of normal with genetically diabetic mice. Am. J. Physiol., 217:1298–1304, 1969.

Comstock, G. W. and Stone, R. W.: Changes in body weight and subcutaneous fat thickness related to smoking habits. Arch. Environm. Health, 24:271–276, 1972.

Coons, E. E., Levak, M. and Miller, N. E.: Lateral hypothalamus: Learning of foodseeking response motivated by electrical stimulation. Science, 150:1320–1321, 1965.

Corbit, J. D. and Stellar, E.: Palatability, food intake and obesity in normal and hyperphagic rats. J. Comp. Physiol. Psychol., 58:63–67, 1964.

Davis, J. D., Gallagher, R. J., Ladove, R. F. and Turansky, A. J.: Inhibition of food intake by a humoral factor. J. Comp. Physiol. Psychol., 67:407–417, 1969.

Davis, J. D., Campbell, C. S., Gallagher, R. J. and Zurakov, M. A.: Disappearance of a humoral satiety factor during food deprivation. J. Comp. Physiol. Psychol., 75:476–482, 1971.

Davis, J. D., Collins, B. J. and Levine, M. W.: Peripheral control of meal size: The interaction of gustatory stimulation and postingestial feedback. In: Hunger: Basic Mechanisms and Clinical Implication; (Novin, D., Wyrwicka, W. and Bray, G. A., eds.), New York, Raven Press, 1975.

Debons, A. F., Krimsky, I. and From, A.: A direct action of insulin on the hypothalamic satiety center. Am. J. Physiol., 219:938–943, 1970.

Debons, A. F., Krimsky, I., Likuski, H. J., From, A. and Cloutier, R. J.: Gold thioglucose damage to the satiety center: Inhibition in diabetes. Am. J. Physiol., 214:652–658, 1968.

Debons, A. F., Silver, L., Cronkite, E. P., Johnson, H. A., Brecher, G., Tenzer, D. and Schwartz, I. L.: Localization of gold in mouse brain in relation to gold thioglucose obesity. Am. J. Physiol., 202:743–750, 1962.

Debons, A. F., Krimsky, I., From, A. and Cloutier, R. J.: Rapid effects of insulin on the hypothalamic satiety center. Am. J. Physiol., 217:1114–1118, 1969.

Delgado, J. M. R. and Anand, B. K.: Increase of food intake induced by electrical stimulation of the lateral hypothalamus. Am. J. Physiol., 172:162–168, 1953.

Emmons, L. and Hayes, M.: Accuracy of 24-hour recalls of young children. J. Am. Diet. Assoc., 62:409–415, 1973.

Epstein, A. N.: Reciprocal changes in feeding behavior produced by intrahypothalamic chemical injections. Am. J. Physiol., 199:969–974, 1960.

Epstein, A. N.: Oropharyngeal factors in feeding and drinking. Handbook of Physiolgy, Sect. 6, Vol. 1, 1967, pp. 197–218.

Epstein, A. N. and Teitelbaum, P.: Specific loss of the hypoglycemic control of feeding in recovered lateral rats. Am. J. Physiol., 213:1159–1167, 1967.

Erdheim, J.: Uber Hypophysenganggeschwulste und Hirncholesteatome. Sitzungsb. Akad. Wissenschaften Wien., 113:537–726, 1904.

Ferguson, N. B. L. and Keesey, R. E.: Comparison of ventromedial hypothalamic lesion effects upon feeding and lateral hypothalamic self-stimulation in the female rat. J. Comp. Physiol. Psychol., 74:263–271, 1971.

Fleming, D. G.: Food intake studies in parabiotic rats. Ann. N.Y. Acad. Sci., 157:985–1002, 1969.

Fonberg, E. and Delgado, J. M.: Avoidance and alimentary reactions during amygdala stimulation. J. Neurophysiol., 24:651–664, 1961.

Fonberg, E.: The relation between alimentary and emotional amygdalar regulation. In: Hunger: Basic Mechanisms and Clinical and Implications; (Novin, D., Wyrwicka, W. and Bray, G. A., eds.), New York, Raven Press, 1975.

Forbes, G. B. and Reina, J. C.: Adult lean body mass declines with age: Some longitudinal observations. Metabolism, 19:653–663, 1970.

Fröhlich, A.: Ein Fall von Tumor der Hypophysis cerebri ohne Akromegalie. Wie. Klin. Fund., *15*:883–886, 1901.

Frohman, L. A. and Bernardis, L. L.: Growth hormone and insulin levels in weanling rats with ventromedial hypothalamic lesions. Endocrinology, *82*:1125–1132, 1968.

Frohman, L. A., Bernardis, L. L. and Kant, K. J.: Hypothalamic stimulation of growth hormone secretion. Science, *162*:580–582, 1968.

Frohman, L. A., Bernardis, L. L., Schnatz, J. D. and Burck, L.: Plasma insulin and triglyceride levels after hypothalamus lesions in weanling rats. Am. J. Physiol., *216*:1496–1501, 1969.

Garcia, J. and Koelling, R. A.: Handbook of sensory physiology, Vol. 4. The chemical senses. L. M. Beidler (ed.), Berlin, Springer-Verlag, 1971.

Garrow, J.: Energy Balance and Obesity in Man. North-Holland Publishing Company, Ltd., London, 1974.

Gibbs, J., Young, R. C. and Smith, G. P.: Cholecystokinin decreases food intake in rats. J. Comp. Physiol. Psychol., *84*:488–495, 1973a.

Gibbs, J., Young, R. C. and Smith, G. P.: Cholecystokinin elicits satiety in the rat with open gastric fistulas. Nature, *245*:323–325, 1973b.

Gibson, W. R. and Nalbandov, A. V.: Lipid mobilization in obese hypophysectomized cockerels. Am. J. Physiol., *211*:1345–1351, 1966.

Glacheva, L., Manchando, S. K., Box, B. and Stevenson, J. A. F.: Gastric motor activity during feeding induced by stimulation of the lateral hypothalamus in the rat. Canad. J. Physiol. Pharmacol., *50*:1091–1098, 1972.

Glick, Z. and Mayer, J.: Hyperphagia caused by cerebral ventricular infusion of phloridzin. Nature, *219*:1374, 1968.

Gold, R. M.: Hypothalamic obesity: The myth of the ventromedial nucleus. Science, *182*:488–489, 1973a.

Gold, R. M.: Hypothalamic obesity following knife cuts that minimize arterial damage. Physiol. Behav., *10*:403–406, 1973b.

Gold, R. M., Kapatos, G. and Carey, R. J.: A retracting wire knife for stereotaxic brain surgery made from a microliter syringe. Physiol. Behav., *10*:813–815, 1973.

Goldman, R., Jaffa, M. and Schachter, S.: Yom Kippur, Air France, dormitory food, and the eating behavior of obese and normal person. J. Pers. Soc. Psychol., *10*:117–123, 1968.

Goodner, C. J., Ogilvie, J. T. and Koerker, D. T.: The metabolism of glycerol by hypothalamic and pituitary tissues *in vitro* in the rat. Proc. Soc. Exp. Biol. Med., *143*:616–622, 1973.

Gordon, T. and Kannel, W. B.: The effects of overweight on cardiovascular diseases. Geriatrics, *28*:80–88, 1973.

Grinker, J.: Sensory and cognitive factors in food intake. *In*: Obesity in Perspective, Fogarty International Center Series on Preventive Medicine, Vol. II, Part 1 and Part 2, (Bray, G. A., ed.), Washington, D.C., U.S. Government Printing Office, 1975.

Grossman, S. P.: Neurophysiologic aspects: Extrahypothalamic factors in the regulation of food intake. Adv. Psychosom. Med., 7:49–72, 1972.

Grossman, S. P.: Neuroanatomy of food and water intake regulation: Some recent observations. *In*: Hunger: Basic Mechanisms and Clinical Implications; (Novin, D., Wyrwicka, W. and Bray, G. A., eds.), New York, Raven Press, 1975.

Grossman, S. P. and Grossman, L.: Food and water intake in rats with parasagittal knife cuts medial or lateral to the lateral hypothalamus. J. Comp. Physiol. Psychol., 74:148–156, 1968.

Grossman, S. P.: Hypothalamic and limbic influences on food intake. Fed. Proc., 27:1349–1358, 1969.

Grossman, S. P.: Eating and drinking elicited by direct adrenergic or cholinergic stimulation of hypothalamus. Science, *132*:301–302, 1960.

Hales, C. N. and Kennedy, G. C.: Plasma glucose, non-esterified fatty acids and insulin concentrations in hypothalamic-hyperphagic rats. Biochem. J., *90*:620–624, 1964.

Hamilton, C. L.: Long term control of food intake in the monkey. Physiol. Behav., 9:1–6, 1972.

Hamilton, C. L.: Physiologic control of food intake. J. Am. Diet. Assoc., 62:35–40, 1973.

Hamilton, C. L. and Brobeck, J. R.: Hypothalamic hyperphagia in the monkey. J. Comp. Physiol. Psychol., 57:271–278, 1964.

Hamilton, C. L. and Brobeck, J. R.: Food intake and temperature regulation in rats with rosteral hypothalamic lesions. Am. J. Physiol., 207:291–297, 1964.

Hamilton, C. L. and Brobeck, J. R.: Food intake and activity of rats with rostral hypothalamic lesions. Proc. Soc. Exptl. Biol. Med., 122:270–272, 1966.

Hamilton, C. L., Kuo, P. T. and Feng, L. Y.: Experimental production of syndrome of obesity, hyperinsulinemia and hyperlipidemia in monkeys. Proc. Soc. Exp. Biol. Med., 140:1005–1008, 1972.

Han, P. W. et al.: Hypothalamic obesity in weanling rats. Am. J. Physiol., 209:627–631, 1965.

Han, P. W.: Hypothalamic obesity in rats without hyperphagia. Trans. N.Y. Acad. Sci., 30:229–243, 1967.

Han, P. W.: Energy metabolism of tube-fed hypophysectomized rats bearing hypothalamic lesions. Am. J. Physiol., 215:1343–1350, 1968.

Han, P. W. and Liu, A. C.: Obesity and impaired growth of rats force fed 40 days after hypothalamic lesions. Am. J. Physiol., 211:229–231, 1966.

Harper, A. E.: Protein and amino acids in the regulation of food intake. In: Hunger: Basic Mechanisms and Clinical Implications. (Novin, D., Wyrwicka, W. and Bray, G. A., eds.), New York, Raven Press, 1975.

Hashim, S. A. and Van Itallie, P. B.: Studies in normal and obese subjects with a monitored food dispensing service. Ann. N.Y. Acad. Sci., 131:654–661, 1965.

Hervey, G. R.: The effects of lesions in the hypothalamus in parabiotic rats. J. Physiol., 145:336–352, 1959.

Hervey, G. R.: Regulation of energy balance. Nature, (London) 222:629–631, 1969.

Hervey, G. R.: Physiological mechanisms for the regulation of energy balance. Proc. Nutr. Soc., 30:109–116, 1971.

Hervey, G. R.: Physiological mechanisms in the regulation of energy balance. In: Anorexia Nervosa and Obesity. (Robertson, R. F., ed.) Publ No. 42, R. C. P., Edinburgh, pp. 7–17, 1973.

Hess, W. R.: The functional organization of the diencephalon. Hughes, J. R. (ed.) New York, Grune and Stratton, 1951.

Hetherington, A. W.: Non-production of hypothalamic obesity in rat by lesions rostral or dorsal to ventromedial hypothalamic nuclei. J. Comp. Neurol., 80:33–45, 1944.

Hetherington, A. W. and Ranson, S.: Effect of early hypophysectomy on hypothalamic obesity. Endocrinol., 31:30–34, 1942a.

Hetherington, A. W. and Ranson, S. W.: The spontaneous activity and food intake of rats with hypothalamic lesions. Am. J. Physiol., 136:609–617, 1942b.

Hirsch, J.: The regulation of food intake. (Discussion) Adv. Psychosom. Med., 7:229–242, 1972.

Hoebel, B. G.; Hypothalamic lesions by electrocauterization: disinhibition of feeding and self-stimulation. Science, 149:452–453, 1965.

Hoebel, B. G.: Feeding: Neural control of intake. Ann. Rev. Physiol., 33:533–568, 1971.

Hoebel, B. G. and Teitelbaum, P.: Hypothalamic control of feeding and self stimulation. Science, 135:375–377, 1962.

Hoebel, B. G. and Teitelbaum, P.: Weight regulation in normal and hypothalamic hyperphagic rats. J. Comp. Physiol. Psychol., 61:189–193, 1966.

Hoebel, B. G. and Thompson, R. D.: Aversion to lateral hypothalamic stimulation caused by intragastric feeding or obesity. J. Comp. Physiol. Psychol., 68:536–543, 1969.

Hustfelt, B. E. and Lovo, A.: Correlation between hyperinsulinemia and hyperphagia in rats with ventromedial hypothalamic lesion. Acta Physiol. Scand., 84:29–33, 1972.

Ingram, W. R., Barris, R. W., and Ranson, S. W.: Catalepsy: An experimental study. Arch. Neurol. Psychiat., 35:1175–1197, 1936.

Jacobs, H. L. and Sharma, K. N.: Taste versus calories: Sensory and metabolic signals in the control of food intake. Ann. N.Y. Acad. Sci., 157:1084–1125, 1969.

Janowitz, H. D. and Grossman, M. I.: Some factors affecting food intake of normal dogs and dogs with oesophagostomy and gastric fistulas. Am. J. Physiol., 159:143–148, 1949a.

Janowitz, H. D. and Grossman, M. I.: Effect of variations in nutritive density on intake of food of dogs and rats. Am. J. Physiol., 158:184–193, 1949b.

Jansen, G. R. and Hutchison, C. F.: Production of hypothalamic obesity by micro-surgery. Am. J. Physiol., 217:487–493, 1969.

Johnson, M. L., Burke, B. S. and Mayer, J.: Relative importance of inactivity and over-eating in the energy balance of obese high school girls. Am. J. Clin. Nutr., 4:37–44, 1956.

Jordan, H. A.: Voluntary intragastric feeding: Oral and gastric contributions to food intake and hunger in man. J. Comp. Physiol. Psychol., 68:498–506, 1969.

Jordan, H. A.: In defense of body weight. J. Am. Diet. Assoc., 62:17–21, 1973a.

Jordan, H. A.: Weight regulation in man: Physiological and psychological factors. Obesity & Baria. Med., 2:42–48, 1973b.

Kakolewski, J., Deaux, E., Christensen, J., and Case, B.: Diurnal patterns in water and food intake and body weight changes in rats with hypothalamic lesions. Am. J. Physiol., 221:711–718, 1971.

Kannel, W. B. and Gordon, T.: Obesity and cardiovascular disease. The Framingham Study on Obesity. In: Obesity. (Burland, W. L., Yudkin, J. and Samuel, P., eds.) Servier Inst. Monograph. Edinburgh, Churchill Livingston Publishers, 1974.

Kapatos, G. and Gold, R. M.: Evidence for ascending noradrenergic mediation of hypothalamic hyperphagia. Pharmacol. Biochem. Behav., 1:81–87, 1973.

Keesey, R. E.: The role of the lateral hypothalamus in determining of body weight set point. In: Hunger: Basic Mechanisms and Clinical Implications; (Novin, D. Wyrwicka, W. and Bray, G. A., eds.), New York, Raven Press, 1975.

Kennedy, G. C.: The hypothalamic control of food intake in rats. Proc. Roy. Soc. Biol., 137:535–549, 1950.

Kennedy, G. C.: The role of depot fat in the hypothalamic control of food intake in the rat. Proc. Roy. Soc. Biol. (London), 140:578–592, 1953.

Kennedy, G. C.: Food intake, energy balance and growth. Brit. Med. Bull., 22:216–220, 1966.

Kennedy, G. C.: The regulation of food intake. Adv. Psychosom. Med., 7:91–99, 1972.

Kennedy, G. C and Parrott, D. M. V.: The effect of increased appetite and of insulin on growth in the hypophysectomized rat. J. Endocrinol., 17:161–166, 1958.

Kent, M. A. and Peters, R. H.: Effects of ventromedial hypothalamic lesions on hunger-motivated behavior in rats. J. Comp. Physiol. Psychol., 83:92–97, 1973.

Keys, A., Brozek, J., Henschel, A., Mickelsen, O. and Taylor, H. L.: The Biology of Human Starvation. Minneapolis, University of Minnesota Press, 1950.

Khairy, M., Morgan, T. B. and Yudkin, J.: Choice of diets of differing caloric density by normal and hyperphagic rats. Brit. J. Nutr., 17:557–568, 1963.

Larsson, S.: On hypothalamic organization of nervous mechanism regulating food intake. Acta Physiol. Scand. (Suppl. 89), 32:1–250, 1954.

Leibowitz, S. F.: Hypothalamic beta adrenergic "satiety" system antagonises an alpha-adrenergic hunger system in the rat. Nature (London), 226:963–964, 1970a.

Leibowitz, S. F.: Reciprocal hunger-regulating circuits involving alpha- and beta-adrenergic receptors located, respectively, in the ventromedial and lateral hypothalamus. Proc. Nat. Acad. Sci., 67:1063–1070, 1970b.

Leibowitz, S. F.: Brain catecholaminergic mechanisms for control of hunger. In: Hunger: Basic Mechanisms and Clinical Implications; (Novin, D., Wyrwicka W. and Bray, G. A., eds.), New York, Raven Press, 1975.

Le Magnen, J.: Habits and food intake. In: Code and Hadel (eds.) Handbook of Physiology, Section 6, Alimentary canal, Vol. 1, 1967, pp. 11–30.

LeMagnen, J., Devos, M., Gaudillere, J. P., Louis-Sylvestre, J. and Tollon, S.: Metabolic substrates in the short-term regulation of food intake in rats. In: Energy Balance in Man. (Apfelbaum, M., ed.) Paris, Masson et cie, pp. 13–25, 1973.

Lepkovsky, S.: Hypothalamic-adipose tissue interrelationships. Fed. Proc., 32:1705–1708, 1973a.

Lepkovsky, S.: Newer concepts in the regulation of food intake. Am. J. Clin. Nutr., 26:271–284, 1973b.

Levison, M. J., Frommer, G. P. and Vance, W. B.: Palatability and caloric density as determinants of food intake in hyperphagic and normal rats. Physiol. Behav., 10:455–462, 1973.

Liebelt, R. A., Ichinoe, S. and Nicholson, N.: Regulatory influences of adipose tissue on food intake and body weight. Ann. N.Y. Acad. Sci., 131:559–582, 1965.

Linton, P. H., Conley, M., Kuechenmeister, C. and McClusky, H.: Satiety and obesity. Am. J. Clin. Nutr., 25:368–370, 1972.

Lipton, J. M., Jr.: Effects of high fat diets on caloric intake, body weight, and heat-escape responses in normal and hyperphagic rats. J. Comp. Physiol. Psychol., 68:507–515, 1969.

Lusk, G.: The Elements of the Science of Nutrition. 4th ed. Philadelphia, W. B. Saunders Co., 1928.

MacKay, E. M., Calloway, J. W. and Barnes, R. H.: Hyperalimentation in normal animals produced by protamine insulin. J. Nutr., 20:59–66, 1940.

Mann, G. V., Tell, K. and Hayes, O.: Exercise in the disposition of dietary calories: Regulation of serum lipoprotein and cholesterol in human subjects. New. Engl. J. Med., 253:349–355, 1955.

Margules, D. L. and Dragovich, J.: Studies on phentolamine-induced overeating and finickiness. J. Comp. Physiol. Psychol., 84:644–651, 1973.

Margules, D. L. and Olds, J.: Identical "feeding" and "rewarding" systems in the lateral hypothalamus of rats. Science, 135:374–375, 1962.

Marks, H. E. and Remley, N. R.: The effects of type of lesion and percentage body weight loss on measures of motivated behavior in rats with hypothalamic lesions. Behav. Biol., 7:95–111, 1972.

Marr, J. W.: Individual dietary surveys: Purposes and methods. World Rev. Nutr. Diet., 13:105–164, 1971.

Marrazzi, M. A.: Hypothalamic glucoreceptor response—Biphasic nature of unit potential change. In: Hunger: Basic Mechanisms and Clinical Implications; (Novin, D., Wyrwicka, W. and Bray, G. A., eds.), New York, Raven Press, 1975.

Marshall, N. B., Barnett, R. J. and Mayer, J.: Hypothalamic lesions in gold thioglucose injected mice. Proc. Soc. Exptl. Biol. Med. (NY), 90:240–244, 1955.

Martin, F. H. and Baile, C. A.: Feeding elicited in sheep by intrahypothalamic injections of PGE_1. Experientia, 29:306–307, 1973.

Mayer, J.: Some aspects of the problem of regulating food intake and obesity. In: Anorexia and Obesity. (Rowland, C. V., ed.) Vol. 7, Boston, Little, Brown and Co., 1970, pp. 255–334.

Mayer, J.: Glucostatic mechanism of regulation of food intake. New. Engl. J. Med., 249:13–16, 1953.

Mayer, J. and Arees, E. A.: Ventromedial glucoreceptor system. Fed. Proc., 27:1345–1348, 1968.

Mayer, J. and Sudsaneh, S.: Mechanism of hypothalamic control of gastric contractions in the rat. Am. J. Physiol., 197:274–280, 1959.

Mayer, J. and Thomas, D. W.: Regulation of food intake and obesity. Science, 156:328–337, 1967.

McCance, R. A.: Food, growth and time. Lancet, 2:671–676, 1962.

Mellinkoff, S. M., Frankland, M., Boyle, D. and Greipel, M.: Relationship between serum amino acid concentration and fluctuations in appetite. J. Appl. Physiol., 8:535–538, 1956.

Mickelsen, O., Takahashi, H. and Craig, C.: Experimental obesity: I. Production of obesity in rats by feeding high fat diets. J. Nutr., 57:541–554, 1955.

Miller, N. E., Bailey, C. J. and Stevenson, J. A. F.: Decreased "hunger" but increased food intake resulting from hypothalamic lesions. Science, 112:256–259, 1950.

Mogenson, G. J.: Neural mechanisms of hunger: Current status and future prospects. In: Hunger: Basic Mechanisms and Clinical Implications; (Novin, D., Wyrwicka, W. and Bray, G. A., eds.), New York, Raven Press, 1975.

Monello, L. F. and Mayer, J.: Hunger and satiety sensations in men, women, boys and girls. Am. J. Clin. Nutr., 20:253–261, 1967.

Montemurro, D. G.: Inhibition of hypothalamic obesity in the mouse with diethylstilbestrol. Can. J. Physiol. Pharmacol., 49:554–558, 1971.

Morgane, P. J. and Kosman, A. J.: A rhinencephalic feeding center in the rat. Am. J. Physiol., 197:158–162, 1959.

Morgane, P. J. and Kosman, A. J.: Relationship of the middle hypothalamus to amygdalar hyperphagia. Am. J. Physiol., 198:1315–1318, 1960.

Morgane, P. J.: Electrophysiological studies of feeding and satiety centers in the rat. Am. J. Physiol., 201:838–844, 1961.

Myers, R. D., Bender, S. A. and Cristic, M. K.: Feeding produced in the satiated rat by elevating the concentration of calcium. Science, 176:1124–1125, 1972.

Naito, C., Yoshitoshi, Y., Higo, K. and Ookawa, H.: Effects of long-term administration of 2-deoxy-D-glucose on food intake and weight gain in rats. J. Nutr., *103*:730–737, 1973.

Niijima, A.: Afferent impulse discharge from glucoreceptors in the liver of the guinea pig. Ann. N.Y. Acad. Sci., *157*:690–700, 1969.

Nisbett, R. E.: Determinants of food intake in obesity. Science, *159*:1254–1255, 1968a.

Nisbett, R. E.: Taste, deprivation and weight determinants of eating behavior. J. Pers. Soc. Psychol., *10*:107–116, 1968b.

Nisbett, R. E.: Hunger, obesity and the ventromedial hypothalamus. Psychol. Rev., 79:433–458, 1972.

Novin, D.: Visceral mechanisms in the control of feeding. *In*: Hunger: Basic Mechanisms and Clinical Implications; (Novin, D., Wyrwicka, W. and Bray, G. A., eds.), New York, Raven Press, 1975.

Novin, D., VanderWeele, D. A. and Rezek, M.: Infusion of 2-deoxy-D-glucose into the hepatic portal system causes eating: evidence for peripheral glucoreceptors. Science, *181*:858–860, 1973.

Nutrition Canada National Survey. 1973 Ottawa, Canada p. 84.

Olney, J. W.: Brain lesions. Obesity and other disturbances in mice treated with monosodium glutamate. Science, *64*:719–721, 1969.

Oomura, Y., Ooyama, H., Yamamoto, T. and Naka, F.: Reciprocal relationship of the lateral and ventromedial hypothalamus in the regulation of food intake. Physiol. Behav., 2:97–115, 1967.

Oomura, Y.: Effects of glucose and free fatty acid in chemosensitive neuron in the rat hypothalamus. *In*: Hunger: Basic Mechanisms and Clinical Implications; (Novin, D., Wyrwicka, W. and Bray, G. A., eds.), New York, Raven Press, 1975.

Paintal, A. S.: A study of gastric stretch receptors. Their role in the peripheral mechanism of satiation of hunger and thirst. J. Physiol, (London), *126*:255–270, 1954.

Panksepp, J.: Hypothalamic radioactivity after intragastric glucose-¹⁴C in rats. Am. J. Physiol., *223*:396–401, 1972.

Panksepp, J.: Reanalysis of feeding patterns in the rat. J. Comp. Physiol. Psychol., 82:78–94, 1973.

Panksepp, J.: Hypothalamic regulation of energy balance and feeding behavior. Fed. Proc., *33*:1150–1165, 1974.

Peng, Y., Tews, J. K. and Harper, A. E.: Amino acid imbalance, protein intake, and changes in rat brain and plasma amino acids. Am J. Physiol., *222*:314–321, 1972.

Pfaff, D.: Histological differences between ventromedial hypothalamic neurones of well fed and underfed rats. Nature, *223*:77–78, 1969.

Polin, D. and Wolford, J. H.: Factors influencing food intake and caloric balance in chickens. Fed. Proc., *32*:1720–1726, 1973.

Porter, J. and Allen, J.: Food motivated performance as a function of weight loss in hypothalamic hyperphagic rats. Psychonomic Sci., *28*:285–288, 1972.

Powley, T. L. and Keesey, R. E.: Relationship of body weight to the lateral hypothalamic feeding syndrome. J. Comp. Physiol. Psychol., *70*:25–36, 1970.

Quaade, F.: On the "glucostatic" therapy of appetite regulation. I: Capillovenous glucose difference in normal obese and diabetic persons during hunger and satiety. Am. J. Med. Sci., *243*:427–437, 1962.

Recommended Dietary Allowances, Washington, National Academy of Sciences, 1974.

Reed, R. B. and Burke, B. S.: Collection and analysis of dietary intake data. Am. J. Publ. Hlth., *44*:1015–1026, 1954.

Reeves, A. G. and Plum, F.: Hyperphagia, rage and dementia accompanying a ventromedial hypothalamic neoplasm. Arch. Neurol., *20*:616–624, 1969.

Rehovsky, D. A. and Wampler, R. S.: Failure to obtain sex differences in development of obesity following ventromedial hypothalamic lesions in rats. J. Comp. Physiol. Psychol., 78:102–112, 1972.

Revusky, B. T.: Failure to support the hypothesis that eating is anticipatory of need. Psychol. Rep., *27*:199–205, 1970.

Richter, C. P.: Total self-regulatory functions in animals and human beings. Harvey Lect., *38*:63–103, 1943.

Rodin, J.: Responsiveness of the obese to external stimuli. *In*: Obesity in Perspective. Fogarty International Center Series on Preventive Medicine, Vol. II, Part 1 and Part 2 (Bray, G. A., ed.), Washington, D.C., U.S. Government Printing Office, 1976.

Rogers, Q. R. and Leung, P. M. B.: The influence of amino acids on the neuroregulation of food intake. Fed. Proc., 32:1709–1719, 1973.

Ross, L. D., Pliner, P. , Nisbett, P. and Schachter, S.: Patterns of externality and internality in the eating behavior of obese and normal college students. Unpublished manuscript, Columbia Univ. Cited in S. Schachter: Emotion, Obesity and Crime, New York, Academic Press, 1971.

Russek, M.: Participation of hepatic glucoreceptors in the control of intake of food. Nature, 197:79–80, 1963.

Russek, M.: Mathematics and satiety. In: Hunger: Basic Mechanisms and Clinical Implications (Novin, D., Wyrwicka, W. and Bray, G. A., eds.), New York, Raven Press, 1975.

Rutman, M. N., Lewis, F. S. and Bloomer, W.: Metabolic investigations during the development of obesity in bipiperidyl mustard treated mice. Trans. N.Y. Acad. Sci., 30:244–255, 1967.

Schachter, S.: Obesity and eating. Internal and external cues differentially effect the eating behavior of obese and normal subjects. Science, 161:751–756, 1968.

Schachter, S., Goldman, R. and Gordon, A.: Effects of fear, food deprivation, and obesity on eating. J. Personality Soc. Psychol., 10:91–97, 1968.

Schachter, S. and Gross, L. P.: Manipulated time and eating behavior. J. Personality Soc. Psychol., 10:98–106, 1968.

Schachter, S. and Rodin, J.: Obese Humans and Rats. (Festinger, L. and Schachter, S., eds.) Potomac, Maryland, Lawrence Erlbaum Associates, 1974.

Schachter, S.: Some extraordinary facts about obese humans and rats. Am. Psychol., 26:129–144, 1971.

Schemmel, R., Mickelsen, O. and Gill, J. L.: Dietary obesity in rats: body weight and fat accretion in seven strains of rats. J. Nutr., 100:1041–1048, 1970.

Sclafani, A.: Neural pathways involved in the ventromedial hypothalamic lesion syndrome in the rat. J. Comp. Physiol. Psychol., 77:70–96, 1971.

Sclafani, A.: Appetite and hunger in experimental obesity syndromes. In: Hunger: Basic Mechanisms and Clinical Implications. (Novin, D., Wyrwicka, W. and Bray, G. A., eds.), New York, Raven Press, 1975.

Sclafani, A., Berner, C. H. and Maul, G.: Feeding and drinking pathways between medial and lateral hypothalamus in the rat. J. Comp. Physiol. Psychol., 85:29–51, 1973.

Sclafani, A. and Grossman, S. P.: Reactivity of hyperphagic and normal rats to quinine and electric shock. J. Comp. Physiol. Psychol., 74:157–166, 1971.

Shapiro, N., Robinson, B., Godchalk, M., Heller, E. D. and Perek, M.: The effect of intrahypothalamic administration of sodium pentobarbital on eating behavior and feed intake in chickens. Physiol. Behav., 19:97–100, 1973.

Share, I., Martyniuk, E. and Grossman, M. I.: Effect of prolonged intragastric feeding on oral food intake in dogs. Am. J. Physiol., 169:229–235, 1952.

Sharma, K. N., Anand, B. K., Dua, S. and Singh, B.: Role of stomach in regulation of activities of hypothalamic feeding centers. Am. J. Physiol., 201:593–598, 1961.

Sims, E. A. H., Danforth, E., Jr., Horton, E. S., Bray, G. A., Glennon, J. A. and Salans, L. B.: Endocrine and metabolic effects of experimental obesity in man. Recent Progr. Horm. Res., 29:457–487, 1973.

Sims, E. A. H., Goldman, R. F., Gluck, C. M., Horton, E. S., Keleher, D. C. and Rowe, D. W.: Experimental obesity in man. Trans. Assoc. Am. Physicians, 81:153–170, 1968.

Singh, D.: Effects of preoperative training on food-motivated behavior of hypothalamic hyperphagic rats. J. Comp. Physiol. Psychol., 84:47–52, 1973.

Smith, G. P. and Epstein, A. N.: Increased feeding in response to decreased glucose utilization in the rat and monkey. Am. J. Physiol., 217:1083–1087, 1969.

Smith, O. A., Jr., McFarland, W. L. and Teitelbaum, H.: Motivational concomitants of eating elicited by stimulation of the anterior thalamus. J. Comp. Physiol. Psychol., 54:484–488, 1961.

Snowden, C. T.: Gastro-intestinal sensory and motor control of food intake. J. Comp. Physiol. Psychol., 71:68–76, 1970.

Sohar, E., Scapa, E. and Ravid, M.: Constancy of relative body weight in children. Arch. Dis. Child, 48:389–392, 1973.

Soulairac, A.: Control of carbohydrate intake. In: Handbook of Physiology. Chapter 28, pp. 387–398, 1967.

Spector, N. H., Brobeck, J. R. and Hamilton, C. L.: Feeding and core temperature in albino rats; Changes induced by preoptic heating and cooling. Science, 161:286–288, 1968.

Spiegel, T. A.: Caloric regulation of food intake in man. J. Comp. Physiol. Psychol., 84:24–37, 1973.

Steffens, A. B.: Blood glucose and FFA levels in relation to the meal pattern in the normal rat and the VMH hypothalamic lesion rat. Physiol. Behav., 4:212–225, 1969.

Steffens, A. B.: The influence of reversible obesity on eating behavior, blood glucose and insulin in the rat. Am. J. Physiol. 1975.

Steinbaum, E. A. and Miller, N. E.: Obesity from eating elicited by daily stimulation of hypothalamus. Am. J. Physiol., 208:1–5, 1965.

Stevenson, J. A. F.: Neural control of food and water intake. In: The Hypothalamus (Haymaker, W., Anderson, E. and Nauter, W. J. H., eds.) Springfield, Ill., Charles C Thomas, 1969, pp. 524–621.

Stricker, E. M. and Zigmond, M. J.: Brain catecholamines and the lateral hypothalamic syndrome. In: Hunger: Basic Mechanisms and Clinical Implications. (Novin, D., Wyrwicka, W. and Bray, G. A., eds.) New York, Raven Press, 1975.

Strominger, J. L. and Brobeck, J. R.: Mechanism of regulation of food intake. Yale J. Biol. Med., 25:383–390, 1953.

Stunkard, A. J., Van Itallie, T. B. and Reis, B. B.: The mechanism of satiety: Effect of glucagon on gastric hunger contractions in man. Proc. Soc. Exp. Biol. Med., 89:258–261, 1955.

Stunkard, A. J. and Wolff, H. G.: Studies on the physiology of hunger. I. The effect of intravenous administration of glucose on gastric hunger contractions in man. J. Clin. Invest., 35:954–963, 1956.

Stunkard, A. J. and Fox, S.: The relationship of gastric motility and hunger: A summary of the evidence. Psychosom. Med., 33:123–134, 1971.

Sudsaneh, S. and Mayer, J.: Relation of metabolic events to gastric contractions in the rat. Am. J. Physiol., 197:269–273, 1959.

Sullivan, L. W. and Smith, T. C.: Influence of estrogens on body growth and food intake. Proc. Soc. Exp. Biol. Med., 96:60–64, 1957.

Sutin, J.: Neural factors in the control of food intake. In: Obesity in Perspective. Fogarty International Center Series on Preventive Medicine, Vol. II, Part 1 and Part 2 (Bray, G. A., ed.), Washington, D.C., U.S. Government Printing Office, 1976.

Szabo, O. and Szabo, A. J.: Evidence for an insulin-sensitive receptor in the central nervous system. Am. J. Physiol., 223:1349–1353,1972.

Tanner, J. M. and Whitehouse, R. H.: The effect of growth hormone on subcutaneous fat thickness in hyposomatotrophic and panhypopituitary dwarfs. J. Endocrinol., 39:263–275, 1967.

Tartellin, M. F. and Gorski, R. A.: Variations in food and water intake in the normal and acyclic female rat. Physiol. and Behav., 7:847–852, 1971.

Teitelbaum, P., Cheng, M. F. and Rozin, P.: Development of feeding parallels its recovery after hypothalamic damage. J. Comp. Physiol. Psychol., 67:430–441, 1969a.

Teitelbaum, P., Cheng, M. F. and Rozin, P.: Stages of recovery and development of lateral hypothalamic control of food and water intake. Ann. N.Y. Acad. Sci., 157:849–860, 1969b.

Teitelbaum, P.: Sensory control of hypothalamic hyperphagia. J. Comp. Physiol. Psychol., 48:156–163, 1955.

Ten State Nutrition Survey 1968–1970. DHEW Publication No. (HSM) 72–8131, 1972.

ter Haar, M. B.: Circadian and estrual rhythms in food intake in the rat. Hormones and Behav., 3:213–220, 1972.

Thomson, A. M., Billewicz, N. Z. and Passmore, R.: The relation between caloric intake and body-weight in man. Lancet, 1:1027–1028, 1961.

Traczyk, W.: Feeding and escape reactions in rabbits caused by hypothalamic stimulation. Acta Physiol. Pol., 13:239–251, 1962.

Underwood, P. J., Belton, E. and Hulme, P.: Aversion to sucrose in obesity. Proc. Nutr. Soc., 32:92A–93A, 1973.

Ungerstedt, U.: Stereotaxic mapping of the monoamine pathways in the rat brain. Acta Physiol. Scand. (Suppl), 367:1–122, 1971.

Valenstein, E. S., Cox, V. C. and Kakolewski, J. W.: Sex differences in hyperphagia and body weight following hypothalamic damage. Ann. N.Y. Acad. Sci., 157:1030–1046, 1969.

Van den Berg, A. S. and Mayer, J.: Comparison of one-day food record and research, dietary history on a group of obese pregnant women. J. Am. Diet. Assoc., 30:1239–1244, 1954.

Wade, G. N. and Zucker, I.: Modulation of food intake and locomotor activity in female rats by diencephalic hormone implants. J. Comp. Physiol. Psychol., 72:328–336, 1970.

Wade, G. N.: Gonadal hormones and behavioral regulation of body weight. Physiol. Behavior, 8:523–534, 1972.

Wagner, J. W. and De Groot, J.: Changes in feeding behavior after intracerebral injections in the rat. Am. J. Physiol., 204:483–487, 1963.

Walike, B. C., Jordan, H. A. and Stellar, E.: Preloading and the regulation of food intake in man. J. Comp. Physiol. Psychol., 68:327–333, 1969.

Wendt, R. and Olds, J.: Relations of drive and reward systems in the hypothalamus. Fed. Proc., 16:136, 1957.

Wolgin, D. L., Cytawa, J. and Teitelbaum, P.: The role of activation in the regulation of food intake. In: Hunger: Basic Mechanisms and Clinical Implications; (Novin, D., Wyrwicka, W. and Bray, G. A., eds), New York, Raven Press, 1975.

Woods, S. C., Decke, E. and Vasselli, J. R.: Metabolic hormones and regulation of body weight. Psychol. Rev., 81:26–43, 1974.

Wooley, S. C. and Wooley, O. W.: Salivation to the sight and thought of food: A new measure of appetite. Psychosom. Med., 35:136–142, 1973.

Wooley, S. C., Wooley, O. W. and Dunham, R. B.: Can calories be perceived and do they affect hunger in obese and nonobese humans. J. Comp. Physiol. Psychol., 80:250–258, 1972.

Yamamoto, S., Mizutani, T. and Kaneuchi, G.: Obesity induced in mice injected intracerebrally with 4-nitroquinoline 1-oxide or 4-hydroxyamino-quinoline 1-oxide. Proc. Soc. Exp. Biol. Med., 133:303–306, 1970.

York, D. A. and Bray, G. A.: Dependence of hypothalamic obesity on insulin, the pituitary and the adrenal gland. Endocrinology, 90:885–894, 1972.

CHAPTER 3

PATHOGENESIS OF OBESITY: COMPOSITION AND METABOLISM OF ADIPOSE TISSUE

The most obvious characteristic of the obese patient is the increased quantity of fat. As analytical techniques have improved, considerable attention has been focused on the role that adipose tissue plays as a depository of stored energy, and the way in which this storage of energy might contribute to the development or perpetuation of obesity. It is conceivable, for example, that metabolic defects in the breakdown of fat stored in adipose tissue might lead to increased food intake to compensate for a shortage of available energy released from adipose tissue. Alternatively, increased rates of fat storage might lead to obesity.

Some indication of the importance of adipose tissue in the body economy is presented in Table 3–1. These data are calculated for the normal weight 70 kg man and for the obese 100 kg man whose body

TABLE 3–1. *Total Energy Available from Various Storage Depots*

	NORMAL		OBESE	
	KG	KCAL	KG	KCAL
Body weight	70		100	
Fat (Adipose triglyceride)*	15	135,000	40	360,000
Protein (Muscle)*	6	24,000	7	28,000
Glycogen				
Liver	0.07	280	0.07	280
Muscle	0.12	480	0.14	560
Glucose	0.020	80	0.25	100

*Caloric equivalent of protein 4 Cal/g; fat 9 Cal/g; glucose and glycogen 4 Cal/g.

94

composition was depicted in Chapter 1 (Table 1–6). In the normal weight man, fat represents nearly 85 percent of the total stored energy. When body weight rises to 100 kg, the energy stored in fat increases more than 2.5-fold and represents more than 90 percent of the stored calories. Although energy is stored in protein and glycogen, it is clear from Table 3–1 that these components contain only a small fraction of total energy stored in the body.

In this chapter some of the aspects of the storage and release of fat from this tissue will be examined, including morphologic characteristics of adipose tissue, its biochemical and physiological function, and breakdown of the triglycerides stored in fat cells. More detailed discussion of these topics can be found elsewhere (Jeanrenaud and Hepp, 1970; Vague and Boyer, 1974; Galton, 1971).

COMPOSITION AND MORPHOLOGY OF ADIPOSE TISSUE

Composition of Adipose Tissue

Triglycerides are composed of free fatty acids attached to a molecule of glycerol in an ester linkage (Table 3–2). Fatty acids generally differ by two carbon units and range from 10 to 18 carbons in length. The fatty acids most frequently found in triglycerides have 16 or 18 carbons. Fatty acids of 10 to 16 carbons in length are most frequently saturated (i.e., they have no double bonds). Stearic acid, the saturated 18 carbon fatty acid, is present as 3.2 percent of triglycerides in homeotherms because at 37° it is a solid with a melting point of 69.4° C. Tristearin, the triglyceride with 3 stearic acids, is also a solid which melts at 54.5° C, well above body temperature. Oleic acid, which has one double bond, is a liquid at room temperature and has a melting point of 14° C (57° F). Thus triglycerides containing oleic or other liquid fatty acids are liquid at room temperature.

The relationship between fatty acids of various lengths and their frequency in biological triglycerides is shown in Figure 3–1. This figure plots the ratio of saturated to unsaturated fatty acids in relation to the length of the carbon chains in the triglycerides (Jacob and Grimmer, 1968). The saturated fatty acids with carbon lengths of 14 or less occur 6 or more times as often as the unsaturated ones. Triglycerides, however, contain almost no saturated fatty acids with a carbon length of 18.

The fatty acid composition of triglycerides from adipose tissue of obese and normal subjects has been investigated by Heffernan (1964), Hirsch et al. (1960), and Baker (1969). It was found that adipose tissue from obese subjects contained percentages of saturated and unsaturated fatty acids comparable to adipose tissue from lean subjects (Table 3–3). The ratio of the monounsaturated to saturated acids, how-

TABLE 3–2. *Chemical Structures of the Lipid Components of Adipose Cells*

Triglyceride

$$H_2C-O-FA_1$$
$$H-C-O-FA_2$$
$$H_2C-O-FA_3$$

FA$_1$, FA$_2$, FA$_3$ represent different fatty acids

Fatty Acids

Palmitic	$C_{16:0}$	$CH_3(CH_2)_{14}-COOH$
Stearic	$C_{18:0}$	$CH_3(CH_2)_{16}-COOH$
Oleic	$C_{18:1}^{\Delta 9}$	$CH_3-(CH_2)_7-\underset{10}{CH}=\underset{9}{CH}-(CH_2)_7-COOH$
Linoleic	$C_{18:2}^{\Delta 9,12}$	$CH_3-(CH_2)_4-\underset{13}{CH}=\underset{12}{CH}-CH_2-\underset{11}{CH}=\underset{10}{CH}_2-CH_2=\underset{9}{CH}-(CH_2)_7-COOH$
Linolenic	$C_{18:3}^{\Delta 9,12,15}$	$CH_3-CH_2-\underset{16}{CH}=\underset{15}{CH}-CH_2-\underset{14}{CH}=\underset{13}{CH}-CH_2-\underset{12}{CH}=\underset{11}{CH}-CH_2-\underset{10}{CH}=\underset{9}{CH}-(CH_2)_7-COOH$

Cholesterol

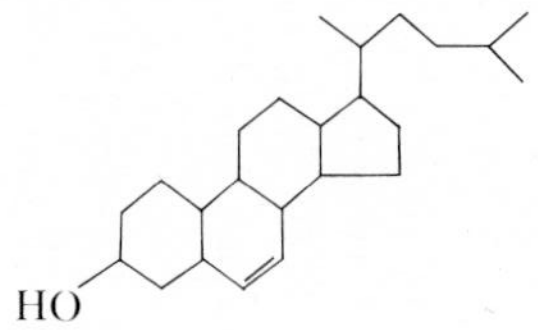

Phospholipids

$$H_2C-O-FA_1$$
$$H-C-O-FA_2$$
$$H_2C-O-PO_3R$$

	R
Phosphatidic acid	= H
Phosphatidylserine	= serine
Phosphatidylethanolamine	= ethanolamine

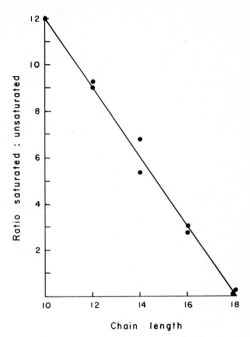

Figure 3–1. Frequency of fatty acids in triglyceride. As the chain length increased the frequency of saturated fatty acids decreased. (Reprinted from Jacob and Grimmer: J. Lipid Research, 9:730–732, 1968, with permission.)

ever, was higher in the obese subjects than in the lean ones. In addition, the percentage of various fatty acids was similar in fat from several regions of the body (Hirsch et al., 1960).

The predominant component of adipose tissue is the triglyceride droplet (Bjorntorp et al. 1966b). Martinsson (1967) found that lipids represent 90.3 mg/100 mg wet weight of adipose tissue or just over 90 percent of the total tissue weight. The majority of the lipid was triglyceride (Table 3–4). Cholesterol accounts for 0.16 percent and phos-

TABLE 3–3. *Fatty Acids in Triglycerides from Human Gluteal Adipose Tissue Obtained by Needle Aspiration**

FATTY ACID	LENGTH: SATURATION	PERCENT COMPOSITION OBESE	NORMAL
Lauric	12:0	0.4	0.7
Myristic	14:0	3.2	3.5
	14:1	0.8	1.1
	15:0	0.5	0.6
Palmitic	16:0	21.1	20.0
Palmitoleic	16:1	10.6	10.7
Stearic	18:0	3.2	3.4
Oleic	18:1	53.4	53.0
Linoleic	18:2	7.3	7.1

*Adapted from Heffernan: Am. J. Clin. Nutr., *15*:5, 1964, with permission.

pholipid for 0.15 percent (.15 mg/100 mg tissue) (Table 3–4). The volume occupied by the triglyceride and other lipids is reflected in the small quantity of intracellular water and proportionally greater quantity of extracellular water (Bjorntorp et al. 1966a). Intracellular water comprises about 60 percent of the weight of most cells. In the fat cell, however, it is about 54 percent (53.9 ml/kg) of adipose tissue weight in normal and 52 percent (52.2 ml/kg) of fat tissue weight in obese subjects (Englehardt et al., 1971).

The extracellular water is approximately three times as much as the intracellular water and represents 139.2 to 144 ml/kg for normal and 142.3 to 143.9 ml/kg for the obese. The nitrogen content of fat tissue is 26 mg/100 mg wet weight (Gelhorn and Marks, 1961; Hirsch and Goldrick, 1964; Vague,1974). Martinsson observed positive correlations between deoxyribonucleic acid (DNA) and nitrogen content, and between nitrogen and phospholipids. However, DNA content and the total lipids are inversely related. Thus an increase in the size of fat cells in adipose tissue, while not associated with an increase in the quantity of DNA per fat cell, is associated with an increase in the quantity of water, triglyceride, phospholipid, and nitrogen in each cell.

Morphology of Adipose Tissue

The development of fat cells in adipose tissue has been recently reviewed by Slavin (1972). The precise stem cell from which the adipocyte develops remains unsettled, but it appears to be of mesodermal origin and to have a perivascular location. Napolitano (1963) followed the development of adipocytes in the epididymal fat organ of the rat for the first nine days of life. The first visible lipid droplets (i.e., those stained with osmium tetroxide) were termed "preadipose fibroblasts." It was found that the number of droplets increases with the passage of time and that the cell loses its cytoplasmic extensions and becomes more ovoid. As lipid deposition continues, smooth sur-

TABLE 3–4. *Composition of Subcutaneous Human Adipose Tissue**

COMPONENT	N	PERCENT	
Wet weight	23	100	
Dry weight	23	91.1	± 0.63
Total lipid	23	90.3	± 0.92
Triglycerides	12	86.0	± 1.67
Cholesterol	23	0.16	± 0.01
Phospholipid	23	0.15	± 0.01
Nitrogen	23	0.26	± 0.02
Deoxyribonucleic acid	11	0.0074	± 0.001

*Adapted from Martinsson: Acta Med. Scand., *182*:795, 1967, with permission.

face vesicles appear in these small droplets. The numerous lipid droplets coalesce into a larger fat droplet and a stage called "mid-differentiation" is reached. With the continued growth of the fat droplet, there is continuing reduction in the volume of the cytoplasmic structures, including the endoplasmic reticulum and Golgi apparatus.

According to Napolitano (1963) there is no clear cut cellular organelle which has an intimate relationship with the developing fat droplet. As animals grow, the size and number of adipocytes increases. The multiplication of adipocytes occurs during a finite and limited fraction of the life span of most animals . However, in rats the number of adipocytes in the epididymal fat organ appears to reach its maximum before 14 weeks of age (Hirsch and Han, 1969). But important species differences exist (DiGirolamo and Mendlinger, 1971). During the adult life of rats and hamsters, the accretion of fat occurs primarily by increasing the size of adipoctyes; there is little change in adipocyte number, which is largely determined by the time the animal reaches maturity. In the guinea pig, on the other hand, the number of fat cells in the epididymal fat organ increases 12-fold during the adult life of the animal.

Adipocytes from most adult animals range between 100 and 120 microns in diameter. They appear as large oval cells of which the major component is the central droplet. Mature adipocytes apparently do not divide. This has been concluded from two kinds of experiments: studies in rats with hypothalamic obesity, and studies on synthesis and turnover of deoxyribonucleic acid (DNA) in the nucleus of the fat cell. In adult animals with hypothalamic hyperphagia (see Chapters 2 and 5), the adipocytes increase markedly in size but the total number in the epididymal fat pad remains unchanged in spite of the marked increase in weight of the fat pad (Hirsch and Han, 1969). The turnover of DNA has been studied by Hollenberg, Vost, and Patten (1971) and by Greenwood and Hirsch (1974). The technique involves labeling the DNA with radioactive thymidine, one of the nucleic acids which is incorporated into the DNA of the nucleus during cell division. The radioactivity remaining after its incorporation in the DNA of the fat cells may be examined after weight loss or gain.

Experiments have shown that in the mature animal, the ratio of radioactively-labeled DNA to unlabeled DNA in adipocytes does not change during either of these nutritional manipulations. A loss of labeled adipoctyes would increase the ratio, and the appearance of new unlabeled adipocytes would reduce the ratio of labeled to unlabeled DNA. Since no change occurs, it can be concluded that the number of adipocytes remains stable. These two experimental approaches indicate that in the normal adult rat an adipocyte is a mature cell which does not divide and which has a very long life span. These data obtained in rats have been extrapolated to other species, including man. However, there is some data (Lemonnier, 1972, 1974) to suggest that under special conditions the number of adipocytes in some fat organs may continue to increase throughout life.

THE SIZE AND NUMBER OF ADIPOCYTES

Methods of Measurement

To determine the size and number of adipocytes, two measurements are needed: the size of fat cells, and the total quantity of body fat (methods for measuring the latter are described in detail in Chapter 1). Three general methods are in use for measuring the size of individual adipocytes. 1. The microscopic method measures the diameter of the adipocyte in fixed tissue (Bjurlf, 1959) or fixed-frozen tissue (Sjostrom, Bjorntorp and Vrana, 1971). 2. The diameter of individual fat cells which have been isolated from an adipose tissue depot can be measured optically after treating the tissue with collagenase. This enzyme breaks down the intercellular collagen bridges and releases free adipocytes (Zinder and Shapiro, 1971; Gliemann, 1967; Goldrick, 1967; Bray, 1970a; DiGirolamo, Mendlinger and Fertig, 1971). The diameter of the adipocyte can then be converted to fat cell volume using mathematical formulas (Goldrick, 1967). 3. Finally, osmium-fixed fat cells can be prepared and the number of such cells in a preweighed piece of tissue can be counted by use of an electronic particle counter (Hirsch and Gallian, 1968).

The first two histologic methods have advantages of economy and simplicity but have two major disadvantages (Smith et al., 1972). First, it is tedious to optically measure the dimensions of individual fat cells. Moreover, the optical methods measure only one dimension (diameter) of a cell. Small errors in this measurement will be amplified in calculating volume because volume = $\pi/6(d)^3$. Thus the variance is large and reliability of the optical methods is less than those that count fat cells as particles. The osmium-fixed method (Hirsch and Gallian, 1968) has the advantage of counting large numbers of particles and eliciting a good frequency distribution. Its major disadvantage is the lower limit of size which can be counted. The optical method can detect all visible particles but the electronic counting methods usually have a lower limit of 25 microns. Cells smaller than this are present in the animal as it grows and after profound weight loss. A second disadvantage with the electronic counter is the expense of the osmium tetroxide and the electronic counter itself.

Genetic Factors

Both genetic and environmental factors influence the size and number of adipocytes. The genetic factors include differences in species and strains of animals, differences due to sex, and differences in anatomic location of fat deposits. The differences in the effects of age on the number of epididymal fat cells in rats and guinea pigs (DiGirolamo and Mendlinger, 1971) have been discussed. A second difference in adipose cell number and cell size has been found in genetically transmitted obesity in rodents (Chapter 5).

The increased amount of stored triglyceride in the obese animal is obvious. Such deposition of triglyceride can occur by increasing the size of fat cells that already exist, or by increasing the total number of such fat cells. The size and number of fat cells has now been measured in most forms of experimental obesity (Johnson and Hirsch, 1972; Lemonnier and Alexiu, 1974; Johnson, et al., 1971; Stern and Greenwood, 1974; Bray and York, 1971). Table 3–5 lists several of the experimental forms of obesity and the changes in size and number of adipocytes. In all of these forms of obesity, the size of the adipocytes was increased but not the total number of fat cells. Increased numbers of fat cells occurred in the obese (ob/ob) mouse and in the fatty rat, two strains in which obesity is transmitted as autosomal recessive Mendelian trait.

Among rodents made obese by injecting gold thioglucose, by destroying the ventromedial hypothalamic nuclei (Chapter 2), or by changing nutritional status, obesity results almost entirely from an increase in the size of the individual adipocytes and not in the number of these cells. The interaction of genetic and nutritional components in animals with hypercellular obesity has been examined. Johnson et al. (1973) studied fatty rats with hyperplasia of the adipose organ. During the first 30 days of life, nutrition had a major effect on the increase in cell number. If dietary intake was reduced, cell prolifera-

TABLE 3–5. *Size and Number of Adipocytes from Dorsal Subcutaneous Fat of 26 Week Old Male Animals.**

Species	Type of Animal	Body Weight (g)	Cell Size μg lipid/cell	p	Number of Fat Cells 10^6	p
Rat	Lean	432	0.16	–	16.4	–
	Fatty (fa/fa)	705	1.26	<.05	41.0	<.05
	Hypothalamic lesion (VMH)	593	1.03	<.05	18.2	N.S.
Mouse	Lean	29.6	0.07	–	2.05	–
	Yellow-obese (A^{y}a)	42.5	0.28	<.05	3.11	N.S.
	Gold thioglucose obese	40.7	0.35	<.05	2.85	N.S.
	Obese (ob/ob)	53.6	0.70	<.05	2.80	<.05
	Diabetes (db/db)	50.3	0.92	<.05	1.93	N.S.

*Adapted from Stern and Greenwood (1974). For a discussion of various types of obesity consult Chapter 5.

tion was diminished. After 30 days, however, genetic factors became more important than nutritional factors in determining cellularity of the adipose tissue.

The difference between sexes is also genetically and hormonally controlled. In experimental animals the development of estrus cycles is accompanied by cyclic changes in food intake. Female rats have a lower body fat content than male rats.

The size and number of fat cells in men and women was studied by Sjostrom et al. (1975) in Table 3–6. Body fat in the men and women of this study was lower than is usually seen (see Chapter 1). Nonetheless, the difference in total number of adipocytes and regional differences between the sexes are clearly evident. Epigastric and femoral regions showed important differences, but did not show any differences between men and women.

Environmental Factors

Environmental factors also play an important role in modifying the size and number of adipocytes. If rodents are fed a diet restricted in calories, they will have fewer adipocytes than littermates exposed to optimal nutrition (Knittle and Hirsch, 1968). Widdowson and McCance (1960) found that 4 rats suckled with one mother grow more rapidly and weigh more than animals suckled 20 per mother. The animals from these large litters have a smaller number of adipocytes in all depots than animals fed 4 per mother (Knittle and Hirsch, 1968; Hirsch, 1972).

Dietary surpluses may also increase the number of fat cells (Knittle, 1972b; Lemonnier, 1972; Lemonnier and Alexiu, 1974). Lemonnier showed that 32 week old female mice fed a high fat diet had an increase in the number of fat cells in the perimetrial and perirenal depots, but not in the subcutaneous depot. Female rats fed a high fat

TABLE 3–6. *Comparison of Fat Cell Numbers in Men and Women**

	MEN	WOMEN	p
Age (years)	23	22	N.S.
Height (cm)	180	171	<.001
Weight (kg)	72	64	<.001
Body Fat (kg)	4.8	11.8	<.001
%	6.7	18.5	
Fat cell number ($\times 10^{-9}$)	17.5	41.4	<.001
Regional fat cell number ($\times 10^{-3}$)			
Epigastric	39	53	<.025
Femoral	17	28	<.001
Gluteal	35	46	N.S.

*Adapted from Sjostrom et al. (1975).

diet from age 5 months to one year also showed a significant increase in the number of fat cells in the perirenal depot. One attempt to increase the number of fat cells by injecting insulin from an early age has not been successful (Salans, Zarnowski and Segal, 1972).

Exercise has been found to reduce the total number of adipocytes (Oscai, Spirakis, Wolff and Beck, 1972), while vigorously exercised growing rats increase their food consumption. The caloric requirements for exercise reduce the number of calories available for synthesis of new cells, and the production of new adipocytes is decreased. In this study the exercising rats were lighter than control animals which were not exercising. To establish control for this difference in weight, a third group of animals was restricted in food intake so that their weight gain was the same as the exercising rats. The number of adipose cells in the pair-gained group was intermediate (5.72×10^6) between the exercising rats (4.46×10^6) and the animals allowed to eat ad lib. (6.89×10^6). Thus multiplication of fat cells requires availability of substrate at the appropriate time, and this supply can be reduced by vigorous exercise.

Exposure to cold is a third factor which influences the number of adipocytes. When rats are chronically exposed to the cold, they increase heat production and convert increased quantities of ingested energy to maintain body temperature. A low environmental temperature ($5° C$) has been found to increase the number of adipocytes in one fat pad of these rats (Therriault and Mellin, 1971). These studies on environment and the number of fat cells indicate that the process by which mesodermal precursors are converted into mature adipocytes is under a number of controls.

The Effects of Obesity

Obese humans may have a normal or increased number of fat cells (Knittle 1972a). This distinction was originally noted by Bjurlf (1959) and elaborated by Hirsch and his collaborators (Hirsch, Knittle and Salans, 1966; Hirsch, 1972). This difference has subsequently been observed by many investigators (Bray, 1970; Bjorntorp and Sjostrom, 1971; Stern 1974; Hirsch and Knittle, 1970; Brook, Lloyd and Wolff, 1972; Apfelbaum, Brigant and Duret, 1974). Bjurlf (1959, 1963) examined the number and size of adipocytes in the abdominal panniculus of men at autopsy and found two groups; those with increased size and number of fat cells, and those with only increased size of adipocytes. He concluded from this study that genetic factors are of prime importance in determining an individual's number of fat cells, and that environmental factors such as nutrition are probably the major determining factor in the enlargement of adipocytes in men who do not have an increased number of cells.

The frequency distribution curve for the number and size of

adipocytes from 21 lean and 78 obese subjects studied by Salans, Cushman and Weismann (1973) is shown in Figure 3–2. The adipocytes from the obese patients were almost invariably larger than adipocytes from comparable fat deposits in lean individuals. The number of adipocytes, however, had a bimodal distribution. In one subgroup the frequency distribution was comparable to that of the normal population, and in the other subgroup the frequency distribution was outside the normal distribution. When the number of adipocytes and age of onset of obesity were examined, it was clear that individuals with hypercellular obesity (i.e. increased number of fat cells) became fat before age 15. Those whose obesity began after age 20 showed a normal number of, but enlarged, fat cells (Fig. 3–3) (Salans et al., 1971).

Salans et al. also observed significant variation in the size of fat cells between one depot and another in the same individual, as well as a significant variation between individuals. They concluded that the best estimate of size is obtained by averaging the data from three separate sites of measurement. Brook (1972; Brook, Lloyd and Wolff, 1972) has examined this problem in children and has suggested that most of the hyperplasia of fat cells probably occurs in the first year of life. Although there is not general agreement on this early age (Widdowson and Shaw, 1973), the total number of fat cells probably reaches a maximum before the end of puberty. Although the hyperplastic forms of obesity begin in childhood, it is not clear whether all individuals whose obesity begins in childhood have an increased number of fat cells. Hirsch (personal communication) has suggested that some individuals with childhood onset of their obesity may not have an increased number of fat cells.

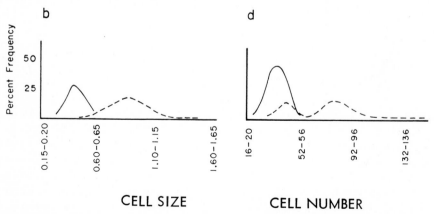

CELL SIZE   **CELL NUMBER**

Figure 3–2. The size and number of fat cells from lean and obese subjects. The distribution of fat cells in lean subjects is shown by the solid line (——). The broken line (----) shows data for the obese patients. Note the bimodal distribution of fat cell number for the obese patients while the cell size is unimodally distributed. (Reprinted from Salans et al.: J. Clin. Invest., 52:929–941, 1973, with permission.)

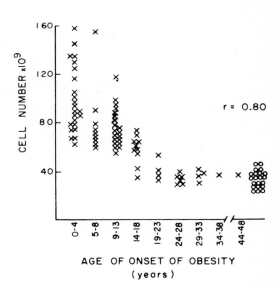

Figure 3–3. Relation between the onset of obesity and the number of fat cells. The number of fat cells in 21 normal weight patients is shown on the right with open circles (○). The obese subjects are shown as crosses (×). All patients whose obesity began before age 13 had increased numbers of fat cells. Those whose obesity began after age 24 had normal numbers of fat cells. (Reprinted from Salans et al.: J. Clin. Invest., 52:929–941, 1973, with permission.)

TRIGLYCERIDE FORMATION (LIPOGENESIS)

The fat droplet of the adipocytes is composed almost entirely of triglycerides. In this section the source of the fatty acids and the glycerol from which the triglycerides are made will be examined. For a more detailed review of the control of fatty acid synthesis, the reader may consult Hollenberg and Angel (1967); Jeanrenaud (1968); Jeanrenaud and Hepp (1970), Galton (1971) and Bjorntorp (1974).

Source of the Fatty Acids

The fatty acids used for synthesis of triglyceride in adipose tissue are derived from 3 sources. These are: (1) the free fatty acids which circulate in the plasma attached to albumin; (2) the fatty acids of lipoprotein triglyceride which can be released near the adipocyte by the enzyme, lipoprotein lipase; and (3) the fatty acids formed within the adipocyte. A schematic diagram of an adipocyte is shown in Figure 3–4. Fatty acids bound to albumin can be incorporated into adipose tissue triglycerides (Galton, Wilson and Kissebah, 1971). In this study the uptake of palmitate into neutral lipid per mg of tissue weight was similar in fat from lean and obese individuals.

Lipoproteins which circulate in plasma can also provide fatty acids for adipose tissue. When adipose tissue is incubated with lipoproteins, the fatty acids are taken into adipose tissue and incorporated

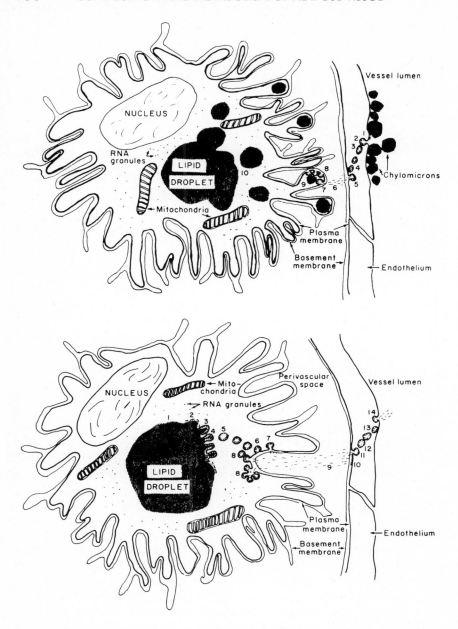

Figure 3–4. Schematic diagram of an adipocyte. Lipogenesis is shown on the top and lipolysis below. Top Panel: Numbers 1 through 5 are the steps involved in hydrolysis of triglyceride in lipoproteins. Numbers 7 through 10 are the process of reesterification and migration of the droplet to the large central droplet. Lower panel: Numbers 1 through 8 are the action of hormone sensitive and monoglyceride lipase along with migration to the plasma membrane. Numbers 9 through 14 are the release of free fatty acids and their migration to the albumin receptors in plasma. (Reprinted from Stein, B. G.: Int. Rev. Cytol., *33*:297–334, 1972, with permission.)

into triglycerides (Wilson, Gutman and Galton, 1973). This process involves the breakdown of the triglyceride in the lipopoptein into fatty acids and glycerol. The glycerol is not, but the fatty acids are, incorporated into adipose tissue triglycerides. Thus when lipoproteins labeled with radioactivity in the glyceride part of the molecule are used for these studies, essentially no radioactivity appears in the glycerides of adipose tissue.

Lipoprotein lipase is an essential enzyme for the release of fatty acids from lipoproteins. This enzyme is probably synthesized in fat cells, and stored there and in the endothelial cells lining capillaries. Its formation is stimulated by insulin and glucose and inhibited by cyclic AMP. Heparin in vivo or in vitro activates this enzyme. The activity of lipoprotein lipase in human adipose tissue has been observed under a variety of conditions. It is present in low activity when compared to the lipoprotein lipase in adipose tissue from rats (Zinder and Bray, 1975). After an overnight fast, lipoprotein lipase activity is lower in fat from overweight subjects than in normal weight subjects (Persson, 1973).

However, these data are not corrected for the number of fat cells. When the activity of lipoprotein lipase is related to the size of the fat cell, we have observed no differences per fat cell between obese and lean patients (Zinder and Bray, 1975). The release of lipoprotein lipase during incubation of human fat with heparin in vitro, however, showed a positive correlation between enzyme activity and cell size (Guy-Grand and Bigorie, 1974). This is to be expected if the lipoproteins provide a major fraction of the fatty acids incorporated into triglyceride in adipose tissue. The incorporation by adipose tissue of fatty acids from lipoprotein has been compared with the incorporation of albumin-bound fatty acids (Wilson, Gutman and Galton, 1973). Fatty acids from lipoprotein are incorporated more rapidly than albumin-bound fatty acids.

The third source of fatty acids is de novo synthesis within the adipocytes utilizing carbons from glucose or pyruvate. The use of radioactively labeled glucose has made it possible to explore this process in detail. Radioactivity from glucose is incorporated into the glycerol and fatty acid part of the triglyceride molecule. The rate of incorporation of isotope is increased by insulin and reduced in starved animals (Jeanrenaud, 1968; Jeanrenaud and Hepp, 1970).

Although it is clear that fatty acids are rapidly synthesized by adipose tissue of rats and mice, two observations have led some researchers to propose that human adipose tissue may not synthesize fatty acids (Shrago, Glennon and Gordon, 1967, 1971; Gordon, 1970). First, several investigators have found little or no evidence of such synthesis from glucose (Hirsch and Goldrick, 1964; Salans et al., 1968; Galton, 1968; Shrago, Glennon and Gordon, 1971; Shrago, Spennetta and Gordon, 1969). Second, Shrago, Glennon and Gordon (1967) have found that citrate cleavage enzyme, a key enzyme in the formation of fatty acids, is almost absent in human adipose tissue (Shrago, Spennetta and Gordon, 1969).

Several recent observations have, however, unequivocally established that human adipose tissue can synthesize long chain fatty acids utilizing pathways identical to those described for rodents (Sjostrom, 1972). The formation of fatty acids by adipose tissue from rodents depends on whether the animal is gaining or losing weight. Similar effects of positive and negative caloric intake can be demonstrated with fat from human subjects. When obese patients were fed high calorie diets, the conversion of carbon atoms from glucose or pyruvate into fatty acids by pieces of adipose tissue incubated in vitro was readily demonstrated (Bray, 1969, 1970b).

Figure 3–5 shows the conversion of radioactivity from glucose into fatty acids when the previous diet was 3500 or 900 calories/day. With excess calorie intake, the synthesis of fatty acids proceeded linearly with time. Conversely, when the diet was restricted with ensuing weight loss, synthesis of fatty acids was nearly abolished (Bray, 1968; Goldrick and Hirsch, 1964), and triglyceride formation was also depressed (Galton and Wilson, 1970). These studies provided careful control of nutritional conditions prior to obtaining sample fat tissue, which is crucial in this kind of research. When adipose tissue is

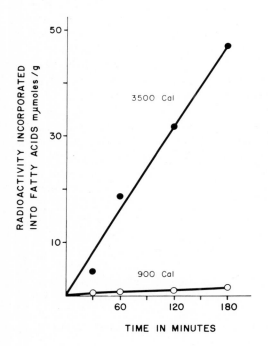

Figure 3–5. Effect of caloric intake on lipogenesis from glucose in human adipose tissue. Fat was removed and studied in vitro. Each line represents the time course for the incorporation of radioactivity from glucose into fatty acids in the presence of insulin. For 2 weeks before each fat biopsy this obese patient was fed 3500 (●) or 900 (○) kcal/day. (Reprinted from Bray, G. A.: J. Clin. Invest., 48:1413–1422, 1969, with permission.)

obtained from obese patients who are ingesting more calories than are needed to maintain body weight, lipogenesis is readily demonstrated. Pyruvate and glucose have been compared, and pyruvate appears to be a better precursor than glucose (Bray, 1972).

Sjostrom, Bjorntorp and Mansson (1973) have examined the conditions under which fatty acids can be synthesized by homogenates of human fat. Carbon from citrate and acetate can be incorporated into fatty acids, mainly myristic and palmitic. Complementing these studies are the observations of Angel, Farkas and Bray (1974) who used tritium-labeled water as a marker for the synthesis of fatty acids. With this approach, the incorporation of fatty acids was readily demonstrated in subcutaneous and omental human fat. The incorporation of radioactivity from tritiated water into fatty acids in vitro was examined in adipose tissue and in slices of human liver. With this data, synthetic rates for the entire body could be calculated. The overall contribution of fat and liver to the synthesis of fatty acids is shown in Table 3–7. In this table the formation of fatty acids by liver was 9 to 13 times greater than by fat. The liver normally weighs 2000 g and body fat ranges between 15 and 25 percent of body weight (10.5 to 17.5 kg in a 70 kg individual). In such an individual the total synthesis of fatty acids would be 10 to 50 percent greater in liver than in fat. However, if the total fat were greater than 20 kg, fat might be the more important tissue.

This interpretation of these experiments is limited by the fact that the incubations were performed in vitro. Extrapolation to the subject supplying the tissue is thus based on questionable assumptions. However, these studies provide the only data comparing lipogenesis in liver and fat from human subjects. They suggest that human fat may be a major tissue for converting glucose carbons to fatty acids. In both tissues the formation of fatty acids was stimulated by the addition of insulin, adding further support to the physiological importance of this study.

Earlier observations about the enzymatic steps in the synthesis of fatty acids in human fat have been re-examined by Goldrick and Gal-

TABLE 3–7. *Fatty Acid Synthesis in Human Liver and in Adipose Tissue*

TISSUE	FATTY ACID SYNTHESIS 10^4 cpm/g/4h	
	Nonobese	Obese
Liver	18.3 ± 10.2	26.4 ± 10.5
Adipose tissue	2.14 ± 0.93	2.06 ± 0.48

*Slices of liver weighing approximately 100 mg and pieces of fat weighing 1000 mg were incubated 4 hours in Krebs-Ringer bicarbonate buffer containing 4 percent albumin, 10 mM glucose and ^3H_2O (Angel, Farkas and Bray—unpublished observations).

ton (1974). They found higher levels of citrate cleavage enzyme in human adipose tissue than were originally observed. The principal difficulty in the earlier studies (Shrago et al., 1967) was the conditions under which the enzyme was assayed. The pH optimum for the citrate cleavage enzyme from human fat appears to differ from that obtained from rat adipose tissue.

In summary, human adipose tissue, like fat tissue of rats and other rodents, can synthesize fatty acids from glucose and pyruvate in vitro. The intracellular pathways by which this process occurs seem to be the same as in other mammals where the process has been studied in detail.

The question which remains to be answered is the relative role of fatty acid synthesis de novo as compared with the supply of fatty acids from circulating lipoproteins. Since human tissues cannot manufacture linoleic or linolenic acid, it seems possible to use the rate at which these fatty acids accumulate in adipose tissue while using a corn oil diet as an indicator for the rate of fatty acid turnover. Utilizing this technique Hirsch et al. (1960) found that the turnover of linoleic acid (18:2) ranged between 350 and 750 days, indicating the slow turnover of triglycerides in the large fat droplet of the fat cell.

Turnover of fatty acids in triglycerides of adipose tissue can also be assessed by labeling the triglyceride fatty acids. Glucose can be injected in vivo for this purpose (Gordis, 1965), or an epididymal fat pad can be incubated in vitro with radioactively labeled glucose for a short time, returned to the animal, and removed at a later time (Hollenberg, 1966). These two approaches in the experimental animal have indicated that the triglyceride molecules, once formed, have considerable stability; they are not broken down and resynthesized rapidly.

A similar conclusion has been reached by studies in human volunteers who were fed for long periods of time on diets with fatty acid composition markedly different from the composition of the adipose depots at the initiation of the study. The rate at which the composition of the fatty acids in the depot changed could thus be observed (Hirsch et al., 1960). With this technique Hirsch found that the triglyceride molecules of human fat depots had great stability and that only after a prolonged time on the experimental diet was a change in composition evidenced. Moreover, the composition tended to reflect the diet which was fed. These studies lead to the conclusion that in a diet with a significant fraction of exogenous fat (the average American diet), the principal source of the fatty acids in triglycerides of adipose tissue is obtained from the dietary fatty acids. However, adipose tissue probably plays a role in the short term synthesis and storage of fatty acids derived from dietary carbohydrate. It may well be that fatty acids synthesized in adipose tissue enter a small, rapidly changing pool and are released rapidly during the day (Zinder et al., 1973).

Source of Glycerol

When glycerol is added to adipose tissue, it is not to a significant degree converted into the glyceride esters of triglyceride (Galton, 1969). Glycerokinase, an enzyme which phosphorylates glycerol, is present in very low levels in adipose tissue (Vaughn, 1962). Glycerol 3-phosphate, formed from glucose, is the essential metabolic precursor of the glyceride-glycerol in triglyceride. Addition of glycerol 3-phosphate to an homogenate of adipose tissue will stimulate the incorporation of fatty acids into triglyceride (Margolis and Vaughan, 1962; Howard and Lowenstein, 1965). Under usual conditions in vivo and in vitro, glucose is the principal source of the glycerol 3-phosphate required for the synthesis of triglycerides (Galton, 1968). In the absence of glucose, pyruvate carbons can be converted to glycerol or to glyceride glycerol 3-phosphate) Leveille, 1970; Bray, 1969).

The possibility that the metabolism of glycerol 3-phosphate might be abnormal in obesity was suggested by Galton (1966) and investigated in detail by Galton and Bray (1967). This study showed that the activity of both the mitochondrial glycerophosphate oxidase and soluble glycerophosphate dehydrogenase was reduced in the adipose tissue from obese patients (Fig. 3–6). In contrast, most of the other en-

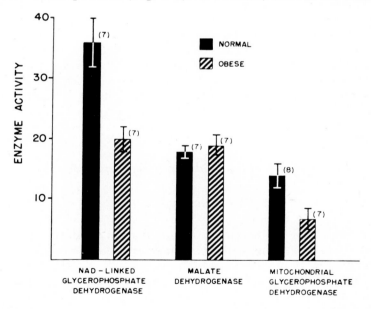

Figure 3–6. Activity of three enzymes in human adipose tissue. Homogenates of human fat from obese and lean subjects were used to measure 3 enzymes and the data is expressed in terms of protein concentration. The activity of the NAD-linked and the mitochondrial glycerophosphate dehydrogenases is significantly reduced but malate dehydrogenase was unchanged. (Adapted from Galton and Bray: J. Clin. Endocr., 27:1573–1580, 1967b.)

zymes which have been measured in human adipose tissue are the same in fat from normal and overweight subjects (Shrago et al., 1967; Bray, 1969, 1970; Galton and Bray, 1967b). Galton and Bray suggested that low levels of the enzymes which metabolize glycerol 3-phosphate might increase the quantity of glycerol 3-phosphate available for the synthesis of triglycerides and thus facilitate the development of obesity.

This interpretation was no longer tenable when it was shown that the activity of these enzymes was *higher* during overfeeding of obese patients (Bray, 1969). A new interpretation was suggested by the observation that the activity of the mitochondrial glycerol 3-phosphate oxidase was increased in fat tissue after two weeks of treatment with triiodothyronine (Bray, 1969). The oxidation of substrate by the enzymes of the glycerophosphate cycle might reduce the production of useful energy. This could occur because the transfer of hydrogen from an extra-mitochondrial to an intra-mitochondrial site by the glycerophosphate cycle skips one step for generating ATP. Thus the glycerophosphate cycle might provide a mechanism for partially uncoupling oxidative phosphorylation.

This possibility was tested by overfeeding normal subjects, a situation in which calories appear to be dissipated (see Chapter 4). If the glycerophosphate cycle was the mechanism for such a loss, then its enzymes should increase in activity. Contrary to this prediction, the enzymatic activity of the glycerophosphate cycle in adipose tissue from normal men fell after they had gained weight (Sims et al., 1973). The glycerophosphate cycle of adipose tissue was thus not the cause of any calorie wastage in these men. Thus the physiological importance of change in the activity of the enzymes in the glycerophosphate cycle which are produced by nutrition and hormones remains to be elucidated.

Factors Which Modify Fatty Acid Synthesis (Lipogenesis)

INSULIN

The addition of insulin to an incubation medium containing adipose tissue or adipose cells accelerates the rate at which glucose is metabolized by these cells (Kahlenberg and Kalant, 1964). This effect of insulin appears to reside in at least two loci. First, insulin enhances the entry of glucose into the fat cell (Crofford et al., 1970; Bjorntorp et al., 1971). In addition, insulin enhances the conversion of carbon from glucose into glycogen and fatty acids. However, there is only a small or minimal effect on the conversion of radioactivity from glucose into the glyceride portion of triglyceride. The effects of insulin on glucose entry can be simulated in part by increasing the concentration of glucose in the incubation medium. In human adipose tissue the glyceride portion of the triglyceride has more than 85 percent of the radioactivity incorporated when tissue is incubated in the presence of radioactive glucose (Hirsch and Goldrick, 1964; Gries. and Steinke, 1967).

The effects of insulin on the metabolism of human adipose tissue have been a source of much debate. Insulin has been found almost uniformly to stimulate the oxidation of glucose with the production of increased quantities of radioactively labeled carbon dioxide ($^{14}CO_2$) (Bjorntorp, 1966; Salans, Knittle and Hirsch, 1968; Bray, 1969; Gries and Steinke, 1967; Goldrick, 1967; Davidson, 1972). The effects on the synthesis of fatty acids, however, are more complex. When isolated fat cells or portions of adipose tissue obtained from aspiration biopsies are used (Hirsch and Goldrick, 1964; Salans, Knittle and Hirsch, 1968; Galton, 1968), a stimulatory effect of insulin on the conversion of radioactivity from glucose into fatty acid carbons may not be detectable. When pieces of fat are used (Gries and Steinke, 1967; Bray, 1969), however, insulin stimulates the conversion of glucose carbon into carbon dioxide of fatty acids. From the work of Martinsson it would appear that the larger the pieces of fat (up to 500 mg) the greater the sensitivity to insulin in vitro. A similar effect was observed by Goldrick (1967), Goldrick, Ashley and Lloyd (1969) and Bray (1969), who found that concentrated fat cells have a much greater response to insulin than fat cells in dilute concentrations.

The effects of insulin are in turn influenced by a number of factors. The pattern of food intake is one of these. When experimental animals eat their food rapidly in one or two large meals, adipose tissue becomes more sensitive to the lipogenic effects of insulin (Leveille, 1970); that is, the rate of incorporation of radioactivity from glucose into fatty acids is greater in animals eating one or two meals than in animals which eat food continuously through the day.

The initial step in the action of insulin on the fat cell is its binding to the plasma membrane. Most of the studies on this phenomenon have used fat from experimental animals. In one study with human fat cells, Olefsky, Jen and Reaven (1974) found two populations of receptors. One population had a high affinity and consisted of 50,000 sites per cell, and the other site was five times as numerous but had a lower affinity for insulin. The relationship of obesity to the binding of insulin by cell membrane has been studied in the experimental animal. In mice with genetically inherited obesity (ob/ob, db/db) and mice with obesity due to treatment with gold thioglucose, there is a decrease in the number of insulin binding sites (Kahn et al., 1975). The binding of insulin has been assessed less directly in obese patients by studying lymphocytes (Archer, Gordon and Roth, 1975). The binding of insulin by lymphocytes (actually monocytes) from obese patients was less than with lymphocytes from lean individuals. Weight loss improved binding and increased the number of insulin binding receptors.

DIET

Rapid ingestion of food by obese human subjects increases the sensitivity of human adipose tissue to insulin. In one study, obese subjects were fed a high carbohydrate diet in one large meal or several small ones (Bray, 1972). The response to insulin and the rate of fatty acid synthesis by adipose tissue in vitro were greater when the subjects consumed the same number of calories in several small meals as opposed to one large meal (Bray, 1972).

Total carbohydrate and calorie intake also influences the responsiveness to insulin (Bray, 1969, 1972). This has been most cogently examined by Salans et al. (1974). They studied the effects of two levels of carbohydrate intake in normal weight and obese human subjects. Subcutaneous biopsies of fat were obtained by needle aspiration after each subject had been on the diet for several weeks. Glucose oxidation to CO_2 was increased more by insulin when the adipocytes were obtained during periods of high carbohydrate intake than when the diet was low in carbohydrate (Fig. 3-7). This was true for both the lean and obese individuals. Similar findings have been obtained in animal studies where diet has been manipulated (Ogundipe and Bray, 1974). The insulin response is enhanced by a high carbohydrate diet. Even

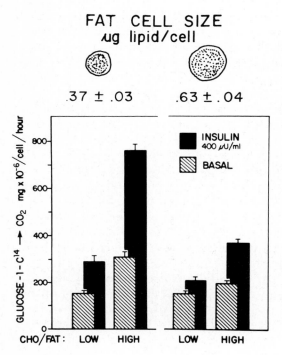

FAT CELL SIZE
µg lipid/cell

Figure 3-7. Effects of insulin on the metabolism of glucose by adipocytes of different sizes. Samples of adipose tissue were obtained from normal volunteers before and after weight gain. The size of the fat cells in these biopsies is shown at the top of the figure. The quantity of glucose converted to CO_2 in the presence and absence of insulin is shown by the bars. The effects of insulin on either diet were reduced after weight gain. However, the effects of insulin on fat cells obtained after ingesting a high carbohydrate diet were greater than the effects of insulin on fat cells obtained during the period on the low carbohydrate diet. (Adapted from Sims et al.: Rec. Prog. Horm. Res., 29:457–487, 1973, with permission.)

the sensitivity of very large adipocytes to insulin can be increased after a short period of overfeeding (Bray, 1969).

SIZE OF FAT CELLS

The size of the adipocyte also modifies the response to insulin and glucose (Brook and Lloyd, 1973). In 1968 Salans, Knittle, and Hirsch showed that enlarged adipocytes from obese subjects were less sensitive to the effects of insulin than small adipocytes obtained from the same subjects after weight loss. They proposed that insulin resistance in obesity is due to the enlarged fat cell. The major effect of weight loss was a fall in basal glucose oxidation, that is, the conversion of glucose to CO_2 in the absence of insulin was reduced in the smaller adipocytes. The addition of insulin increased glucose oxidation to CO_2 to the level obtained in the large adipocytes prior to weight loss. The hypothesis that insulin resistance in obesity might be the result of enlargement of adipocytes is provocative, although many would now interpret the apparent response to insulin as a result of basal changes.

The findings of Bjorntorp (1966) are contrary to those of Salans et al. (Salans and Dougherty, 1971). Bjorntorp found that large adipocytes metabolized glucose more rapidly than smaller fat cells from control subjects. Bjorntorp and Karlsson (1971) developed a method of isolating fat cells of different sizes from the same subject by flotation. Larger cells isolated by this technique had more cholesterol, phospholipid and protein than smaller cells. More importantly, the larger fat cells incorporated more radioactivity from glucose into triglyceride and fatty acids and had higher levels of activity for lactic dehydrogenase and aldolase (Englehardt et al., 1971). Similar results have been obtained by Gliemann (1967) and Gries, Koschinsky and Herberg (1974), who have separated fat cells of different sizes from the same animal.

In a careful study of the effects of insulin resposiveness in adipocytes from lean subjects before and after weight gain and in obese subjects before and after weight loss, Salans et al. (1974) concluded that the size of the adipocyte was one factor in the responsiveness to insulin (Fig. 3–8), but that total caloric intake and the effects of distribution of the calories between carbohydrate and fat were at least as important in determining the responsiveness of these fat cells to insulin. Similar laboratory results with experimental animals were obtained by Ogundipe and Bray (1974). Rats were fed so that carbohydrate intake and the size of fat cells could be studied independently. It was found that sensitivity of the adipocyte to insulin varies with the size of the fat cell and with the composition of the diet.

EXERCISE

Exercise also plays an important role in the response of adipo-cytes to insulin. In rats trained to run on a treadmill five days a week, lipogenesis from glucose was greater than in untrained animals (Palmer and Tipton, 1974). Obese individuals who are exercised show evidence of improved glucose tolerance and decreased insulin levels (Bjorntorp, 1975). Animal studies indicate that the responsiveness of adipocytes to insulin is improved by exercise, suggesting that overall metabolism (including carbohydrate utilization as well as the effects of insulin on this process) may be influenced by exercise.

TRIGLYCERIDE BREAKDOWN (LIPOLYSIS)

Lipolysis is the breakdown of triglyceride molecules into their constituent fatty acids and glycerol. This process is depicted schemat-ically in Figure 3–6. The first fatty acid is removed by a rate limiting step which is controlled by a "hormone sensitive" lipase. Removal of the second and third fatty acids occurs by a monoglyceride lipase which is not rate limiting. Lipolysis can be subdivided into two parts; basal lipolysis or the release of glycerol and free fatty acids in the absence of added hormones, and hormone-stimulated lipolysis.

Basal Lipolysis

The best index of lipolysis is the production of glycerol by adipose tissue, since the enzymes for phosphorylation of glycerol are essentially absent. Whether the fatty acids released during hydrolysis of triglycerides leave the fat cell varies with the experimental condi-tions. When glucose is absent from the incubation medium, essen-tially all of the free fatty acids formed during hydrolysis exit from the cell. Under these conditions three molecules of fatty acids are re-leased with each molecule of glycerol. When glucose is present in the incubation medium, the molar ratio of free fatty acid released is usu-ally less than would be anticipated from the complete hydrolysis of triglycerides. This discrepancy occurs because free fatty acids can be coupled to glycerol 3-phosphate to form new triglyceride molecules. Thus lipolysis is best estimated by measuring the release of glycerol.

Basal lipolysis has been examined in detail and is influenced by a number of factors. The size of the adipose tissue cell is the most interesting and relevant to our discussion of obesity. Many laboratories have shown that larger adipocytes from both experimen-tal animals and man release more glycerol than small adipocytes. This is demonstrated by the positive correlation between the size of the adipocyte and basal lipolysis (Smith, 1972; Zinder and Shapiro, 1971;

Goldrick and McLoughlin, 1969; Gries et al., 1972; Östman, Backman and Hallberg, 1973; Bray and York, 1971; Bjorntorp, Karlsson and Hovden, 1969; Faulhaber et al, 1969).

Figure 3–8 depicts lipolysis in relation to changes of fat cell size with weight loss in obese subjects (solid circles) and after weight gain in lean subjects (open circles). Enhanced glycerol production might be one biological indicator of the size of the fat cell. Since the adipose cell cannot reuse glycerol, it enters the circulation and returns to the liver where it is phosphorylated to glycerol 3-phosphate and is then recycled back to glucose. The increased breakdown and re-esterification of fatty acids by the large adipose cell is also associated with an increased utilization of oxygen.

Activated Lipolysis

A number of chemicals and hormones can activate the hormone sensitive lipase in adipose tissue (Table 3–8).

Activation of lipolysis by catecholamines has been studied in detail. Rizack (1964) demonstrated that the hormone sensitive lipase can be activated in homogenates of adipose tissue by the addition of adenosine'3'5' cyclic monophosphate (cAMP). Butcher et al. (1965) showed that stimulation of lipolysis in adipose tissue by cate-

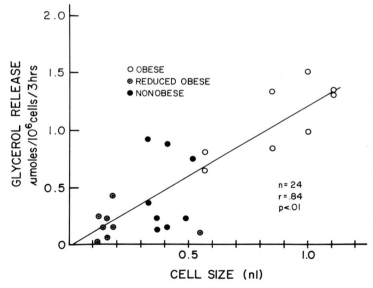

Figure 3–8. Fat cell size and lipolysis. Fat cells from obese patients before (○) and after (●) weight loss and fat cells from nonobese subjects were incubated in vitro without glucose or added hormones. Glycerol release was higher in the big fat cells (r=.84). (From Bray, G. A. et al.: Metabolism of adipose tissue in spontaneous and experimental obesity. In preparation.)

TABLE 3–8. *Effect of Various Substances on Lipolysis*
in Human Fat

STIMULATES LIPOLYSIS	INACTIVE OR UNCERTAIN	INHIBITS LIPOLYSIS
Epinephrine	ACTH	Insulin
Norepinephrine	Growth hormone	Prostaglandins
Isoproterenol	Peptides I and II	
Dibutyryl cyclic AMP	Glucagon	
Theophylline	Placental lactagen	
Thyrotropin	Glucocorticoids	
Lipid mobilizing factor	Secretin	
β lipotropin		

cholamines is accompanied by a rise in the concentration of cyclic AMP in fat cells. Additional evidence suggesting that cyclic AMP is the intracellular mediator of lipolysis has been obtained in studies with derivatives of cyclic AMP added directly to adipose tissue. One such derivative, N^6-2-0′-dibutyryl-cyclic-adenosine-3′5′ cyclic monophosphate (DBC AMP), is an effective stimulator of lipolysis. The fact that drugs which inhibit lipolysis in the presence of catecholamines also block the rise in cyclic AMP provides further support for the role of this nucleotide in lipolysis. The sequence of events in catecholamine-induced lipolysis thus involves an initial rise in the concentration of cyclic AMP which, in turn, activates a protein kinase which activates the hormone sensitive lipase. This cascade is depicted graphically in Figure 3–9.

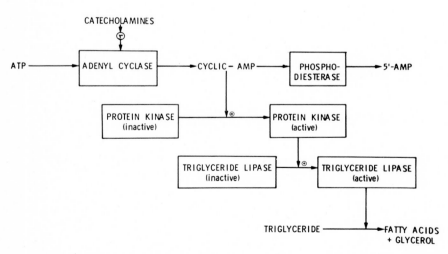

Figure 3–9.   The hormonal control of lipolysis through cyclic-AMP and protein kinase. The catecholamine acts on the adenylcyclase in the plasma membrane to activate the conversion of ATP to cyclic-AMP. Cyclic-AMP continues through a cascade to activate tryglyceride lipase and thus lipolysis. (Reprinted from Steinberg et al.: *In:* Excerpta Medica, J. Vague and J. Boyer, eds., 1974, pp. 61–68, with permission.)

Khoo, Steinberg and Thompson (1973) have recently isolated the hormone sensitive lipase from adipose tissue and demonstrated that it can be activated by a protein kinase (Steinberg, Khoo and Mayer, 1974). The time course for the rise in cyclic AMP and for the activation of lipolysis in human adipose tissue is shown in Figure 3–10. Cyclic AMP rises to a peak concentration by 20 minutes but lipolysis, as measured by glycerol release, continues over a period of hours. The lipolytic effect of norepinephrine is greater than epinephrine, but an even greater effect is seen with isoproterenol. Activation of the hormone sensitive lipase by the addition of catecholamines can be blocked by beta adrenergic blocking drugs, of which propranolol is one example.

In addition to the beta receptor which mediated lipolysis (Östman et al., 1969), subcutaneous human adipose tissue also appears to have an alpha adrenergic receptor which inhibits lipolysis. Several laboratories have shown that the rise in glycerol and the release of free fatty acids after the addition of catecholamines to subcutaneous human adipose tissue can be greatly enhanced if the alpha receptors are blocked. Data showing this phenomenon are presented in Figure 3–11. When phentolamine, an alpha adrenergic blocking drug, is present, the stimulation of lipolysis is significantly enhanced (Burns and Langley, 1971; Östman and Efendic, 1970; Bray and Trygstad, 1972). When propranolol, the beta adrenergic blocking drug, is present, the stimulation of lipolysis with or without phentolamine is inhibited. Thus subcutaneous human adipose tissue appears to contain both beta

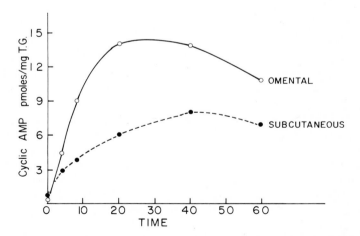

Figure 3–10. Cyclic-AMP formation in human adipose tissue. Pieces of omental and subcutaneous fat were exposed to isoproterenol for various time intervals and the concentrations of cyclic-AMP were then measured. The peak rise in cyclic-AMP was reached later in human fat than in fat from rats. (From Bray, G. A.: Metabolism of omental and subcutaneous adipose tissue from human subjects. Submitted for publication.)

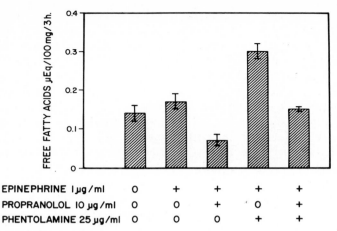

Figure 3–11.   Adrenergic receptors on human fat cells. When human fat was incubated with epinephrine there was a small increase in lipolysis. This effect was blocked by antagonizing the β-receptors with propranolol and enhanced by antagonizing the α-receptors with phentolamine. (Reprinted from Bray, G. A. and Trygstad, O.: Acta Endoc., 70:1–20, 1972, with permission.)

adrenergic receptors and alpha adrenergic receptors which stimulate and inhibit lipolysis respectively.

A number of peptide hormones will also stimulate lipolysis (Table 3–6). ACTH (adrenocorticotropin), which stimulates lipolysis in adipose tissue from rats (Jeanrenaud, 1968), has little or no effect on human fat cells (Mosinger et al., 1965; Galton and Bray, 1967a; Bray and Trygstad, 1972). In contract, thyrotropin (TSH) can stimulate lipolysis in adipocytes from rodents as well as man (Bray and Trygstad, 1972). Growth hormone in the presence of corticosteroids is lipolytic in adipose tissue from rats (Fain, Kovacev and Scow, 1965), but there is contradictory data about this effect in human adipose tissue. Most studies have been unable to detect a lipolytic effect of growth hormone in vitro (Mosinger et al., 1965; Burns et al., 1967; Bray and Trygstad, 1972), but a positive effect has been reported in one study when glucocorticoids were also present (Galton and Bray, 1967a). Glucagon is without effect or is only weakly lipolytic on human adipose tissue. Secretin is probably without effect (Bjorntorp and Östman, 1971).

In addition to the well characterized peptide hormones, there are a number of other lipid mobilizing factors such as beta lipotropin (Li et al., 1965), which is isolated from pig pituitary glands, peptides I and II (Astwood, Barrett and Friesen, 1961) (fraction H of Rudman), lipid mobilizing factor (LMF) (Trygstad and Foss, 1968), and the peptides reported by Burns et al. (1967). Peptides I and II are related to neurophysin. Beta lipotropin (β-LPH) from sheep and pig pituitaries has been purified chemically and contains 90 amino acids. Gamma lipotropin (γ-LPH) is a smaller peptide with 58 amino acids which correspond exactly with the segment 1-58 of β-LPH. Of great interest is that the sequence of β-MSH (melanocyte stimulating hormone) is contained in residues 41-58 of both beta and gamma LPH. The lipolytic properties of all three may thus be synonymous with the activity of β-MSH (Chretien, 1974). The lipid mobilizing factor (LMF) described by Trygstad is present in the pituitary of many species and is active in vitro at concentrations well below 1 μg/ml. Its chemical structure has not been elucidated, nor has the one reported by Burns et al. (1967). However, they appear to be different from other known pituitary peptides. Although there is little doubt that they are effective lipolytic agents, the importance of these pituitary peptide hormones in controlling lipolysis under physiologic conditions is unclear.

The antilipolytic effects of insulin may be as important as its effects on glucose oxidation. In low concentrations insulin will inhibit the lipolytic effect of catecholamine-induced lipolysis. This effect was originally attributed to an increased supply of glucose for re-esterification of fatty acids, until insulin was shown to be antilipolytic when glucose was absent from the incubation medium (Jungas, 1963). Butcher et al. (1966) showed that addition of insulin reduces the concentration of cyclic AMP in the adipocytes, and suggested that the antilipolytic effect of insulin might result from this inhibition of cyclic AMP. Recent data suggest that the antilipolytic effects of insulin are more complex and do not result simply from inhibition of cyclic AMP, but the exact mechanism is not known.

The antilipolytic effect of insulin is of major biological importance because lipolysis is inhibited at lower concentrations of insulin than are required for stimulation of glucose oxidation (Crofford et al. 1970). Insulin is antilipolytic in human adipose tissue (Bjorntorp, 1967; Gries et al., 1968), but whether there is a difference in its antilipolytic effects on large and small adipocytes is unclear.

The effects of obesity on lipolysis are manifested in two ways. First, glycerol release from large adipocytes is increased (see above). Second, the magnitude of the response of large adipocytes to lipid mobilizing agents is enhanced. Goldrick and McLoughlin (1969) and Gries, Berger and Oberdisse (1968) found greater lipolytic response of large adipocytes from obese subjects than smaller adipocytes from nonobese subjects. Similar findings have been obtained by comparing lipolysis in fat cells obtained from lean subjects before and after weight gain (Sims et al., 1973). On the other hand, when obese subjects were reduced in weight, the lipolytic effects of hormones on the smaller adipocytes were diminished compared with effects in the enlarged adipocytes obtained before weight loss (Knittle and Ginsberg-Fellner, 1972; Bray, Sims, Salans and Horton, unpublished observations). The relative carbohydrate and lipid content of the diet had no effect on lipolysis by large or small adipocytes from man (Sims et al., 1973) or experimental animals (Ogundipe and Bray, 1974). Thus lipolysis seems to be influenced largely by cell size and the concentration of lipolytic and antilipolytic hormones.

CHOLESTEROGENESIS IN FAT

Cholesterol is present in adipose tissue in small concentrations (Table 3–4) which range from 0.6 to 1.6 mg/g of weight (Farkas, Angel and Avigan, 1973). Most of the sterols in adipose tissue are cholesterol, and most of the cholesterol is present as free sterol (Angel, 1975). This cholesterol is metabolized slowly, with a half-life in the rat of 27 days. The total quantity of cholesterol as well as its turnover is increased in obesity (see Chapter 7). Table 3–9 shows the relative body weight and quantities of cholesterol metabolized by obese and nonobese subjects. On both an absolute and weight corrected basis, the obese patients metabolized more cholesterol (Miettenen, 1974). Angel et al. (1974) have recently explored the possibility that adipose tissue might be a significant tissue for cholesterol synthesis. In the genetically obese mouse (ob/ob) half or more of the total cholesterol can be synthesized in the adipose tissue if one can extrapolate from in vitro measurements to the entire organism. In man, on the other hand, the liver and gut appear to be the major sources of de novo cholesterol in obese people (Angel, Farkas and Bray, 1974). The adipose tissue in obese patients may account for 15 percent of the total cholesterol synthesis, with liver accounting for most of the rest.

In summary, in the obese patient, fat cells are almost invariably enlarged. In some and possibly all of the patients whose obesity begins in childhood, the total number of fat cells in the body may be increased. The mature fat cell with lipid droplet does not divide, and from all estimates lives for many years. Weight loss and weight gain in adult life are, therefore, accomplished by changing the size of these cells. Formation and breakdown of the triglyceride stored in fat cells is influenced by obesity. The large fat cell consumes more oxygen than the small fat cell. In addition, the breakdown of triglyceride is increased in these larger fat cells. The acceleration of glucose

TABLE 3–9.   *Cholesterol Metabolism in Obese and Nonobese Humans**

	RELATIVE WEIGHT	CHOLESTEROL mg/d	METABOLISM mg/kg
Nonobese	0.96	797	12.7
Obese	1.70	1601	14.9

*Adapted from Miettenen (1974).

metabolism in the presence of insulin is affected by the size of the fat cells. Large fat cells isolated by flotation are more responsive than small ones obtained from the same individual. However, if the small fat cells are obtained by weight reduction, they are more sensitive to the effects of insulin than are larger cells obtained before weight loss. At comparable sizes, however, there is no evidence that fat cells from spontaneously obese subjects are any different from fat cells of normal individuals.

REFERENCES

Angel, A., Farkas, J. and Bray, G. A. (Abs): Enhanced sterol synthesis in obesity: Role of liver, adipose tissue and ileum. Clinical Research, 22:459A, 1974.

Angel, A.: Cholesterol and obesity. In: Obesity in Perspective. Fogarty International Center Series on Preventive Medicine, Vol. II, Part II. (Bray, G. A. ed.) Washington, D.C., U.S. Government Printing Office. 1976.

Angel, A., Farkas, J., Rosenthal, J. and Smigura, F.: Cholesterol storage in adipose tissue. In: The Regulation of the Adipose Tissue Mass. (Vague, J. and Boyer, J. eds.), Excerpta Medica (Amsterdam), 1974, pp. 25–30.

Apfelbaum, M., Brigant, L. and Duret, F.: Relationship between the age of appearance of obesity and adipocyte diameter in 256 obese and 57 non-obese women. In: The Regulation of the Adipose Tissue Mass. (Vague, J. and Boyer, J. eds.), Excerpta Medica (Amsterdam), 1974, pp. 215–218.

Archer, J. A., Gorden, P. and Roth, J.: Defect in insulin binding to receptors in obese man. J. Clin. Invest., 55:166–174, 1975.

Astwood, E. B., Barrett, R. J. and Friesen, H.; Two metabolically active peptides from porcine pituitary glands. Proc. Nat. Acad. Sci., 47:1525–1530, 1961.

Baker, G. L.: Human adipose tissue composition and age. Am. J. Clin. Nutr., 22:829–835, 1969.

Bjorntorp, P.: The effect of insulin in vitro on human adipose tissue from normal and diabetic subjects. Acta Med. Scand., 181:389–402, 1967.

Bjorntorp, P.: Studies on adipose tissue from obese patients with or without diabetes mellitus. II. Basal and insulin-stimulated glucose metabolism. Acta Med. Scand., 179:229–234, 1966.

Bjorntorp, P.: Effects of age, sex, and clinical conditions on adipose tissue cellularity in man. Metabolism, 23:1091–1102, 1974.

Bjorntorp, P.: Effects of physical conditioning in obesity. In: Obesity in Perspective. Fogarty International Center Series on Preventive Medicine, Vol. II, Part II. (Bray, G. A. ed.) Washington, D.C., U.S. Government Printing Office. In press 1976.

Bjorntorp, P., Berchtold, P., Holm, J. and Larsson, B.: The glucose uptake of human adipose tissue in obesity. Europ. J. Clin. Invest., 1:480–485, 1971.

Bjorntorp, P., Hood, B. and Martinsson, A.: The sucrose space of human subcutaneous adipose tissue in obesity. Acta Med. Scand., 180:123–127, 1966a.

Bjorntorp, P. and Karlsson, M.: Triglyceride synthesis in human subcutaneous adipose tissue cells of different size. Europ. J. Clin. Invest., 1:112–117, 1970.

Bjorntorp, P., Karlsson, M. and Hovden, A.: Quantitative aspects of lipolysis and rees-terification in human adipose tissue in vitro. Acta Med. Scand., 185:89–97, 1969.

Bjorntorp, P., Martinsson, A. and Persson, B.: Composition of human subcutaneous adipose tissue in obesity. Acta Med. Scand., 180:117–127, 1966b.

Bjorntorp, P. and Östman, J.: Human adipose tissue dynamics and regulation. Adv. Metab. Disord., 5:277–327, 1971.

Bjorntorp, P. and Sjostrom, L.: Number and size of adipose tissue fat cells in relation to metabolism in human obesity. Metabolism, 20:703–713, 1971.

Bjurlf, P.: Atherosclerosis and body build with special reference to size and number of subcutaneous fat cells. Acta Med. Scand., Suppl. 349, 166:99, 1959.

Bjurlf, P.: Micromorphologic aspects of variation in human body fat. Symposia Swed. Nutr. Found. "Ocurrence, Causes and Prevention of Overnutrition" Edited by G. Blix, 1963.

Bray, G. A.: Effect of diet and triiodothyronine on the activity of sn-glycerol-3-phosphate dehydrogenase and on the metabolism of glucose and pyruvate by adipose tissue of obese patients. J. Clin. Invest., 48:1413–1422, 1969.

Bray, G. A.: Measurement of subcutaneous fat cells from obese patients. Ann. Intern. Med., 73:565–569, 1970a.

Bray, G. A.: Metabolic and regulatory obesity in rats and man. Horm. Metab. Res. (Suppl 2), 2:175–180, 1970b.

Bray, G. A.: Lipogenesis in human adipose tissue: Some effects of nibbling and gorging. J. Clin. Invest., 51:537–548, 1972.

Bray, G. A. and Trygstad, O.: Lipolysis in human adipose tissue: Comparison of human pituitary hormones with other lipolytic agents. Acta Endocr., 70:1–20, 1972.

Bray, G. A. and York, D. A.: Genetically transmitted obesity in rodents. Physiol. Rev., 51:598–646, 1971.

Brook, C. G. D.: Evidence for a sensitive period in adipose-cell replication in man. Lancet, 2:624–627, 1972.

Brook, C. G. D.. and Lloyd, J. K.: Adipose cell size and glucose tolerance in obese children and effects of diet. Arch. Dis. Child. 48:301–304, 1973.

Brook, C. G. D., Lloyd, J. K. and Wolf, O. H.: Relationship between age of onset of obesity and size and number of adipose cells. Br. Med. J., 2:25–27, 1972.

Burns, T. W., Hales, C. N. and Hartree, A. S.: Observations on the lipolytic activity of human serum and pituitary fractions in vitro. J. Endocrinol., 39:213–225, 1967.

Burns, T. W. and Langley, P. E.: Adrenergic receptors and cyclic AMP in the regulation of human adipose tissue lipolysis. Ann. N.Y. Acad. Sci., 185:115–128, 1971.

Butcher, R. W., Ho, R. J., Meng, H. C. and Sutherland, E. W.: Adenosine 3′,5′-monophosphate in biological materials. II. The measurement of adenosine 3′,5′-monophosphate in tissues and the role of the cyclic nucleotide in the lipolytic response of fat to epinephrine. J. Biol. Chem., 240:4515–4523, 1965.

Butcher, R. W., Sneyd, J. G. T., Park, C. R. and Sutherland, E. W.: Effect of insulin on adenosine 3′,5′-monophosphate in the rat epididymal fat pad. J. Biol. Chem. 241:1651–1653, 1966.

Chretien, M.: Obesity and pituitary lipolytic hormones. Triangle, 13:63–71, 1974.

Crofford, O. B., Minemura, T. and Kono, T.: Insulin-receptor interaction in isolated fat cells. Adv. Enzyme Regul., 8:219–238, 1970.

Davidson, M. B.: Effect of obesity on insulin sensitivity of human adipose tissue. Diabetes, 21:6–12, 1972.

Di Girolamo, M. and Mendlinger, S.: Role of fat cell size and number in enlargement of epididymal fat pads in three species. Am. J. Physiol., 221:859–864, 1971.

Di Girolamo, M., Mendlinger, S. and Fertig, J. W.: A simple method to determine fat cell size and number in four mammalian species. Am. J. Physiol., 221:850–858, 1971.

Efendic, S.: Catecholamines and metabolism of human adipose tissue. III. Comparison between the regulation of lipolysis in omental and subcutaneous adipose tissue. Acta Med. Scand., 187:477–483, 1970.

Engelhardt, V. A., Liebermeister, H., Reuter, Th. and Irmscher, K.: Analyse der Wasserräume und des Lipidgehalts des menschlichen subcutanen Fettgewebes. Z. Klin. Chem. Klin. u. Klin. Biochem. 9:356–360, 1971.

Fain, J. N., Kovacev, V. P and Scow, R. O.: Effect of growth hormone and dexamethasone on lipolysis and metabolism in isolated fat cells of the rat. J. Biol. Chem., 240:3522–3529, 1965.

Farkas, J., Angel, A. and Avigan, M. I.: Studies on the compartmentation of lipid in adipose cells. II. Cholesterol accumulation and distribution in adipose tissue components. J. Lipid Res., 14:344–356, 1973.

Faulhaber, J. D., Petruzzi, E. N., Eble, H. and Ditschuneit, H.: In vitro study of lipolysis in isolated human fat cells in relation to size: the effect of epinephrine-induced lipolysis (Ger.) Horm. Metab. Res., 1:80–86, 1969.

Galton, D. J.: An enzymatic defect in a group of obese patients. Brit. Med. J., 2:1498–1500, 1966.

Galton, D. J.: Lipogenesis in human adipose tissue. J. Lipid Res., 9:19–26, 1968.

Galton, D. J.: Regulation of supply of glycerol phosphate for lipogenesis in human adipose tissue. Clin. Sci., 36:505, 1969.

Galton, D. J.: The human adipose cell. London, Butterworth, 1971, p. 220.

Galton, D. J. and Bray, G. A.: Studies on lipolysis in human adipose cells. J. Clin. Invest., 46:621–629, 1967a.

Galton, D. J. and Bray, G. A.: Metabolism of α-glycerol phosphate in human adipose tissue in obesity. J. Clin. Endocr., 27:1573–1580, 1967b.

Galton, D. J. and Wilson, J. P. D.: The effects of starvation on lipogenesis in human adipose tissue. Europ. J. Clin. Invest., 1:94–98, 1970.

Galton, D. J. and Wilson, J. P. D.: The effect of starvation and diabetes on glycolytic enzymes in human adipose tissue. Clin. Sci., 41:545–553, 1971.

Galton, D. J., Wilson, J. P. D. and Kissebah, A. H.: The effect of adult diabetes on glucose utilization and esterification of palmitate by human adipose tissue. Europ. J. Clin. Invest., 1:399–404, 1971.

Gellhorn, A. and Marks, P. A.: The composition and biosynthesis of lipids in human adipose tissue. J. Clin. Invest., 40:925–932, 1961.

Gliemann, J.: Assay of insulin-like activity by the isolated fat cell method. I. Factors influencing the response to crystalline insulin. Diabetologica, 3:382–388, 1967.

Goldrick, R. B.; Effects of insulin on glucose metabolism in isolated human fat cells. J. Lipid Res., 8:581, 1967.

Goldrick, R. B., Ashley, B. C. E. and Lloyd, M. L.: Effects of prolonged incubation and cell concentration on lipogenesis from glucose in isolated human omental fat cells. J. Lipid Res., 10:253–259, 1969.

Goldrick, R. B. and Galton, D. J.: Fatty acid synthesis de novo in human adipose tissue. Clin. Sci. Mol. Med., 46:469–479, 1974.

Goldrick, R. B. and Hirsch, J.: Serial studies on the metabolism of human adipose tissue. II. Effects of caloric restriction and refeeding on lipogenesis and the uptake and release of free fatty acids in obese and non-obese individuals. J. Clin. Invest., 43:1793–1804, 1964.

Goldrick, R. B. and McLoughlin, G. M.: Lipolysis and lipogenesis from glucose in human fat cells of different sizes. Effects of insulin epinephrine and theophylline. J. Clin. Invest., 49:1213–1223, 1969.

Gordis, E.: The long-term stability of triglyceride molecules in adipose tissue. J. Clin. Invest., 44:1978–1985, 1965.

Gordon, E. S.: Metabolic aspects of obesity. Adv. Metab. Dis., 4:229–296, 1970.

Greenwood, M. R. C. and Hirsch, J.: Postnatal development of adipocyte cellularity in the normal rat. J. Lipid Res., 15:474–483, 1974.

Gries, F. A., Berger, M., Neumann, M., Preiss, H., Liebermeister, H., Hesse-Wortmann, C. and Jahnke, K.: Effects of norepinephrine, theophylline and dibutyryl cyclic AMP on in vitro lipolysis of human adipose tissue in obesity. Diabetologia, 8:75–83, 1972.

Gries, F. A., Berger, M. and Oberdisse, K.: Untersuchungen zum antilipolytischen Effekt des Insulins am menschlichen Fettgewebe in vitro. Diabetologia, 4:262–267, 1968.

Gries, F. A., Koschinsky, A. and Herberg, L.: Increased glucose metabolism and insulin sensitivity in large adipocytes. In: Regulation of Adipose Tissue Mass, (Vague, J. and Boyer, J. eds.). Excerpta Medica (Amsterdam) 1974, pp. 89–92.

Gries, F. A. and Steinke, J.: Comparative effects of insulin on adipose tissue segments and isolated fat cells of rat and man. J. Clin. Invest., 46:1413–1421, 1967.

Gries, F. A. and Steinke, J.: Insulin and human adipose tissue in vitro: a brief review. Metab. (Clin. Exp.), 16:693–696, 1967.

Guy-Grand, B. and Bigorie, B.: Lipoprotein lipase activity release by human adipose tissue in vitro: Effect of adipose cell size. In: The Regulation of the Adipose Tissue Mass. (Vague, J. and Boyer, J., eds.). Excerpta Medica (Amsterdam) 1974, pp. 52–57.

Heffernan, A. G. A.: Fatty acid composition of adipose tissue in normal and abnormal subjects. Am. J. Clin. Nutr., 15:5–10, 1964.

Hirsch, J.: Adipose cellularity in relation to human obesity. Adv. Intern. Med., 17:289–300, 1971.

Hirsch, J., Farquhar, J. W., Ahrens, E. H., Jr., Peterson, M. L. and Stoffel, W.: Studies of adipose tissue in man. A microtechnic for sampling and analysis. Am. J. Clin. Nutr., 8:499–511, 1960.

Hirsch, J. and Gallian, E.: Methods for the determination of adipose cell size in man and animals. J. Lipid Res., 9:110–119, 1968.

Hirsch, J. and Goldrick, R. B.: Serial studies on the metabolism of human adipose tissue. I. Lipogenesis and free fatty acid uptake and release in small aspirated samples of subcutaneous fat. J. Clin. Invest., 43:1776–1792, 1964.

Hirsch, J. and Han, P. W.: Cellularity of rat adipose tissue: Effects of growth, starvation, and obesity. J. Lipid Res., 10:77–90, 1969.

Hirsch, J., Knittle, J. L. and Salans, L. B.: Cell lipid content and cell number in obese and nonobese human adipose tissue. J. Clin. Invest., 45:1023, 1966. (abs)

Hirsch, J. and Knittle, J. L.: Cellularity of obese and nonobese human adipose tissue. Fed. Proc., 29:1516–1521, 1970.

Hollenberg, C. H.: The origin and glyceride distribution of fatty acids in rat adipose tissue. J. Clin. Invest., 45:205–216, 1966.

Hollenberg, C. H. and Angel, A.: Adipose tissue metabolism and obesity. Modern Treatment, 4:1083–1095, 1967.

Hollenberg, C. H., Vost, A., and Patten, R. L.: Regulation of adipose mass: Control of fat cell development and lipid content. Recent Prog. Horm. Res., 26:463–503, 1970.

Howard, C. F., Jr. and Lowenstein, J. M.: The effect of glycerol 3-phosphate on fatty acid synthesis. J. Biol. Chem., 240:1470–1475, 1965.

Jacob, J. and Grimmer, G.: Structure and amount of positional isomers of monounsaturated fatty acids in human depot fat. J. Lipid Res., 9:730–732, 1968.

Jeanrenaud, B.: Adipose tissue dynamics and regulation, revisited. Ergebn. Physiol. 60:57–140, 1968.

Jeanrenaud, B. and Hepp, D. (eds.): Adipose tissue: Regulation and metabolic functions. Stuttgart, Georg Thieme Verlag, New York, Academic Press, 1970.

Johnson, P. R. and Hirsch, J.: Cellularity of adipose depots in six strains of genetically obese mice. J. Lipid Res., 13:2–11, 1972.

Johnson, P. R., Zucker, L. M., Cruce, J. A. F. and Hirsch, J.: Cellularity of adipose depots in the genetically obese Zucker rat. J. Lipid Res., 12:706–714, 1971.

Johnson, P. R., Stern, J. S., Greenwood, M. R. C., Zucker, L. M. and Hirsch, J.: Effect of early nutrition on adipose cellularity and pancreatic insulin release in the Zucker rat. J. Clin. Nutr., 103:738–743, 1973.

Jungas, R. and Ball, E. G.: Studies on the metabolism of adipose tissue. The effects of insulin and epinephrine in free fatty acid and glycerol production in the presence and absence of glucose. Biochemistry, 2:383–388, 1963.

Kahlenberg, A. and Kalant, N.: The effect of insulin on human adipose tissue. Canad. J. Biochem., 42:1623–1635, 1964.

Kahn, C. R., Soll, A. H., Neville, D. M., Goldfine, J. D., Archer, J. A., Gorden, P. and Roth, J.: The insulin receptor in obesity and other states of altered insulin sensitivity. In: Obesity in Perspective. Fogarty International Center Series on Preventive Medicine, Vol. II, Part II. (Bray, G. A. ed.) Washington, D.C., U.S. Government Printing Office. 1976.

Khoo, J. C., Steinberg, D. and Thompson, B. et al.: Hormonal regulation of adipocyte enzymes. The effects of epinephrine and insulin on the control of lipase, phosphorylase kinase, phosphorylase and glycogen synthase. J. Biol. Chem., 248:3823–3830, 1973.

Knittle, J. L.: Obesity in childhood: A problem in adipose tissue cellular development. J. Pediatr., 81:1048–1059, 1972a.

Knittle, J. L.: Maternal diet as a factor in adipose tissue cellularity and metabolism in the young rat. J. Nutr., 102:427–434, 1972b.

Knittle, J. L. and Ginsberg-Fellner, F.: Effect of weight reduction on in vitro adipose tissue lipolysis and cellularity in obese adolescents and adults. Diabetes, 21:754–761, 1972.

Knittle, J. L. and Hirsch, J.: Effect of early nutrition on the development of rat epididymal fat pads: Cellularity and metabolism. J. Clin. Invest., 47:2091–2098, 1968.

Lemonnier, D. and Alexiu, A.: Nutritional, genetic and hormonal aspects of adipose tissue cellularity. In: The Regulation of Adipose Tissue Mass. (Vague, J. and Boyer, J. eds.), Excerpta Medica (Amsterdam), 1974, pp. 158–173.

Lemonnier, D.: Effect of age, sex, and site on the cellularity of the adipose tissue in mice and rats rendered obese by a high-fat diet. J. Clin. Invest., 51:2907–2915, 1972.

Leveille, G. A.: Adipose tissue metabolism: Influence of periodicity of eating and diet composition. Fed. Proc., 29:1294–1301, 1970.

Li, C. H., Barnafi, L., Chrétien, M. and Chung, D.: Isolation and amino acid sequence of β-LPH from sheep pituitary glands. Nature (Lond.), 208:1093–1094, 1965.

Margolis, S. and Vaughan, M.: α-Glycerophosphate synthesis and breakdown in homogenates of adipose tissue. J. Biol. Chem., 237:44–48, 1962.

Martinsson, A.: On the composition of human adipose tissue. Acta Med. Scand., 182:795–803, 1967.

Martinsson, A.: Release of glycerol and free fatty acids in human adipose tissue in vitro. Effect of the specimen size. Acta Med. Scand., 182:787–793, 1967.

Miettenen, T. A.: Current view on cholesterol metabolism. Horm. Metab. Res., Suppl. #4, 1974, pp. 37–44.

Mosinger, B., Kuhn, E. and Kujalova, V.; Action of adipokinetic hormones on human adipose tissue in vitro. J. Lab. Clin. Med., 66:380–389, 1965.

Napolitano, L.: The differentiation of white adipose cells. An electron microscope study. J. Cell Biol., 18:663–679, 1963.

Ogundipe, O. and Bray, G. A.: The influence of diet and fat cell size on glucose metabolism, lipogenesis, and lipolysis in the rat. Horm. Metab. Res., 6:351–356, 1974.

Olefsky, J. M., Jen, P. and Reaven, G. M. et al.: Insulin binding to isolated human adipocytes. Diabetes, 23:565–571, 1974.

Oscai, L. B., Spirakis, C. N., Wolff, C. A., and Beck, R. J.: Effects of exercise and of food restriction on adipose tissue cellularity. J. Lipid Res. 13:588–592, 1972.

Östman, J., Backman, L. and Hallberg, D.: Cell size and lipolysis by human subcutaneous adipose tissue. Acta Med. Scand., 193:469–475, 1973.

Östman, J. and Efendić, S.: Catecholamines and metabolism of human adipose tissue. II. Effect of Isopropylnoradrenaline and adrenergic blocking agents on lipolysis in human omental adipose tissue in vitro. Acta Med. Scand., 187:471–476, 1970.

Östman, J., Efendić, S. and Arner, P.: Catecholamines and metabolism of human adipose tissue. I. Comparison between in vitro effects of noradrenaline, adrenaline and theophylline on lipolysis in omental adipose tissue. Acta Med. Scand., 186:241–246, 1969.

Palmer, W. K. and Tipton, C. M.: Effect of training on adipocyte glucose metabolism and insulin responsiveness. Fed. Proc., 33:1964–1968, 1974.

Persson, B.: Lipoprotein lipase activity of human adipose tissue in different types of hyperlipidemia. Acta Med. Scand., 193:447–456, 1973.

Rizack, M. A.: Activation of an epinephrine-sensitive lipolytic activity from adipose tissue by adenosine 3',5'-phosphate. J. Biol. Chem., 239:392–395, 1964.

Salans, L. B., Bray, G. A., Cushman, S. W., Danforth, E., Jr., Glennon, J. A., Horton, E. S. and Sims, E. A. H.: Glucose metabolism and the response to insulin by human adipose tissue in spontaneous and experimental obesity. Effects of dietary composition and adipose cell size. J. Clin. Invest., 53:848–856, 1974.

Salans, L. B., Cushman, S. W. and Weissman, R. E.: Studies of human adipose cell size and number in non-obese and obese patients. J. Clin. Invest., 52:929–941, 1973.

Salans, L. B. and Dougherty, J. W.: The effect of insulin upon glucose metabolism by adipose cells of different size. Influence of cell lipid and protein content, age and nutritional state. J. Clin. Invest., 50:1399–1410, 1971.

Salans, L. B., Horton, E. S. and Sims, E. A. H.: Experimental obesity in man: Cellular character of the adipose tissue. J. Clin. Invest., 50:1005–1011, 1971.

Salans, L. B., Knittle, J. L. and Hirsch, J.: The role of adipose cell size and adipose tissue insulin sensitivity in the carbohydrate intolerance of human obesity. J. Clin. Invest., 47:153–165, 1968.

Salans, L. B., Zarnowski, M. J. and Segal, R.: Effect of insulin upon the cellular character of rat adipose tissue. J. Lipid Res., 13:616–623, 1972.

Shrago, E., Glennon, J. A. and Gordon, E. S.: Studies on enzyme concentration and adaptation in human liver and adipose tissue. J. Clin. Endocrinol. Metab., 27:679–685, 1967.

Shrago, E., Glennon, J. A. and Gordon, E. S.: Comparative aspects of lipogenesis in mammalian tissues. Metabolism, 20:54–62, 1971.

Shrago, E., Spennetta, T. and Gordon, E.: Fatty acid synthesis in human adipose tissue. J. Biol. Chem., 244:2761–2766, 1969.

Sims, E. A. H., Danforth, E., Jr., Horton, E. S., Bray, G. A., Glennon, J. and Salans, L. B.: Endocrine and metabolic effects of experimental obesity in man. Rec. Prog. Horm. Res., 29:457–487, 1973.

Sjostrom, L.: Adult human adipose tissue cellularity and metabolism with special reference to obesity and fatty acid synthesis de novo. Acta Med. Scand. (Suppl. No. 544), pp. 1–52, 1972.

Sjostrom, L., Bjorntorp, P. and Vrana, J.: Microscopic fat cell size measurements on frozen-cut adipose tissue in comparison with automatic determinations of osmium-fixed fat cells. J. Lipid Res., 12:521–530, 1971.

Sjostrom, L., Bjorntorp, P. and Mansson, J. E.: An optimal assay system for subcellular determination of de novo fatty acid synthesis in human adipose tissue. Scand. J. Clin. Lab. Invest., 31:191–204, 1973.

Sjostrom, L., Smith, U., Krotkiewski, M. and Bjorntorp, P.: Cellularity in different regions of adipose tissue in young men and women. Metabolism. In press. 1975.

Slavin, B. G.: The cytophysiology of mammalian adipose cells. Int. Rev. Cytol., 33:297–334, 1972.

Smith, U.: Studies of human adipose tissue in culture. I. Incorporation of glucose and release of glycerol. Anat. Rec., 172:597–602, 1972.

Smith, U., Sjostrom, L. and Bjorntorp, P.: A comparison of two methods for determining adipose cell size. J. Lipid Res., 13:822–824, 1972.

Steinberg, D., Khoo, J. C. and Mayer, S. E.: Mechanisms regulating the mobilization of free fatty acids from human and rat adipose tissue. In: Regulation of Adipose Tissue Mass. (Vague, J. and Boyer, J., eds.), Excerpta Medica, (Amsterdam), 1974, pp. 61–68.

Stern, J. S. and Greenwood, M. R.: A review of development of adipose cellularity in man and animals. Fed. Proc., 33:1952–1955, 1974.

Therriault, D. G. and Mellin, D. B.: Cellularity of adipose tissue in cold-exposed rats and the calorigenic effect of norepinephrine. Lipids, 6:486–491, 1971.

Trygstad, O. and Foss, I.: The lipid mobilizing effect of some pituitary gland preparations. IV Subdivision of a human growth hormone preparation into a somatotrophic and adipokinetic-hyperglycaemic agent. Acta Endocrinol., 58:295–317, 1968.

Vague, J. and Boyer, J. (eds.). The Regulation of the Adipose Tissue Mass. Proceedings of the IV International Meeting of Endocrinology, Marseilles, July 10–12, 1973. Excerpta Medica, (Amsterdam), 1974.

Vaughan, M.: The production and release of glycerol by adipose tissue incubated in vitro. J. Biol. Chem., 237:3354–3358, 1962.

Widdowson, E. M. and McCance, R. A.: Some effects of accelerating growth I. General somatic development. Proc. Roy. Soc. [Biol.] 152:188–206, 1960.

Widdowson, E. M. and Shaw, W. T.: Full and empty fat cells. Lancet, 2:905, 1973.

Wilson, J. P. D., Gutman, R. and Galton, D. J.: Comparison of free fatty acid and glyceride-fatty acid uptake by human adipose tissue. Metabolism, 22:913–921, 1973.

Zinder, O. and Bray, G. A.: Lipoprotein lipase activity in human adipose tissue in obesity. In: Obesity in Perspective. Fogarty International Center Series on Preventive Medicine, Vol. II, Part II. (Bray, G. A. ed.) Washington, D.C., U.S. Government Printing Office. 1976.

Zinder, O., Eisenberg, E. and Shapiro, B.: Compartmentation of glycerides in adipose tissue cells. The mechanism of free fatty acid release. J. Biol. Chem., 248:7673–7676, 1973.

Zinder, O. and Shapiro, B.: Effect of cell size on epinephrine- and ACTH-induced fatty acid release from isolated fat cells. J. Lipid Res., 12:91–95, 1971.

CHAPTER 4

ENERGY EXPENDITURE

The energy required by the body for all metabolic processes can be obtained from ingested food or from the energy stored as fat, glycogen or protein. The energy content of food, as well as that stored in fat, glycogen and protein, is generally expressed in terms of available calories. A calorie is that unit of energy required to heat water by a specified amount.* The proportion of calories stored as protein, carbohydrate and fat in humans was shown in Table 3–1. Fat is obviously the major source of stored energy. In obese humans this depot can become gigantic, holding in reserve enough energy to meet total body energy requirements for over one year! (See section on starvation in Chapter 8.)

The relationship of energy produced by metabolic processes in the body to energy formed by the combustion of foodstuffs or other materials outside the body has been studied by scientists since the days of Lavoisier. In his classic experiments, Lavoisier demonstrated that the quantity of heat produced by animals during metabolism of stored energy (i.e., fat) is the same as the quantity of heat produced by oxidizing the same amount of fat or other source of energy outside of the body. This concept has been explored repeatedly and is now an accepted fact.

Carbohydrates produce approximately four calories for every gram oxidized to carbon dioxide and water, and fats yield approximately 9.1 calories per gram of triglyceride oxidized completely to CO_2 and water. Proteins are more complicated to analyze because metabolism results in the formation of urea plus carbon dioxide and water rather than simply carbon dioxide and water. If one accounts for

---

*The calorie is the quantity of heat required to raise 1 gram of water from 15 to 16° C.

129

the energy remaining in urea, each gram of protein metabolized in the body yields approximately four calories.

Southgate and Durnin (1970) have re-evaluated these factors in human subjects by careful metabolic studies. The average number of kCal produced by metabolism of protein, carbohydrate and fat is shown in Table 4–1. These calories are utilized not only to maintain body temperature but also to perform metabolic and physical work. Biochemists have shown that for most biologic oxidations the energy of foodstuffs is made available through formation of high energy bonds, usually as adenosine triphosphate (ATP). Of the total calories available from the oxidation of glucose, only about 60 percent are stored in phosphate bonds of ATP during metabolism. The remaining third is lost directly as heat and is not available for metabolic needs.

METHODS FOR MEASURING ENERGY EXPENDITURE

Direct Calorimetry

Energy expenditure in man can be measured in two ways. Total heat loss from the body can be assessed by direct calorimetry. This technique has been applied to animal studies (Blaxter, 1971, 1975; Blaxter et al., 1972) and, in a few instances, to human studies (Atwater and Benedict, 1899, 1905). Techniques of direct calorimetry require placing an animal (or human) in a chamber which will measure all of the heat released in the form of thermal energy, radiant energy and energy from vaporization of water from the lungs, as well as the uptake of oxygen and the production of carbon dioxide. This technique has been used principally to validate the measurements of energy expenditure as assessed by indirect methods.

Indirect Methods

One indirect method measures oxygen consumption, carbon dioxide production and nitrogen excretion. If carbohydrate and fat are

TABLE 4–1.   *Caloric Value of Ingested Food Stuffs**

	KCAL	KJ
Protein	3.65 to 3.96	15.3 to 16.6
Fat	8.70 to 9.05	36.4 to 37.9
Carbohydrate	3.89 to 4.05	16.3 to 16.9

*Adapted from Southgate and Durnin: Brit. J. Nutr., 24:517–535, 1970, with permission. The values for each food stuff are the range of mean values for both young and old men and women.

the only substrates being oxidized, the measurement of oxygen uptake and carbon dioxide production is sufficient to quantify energy expenditure; however, when protein is oxidized, a certain fraction of the calories remain stored in urea which is excreted in the urine. Thus for a complete assessment of metabolic rate, we need to measure carbon dioxide production, oxygen uptake, and nitrogen excretion over the same period of time in order to correct for the nitrogenous component of substrate oxidation. This calorimetric technique has proven useful for the study of energy expenditure in normal and abnormal states. (For a more detailed discussion of the methodology of indirect calorimetry, the reader is referred to Consolazio et al., 1963; Astrand and Rodahl, 1970; Durnin and Brockaway, 1959.)

A second indirect approach to estimate energy expenditure has been investigated by Newburgh, who noted a close correlation between total energy expended (as measured by oxygen consumption) and the heat required to vaporize water from the lungs (Johnston and Newburgh, 1942). About 25 percent of the energy expenditure was accounted for this way. This technique, however, has not been utilized widely because it requires special equipment, but it is a potentially valuable technique for studying children (Krieger, 1966).

Measurement of heart rate is yet another indirect approach to estimating energy expenditure. The correlation of heart rate with oxygen uptake is satisfactory however only under rigidly controlled conditions, so the measurements obtained with this method may not be an accurate measure of total energy expenditure (Booyens and Hervey, 1960; Bradfield, 1971; Mayfield, 1971).

BASAL METABOLISM

The energy in ATP (adenosine triphosphate) is used for all of the body's needs including metabolism at rest and during physical activity. Basal metabolism (defined as the sum total of the minimal activity of all tissues of the body under steady-state conditions) provides energy for protein synthesis, brain metabolism, maintenance of ionic balance across cells, and the contraction of the myocardium, gastrointestinal, and other continuously functioning muscle groups. Current estimates suggest that over half of the total basal metabolism is involved in maintenance of ionic equilibrium between intracellular and extracellular components, and for the tubular mechanism controlling reabsorption of ions (Na^+, K^+ Cl^-, HCO_3^-). Careful studies of basal energy expenditure have indicated that it is influenced by a number of factors including body weight, age, sex, climate, hormones and drugs.

Body Weight

Basal energy expenditure increases with body weight. This is most easily seen when comparing energy needs of mammals of different sizes (Table 4–2). In absolute terms the larger animals require more oxygen. However, when expressed in terms of weight, the oxygen consumption rises as body weight falls. When oxygen consumption is expressed in relation to surface area,* the amount of oxygen used by all 5 species of animals was similar.

Sex

When compared by body weight or by surface area, men have a higher BMR than women. DuBois (1936) reviewed the literature and found differences of 5 to 7 percent at all ages over two years of age. However, there was no sex difference in the first two years of life. Boothby et al. (1936) noted a 6 percent difference at 5 years of age, 10 percent in later childhood and early adult life, followed by a fall to 6 percent which persisted through old age. Behnke (1953), on the other hand, compared men and women on the basis of lean body mass and found no significant difference. He concluded that the differences observed by others could be explained by the different proportion of body fat between men and women. Banerjee and Bhattacharjee (1967), however, measured the interrelations of the BMR and body composition in adult male and female medical students and found values of 33.9 cal/m²/hr for males and 28.9 cal/m²/hr for females. The best correlation with BMR was the fat free body and the worst correlation was with body surface area.

---

*Surface area is usually calculated from the equations of DuBois and DuBois. S.A. = .007184 (Ht.)$^{0.725}$ × (Wt.)$^{0.425}$ (Wt. in kg and Ht. in meters) Alternatively a nomogram may be used (Boothby et al. 1936; see Fig. 8–4, Chapter 8.) For animals it is usually calculated as S.A. = 70 × (Wt.)$^{0.75}$

TABLE 4–2. *Comparison of Energy Expenditure in Relation to Body Weight**

| ANIMAL | WEIGHT KG | ENERGY EXPENDITURE | | |
		Total	per Unit Wt kcal/kg	per Unit Area kcal/m²
Horse	441	4990	11.3	948
Man	64.3	2060	32.1	1042
Dog	15.2	784	51.5	1039
Rabbit	2.3	173	75.1	776
Mouse	0.018	3.8	212	1188

*Adapted from Lusk: The Elements of the Science of Nutrition, 4th ed., 1928, p. 123, with permission.

Age

Age also has an important influence on caloric requirements (Fig. 4–1). The caloric needs of rapidly growing children and adolescents are higher than those of adults who are no longer experiencing an active increase in muscle mass (see Table 2–1). At birth caloric requirements are approximately 120 kCal/kg, but they decline by 20 percent by the end of the first year to approximately 100 kCal/kg. These values over the next ten years remain at about 80 kCal/kg until adolescence, when they decline to 50 kCal/kg for males and 35 kCal/kg for females (Recommended Dietary Allowances, 1974).

When corrected for the rising surface area during growth, energy requirements decline throughout life. The fall is most rapid during childhood. Between age 18 and age 20 the rate of decline levels off. In adult life the drop is between 2 and 5 percent per decade (Altman and Dittmer, 1968). For the reference man who is 22 years old and weighs 67 kg. the caloric requirements are set at 3000 kCal or approximately 45 kCal/kg. For the reference female who is 22 years old and weighs 58 kg. the requirements are 2000 kCal or 36 kCal/kg (Recommended Dietary Allowances, 1974). These caloric requirements decline by approximately 5 percent per decade between age 20 and age 35 and by 2 to 3 percent per decade for the next 20 years.

DuBois (1936) noted a great variation in BMR in old people and thought this might be dependent on the degree of senility. In general,

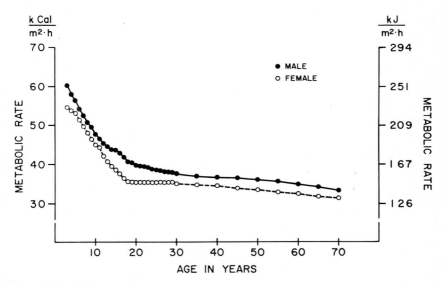

Figure 4–1. Relation of oxygen consumption to age. Males (●) have a significantly higher metabolic rate at all ages than females (○). The decline in metabolism is rapid until age 20, after which the rate of decline slows. (Adapted from Dubois, Altman and Ditmer, eds.: Metabolism. Federation of American Societies of Experimental Biology, Bethesda, Maryland, 1971.)

older people are less active and require less food. Durnin et al. (1961 a,b) found that energy intake and expenditure in 17 females aged 60 to 69 was 1900 cal/day. Matson and Hitchcock (1934) studied eight elderly females ages 77 to 106 and 14 males ages 74 to 92, and found heat productions of 43.6 cal/hr and 50.4 cal/hr respectively. They noted that these values were below the standards of Aub and DuBois (1917). Magnus-Levy (1942) determined his own basal O_2 consumption at age 26 to be 231 ml/min. By age 76 it had fallen to 176 ml/min.

Keys et al. (1973) suggest that studies of BMR with age are inaccurate because they are cross sectional evaluations of the population; such studies do not reflect the true relationship of BMR in an individual over time because of changing diet and body fat content. They studied two groups of men. One group, initially aged 44 to 56, was studied repeatedly over a period of 22 years. In this group body weight increased by an average of only 1 kg and there was no significant change in oxygen consumption. In the second group, initially aged 18 to 26, the BMR fell by 3 percent over 19 years. Weight gain in this group averaged 10.6 kg so that BMR/kg decreased by 9 percent. Keys concluded that there is a reduction in basal metabolism due to aging of only 1 to 2 percent per decade.

Climate and temperature

Climate also influences basal energy needs. As the ambient temperature increases, less heat is needed to maintain body temperature. For each 1° C rise in body temperature, the metabolic rate increases 12 percent (Halmaggi et al., 1974). There is a "thermally neutral zone" from about 27 to 34.7° C where BMR is unaffected by temperature. A lower ambient temperature initiates shivering, which increases metabolic rate, while higher ambient temperatures may increase the body temperature sufficiently to increase the metabolic rate (DuBois, 1936).

Hormones and Drugs

The role of hormones in the control of energy metabolism has been studied intensively. Thyroid hormone is the principal hormone which regulates basal metabolism. Studies at the turn of the century showed that excess thyroid hormone increases body oxygen consumption. It has also been demonstrated that a deficiency of thyroid hormone is accompanied by a reduction of metabolic rate (Pitt-Rivers and Tata, 1959). The mechanism for this effect is not completely understood. One currently attractive hypothesis suggests that thyroid hormone increases the rate of ion transport across cell membranes (Edelman and Ismail-Beigi, 1974). As noted above, ion transport across cell membranes accounts for over half of the energy needs for basal metabolism, so that small changes in the quantity of ionic transport required to maintain ionic equilibrium might be reflected in a significant change of metabolic rate.

At least two other hormones are also calorigenic; that is, they increase metabolic rate. These are catecholamines, especially epinephrine, and growth hormone. Injection of epinephrine produces a significant but short lived increase in metabolic rate (Himms-Hagen, 1967). This rise in metabolic rate with emotional arousal may also be due to the release of epinephrine (Melville and Mezey, 1959). This effect of epinephrine is influenced by the presence and activity of thyroid hormone (Swanson, 1957). In hypothyroidism when thyroid hormone is deficient there is little calorigenic response to epinephrine. With hyperthyroidism, on the other hand, there is an exaggerated response to epinephrine. The underlying mechanism for this interaction of thyroid hormone and catecholamine is unknown.

Growth hormone is also calorigenic. It produces a small but significant effect on basal metabolism in man and animals (Henneman et al., 1960; Bray, 1969a; Evans et al., 1958). The response in obese patients treated with 5 mg/day of human growth hormone is shown in Figure 4–2. All patients showed an increase that was evident after only a few days. This metabolic effect is demonstrable in the absence of thyroid hormone. It may well result from the rise in free fatty acids observable during injections of growth hormone.

At least two drugs are calorigenic. Dinitrophenol uncouples oxidative phosphorylation and was given a brief trial in the treatment

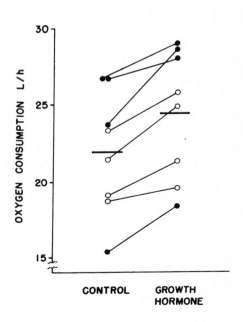

Figure 4–2. Effect of growth hormone on oxygen consumption. Eight obese patients were treated for 8 days with 5 mg/day of human growth hormone. (From Bray, G. A.: J. Clin. Endocrinol. Metab., 29:119–122, 1969a, reprinted with permission.)

of obese patients (see Chapter 9). Salicylates in high doses also un-couple oxidative phosphorylation and raise oxygen consumption. This occurs in both normal and obese subjects (Bray, unpublished observa-tions).

Thermic Effects

The thermic effect of food, also called the "specific dynamic ac-tion," is the caloric expenditure occurring after food ingestion. This phenomenon has been the subject of extensive investigation over the past 50 years or more, but its fundamental basis is not yet fully under-stood (Lusk, 1928; Garrow and Hawes, 1972). There is a rise in caloric expenditure shortly after the ingestion of food, representing 10 per-cent or more of the total calories consumed. Protein may have more effect on caloric expenditure (thermic effect) than carbohydrate or fat (Lusk, 1931), but this has been disputed (Garrow and Hawes, 1972). Buskirk et al. (1957) examined the thermic effects of food and exercise on resting metabolism. Oxygen consumption which was used to measure resting metabolism rose by 12 to 15 percent during the day whether food was ingested or not. The rise after eating was 20 to 22 percent. From these and other studies we can estimate that approxi-mately 10 percent of the ingested calories in food are dissipated as heat and are not available for storage or for conversion into ATP.

Exercise performed after eating a meal results in an additional increment of energy expended as heat when compared to a compara-ble quantity of exercise performed without eating. This phenomenon has been demonstrated in several laboratories (Miller and Mumford, 1966, 1973; Miller et al., 1967; Bradfield et al., 1968; Bray et al., 1974; Whipp et al., 1973). In our studies six normal weight subjects exer-cised by pedaling a stationary cycle adapted to provide variable amounts of resistance to turning the wheel. The actual work done was quantified by measuring oxygen utilization. On one day the cycling was done without breakfast and on another day it was done after a 1000 kCal or 3000 kCal breakfast. In each instance the major energy requirement was related to the quantity of work done to turn the wheel. Exercise after breakfast was associated with a higher oxygen uptake (i.e., higher energy utilization) than on the day with no break-fast. The larger breakfast had no greater effect than the smaller one. Correcting for the thermic effect (SDA) of the breakfast itself did not alter the results.

We concluded that food intake increases by 5 to 10 percent the energy needed for muscular contraction (Bray, Whipp and Koyal, 1974). Although the biochemical explanation is not clear, exercise increases the dissipation of calories as heat at approximately the same rate following a meal as the thermic effect of the food itself, i.e., ap-proximately 10 percent. These two phenomena, the thermic effect of food and the additional thermic effect of exercise after a meal, represent two forms of energy expenditure which are not associated with useful biochemical or physical work.

Physical Activity

Physical activity represents the other major component of total energy expenditure and has been intensively studied by physiologists (Passmore and Durnin, 1955; Astrand and Rodahl, 1970). The energy for physical work is provided by coupling the energy stored in the phosphate bonds of ATP with the contraction process in muscle. The efficiency with which the energy in metabolic substrates is converted to mechanical work by muscle varies between 22 and 30 percent. This difference depends primarily on the method used for this calculation. On a bicycle in the laboratory, the work performed to move the flywheel can be quantitatively related to the oxygen uptake which measures the total energy requirement (Whipp, 1975). If the work required to move the legs is not taken into account, the efficiency is 22 percent. If the energy needed to move the legs is considered, efficiency rises to 30 percent. Thus slightly less than one third of total ingested calories is available for performance of physical work.

The energy required for physical work depends on the amount of physical work being performed. Energy expenditure is increased with body weight. Heavier people require more energy to move than lean ones. (Consolazio and Johnson, 1971). Energy expenditure is also related to the duration and severity of the work. Tables 4–3 and 4–4 show the way in which caloric expenditure is divided between various levels of energy expenditure for men and women. The energy required to walk on a treadmill at 3 miles per hour (5 km/hr) increases in direct proportion to the steepness or grade. Thus it requires more energy to walk up a hill than to walk on a flat surface.

In addition, increasing the rate of walking on any fixed grade

TABLE 4–3. *Distribution of Energy Expenditure Over 24 Hours for a 65 kg Male and a 55 kg Female**

Type of Activity	Duration (Hours)	Low M	Low F	Moderate M	Moderate F	High M	High F
Sleeping	8	500	420	500	420	500	420
Work	8	1100	800	1400	1000	1900	1400
Other	8	1100	780	1100	780	1100	780
Total	24	2700	2000	3000	2200	3500	2600
Range		2300-3100	1800-2200	2600-3400	2000-2400	3100-3900	2400-2700
kcal/kg		42	36	46	40	54	47

To convert kcal to MJ multiply by 4.2×10^{-3}
*Adapted from WHO (1973).

TABLE 4-4.   *Energy Cost of Daily Activities**

TYPE OF ACTIVITY	DURATION (HOURS)	ENERGY EXPENDITURE 70 kg Man kcal/min	kcal	58 kg Woman kcal/min	kcal
Sleeping	8	1.1	540	1.0	480
Sitting	6	1.5	540	1.1	400
Standing	6	2.5	900	1.5	540
Walking	2	3.0	360	2.5	300
Other	2	4.5	540	3.0	360
Total	24	—	2880	—	2080

*Recommended Dietary Allowances (1974).

increases the energy expenditure. Walking 2 km at a rate of 8 km/hr (i.e., walking for 15 minutes) requires more calories than walking 2 km at a rate of 4 km/hr (Fig. 4–3). Loss of energy by friction between muscles provides the best explanation for the disproportionate increase in the energy requirement with walking speed increase. When muscles move more rapidly, the loss of energy as heat may be greater than if they move slowly. Givoni and Goldman (1971) have developed

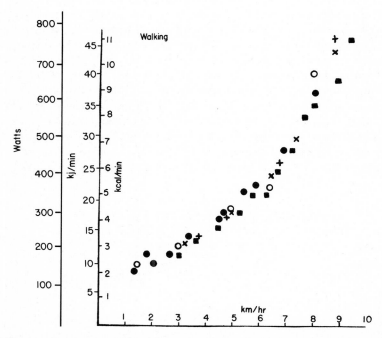

Figure 4–3.   Energy expended walking uphill at different speeds. Note the disproportionate increase in energy expended as the rate of walking increases. (kcal=kilocalories; kj=kilojoules) (From Passmore and Durnin: Physiol. Rev., 35:801–840, 1955, reprinted with permission.)

equations for calculating energy cost in terms of the speed or velocity (V) of walking and the grade (percent). At the lower grades (0 to 10 percent) the calorie requirement for walking faster rises progressively. At very steep grades, however, the energy requirement is nearly linear.

It has been a frequent clinical observation that some individuals require more calories than others for maintenance of a similar body weight. Some people claim to eat anything they like without gaining weight, while others complain that everything they eat "turns to fat." To examine this critically, Rose and Williams (1961) studied 10 male medical students and 2 physicians of the same weight and age who claimed to eat greatly different quantities of food. Those who consumed large quantities of food ate almost double the number of calories of those consuming smaller amounts of food.

Several pairs with different intakes were examined by measuring basal metabolic rate and energy expenditure while performing various levels of physical activity on a bicycle and on a treadmill. The energy expended in spontaneous self-paced tasks, such as climbing stairs and walking a given distance, was also quantified. Basal metabolic requirements and the energy expenditure at constant work rates on a bicycle or treadmill did not differ significantly between the two groups of subjects. In addition, there was no measurable difference in calorie expenditure while sitting or standing. The thermic effect of a meal (SDA) was also the same in both large and small eaters. However, the rate at which subjects performed spontaneous tasks differed significantly. The individuals with the high calorie intake walked at 3.35 mph (5.39 km/h) compared to 2.92 mph (4.69 km/h) for the small eaters (p <.01). Basal pulse rates and the rise in pulse after eating were also significantly greater in the big eaters. Body temperature and total amounts of activity, however, did not differ between the two groups. The higher natural rates of walking in the larger eaters may be an index to general restlessness and higher dissipation of energy.

ENERGY BALANCE IN OBESITY

Basal Metabolism

A reduction in basal metabolic expenditure could provide the imbalance between energy intake and energy expenditure which produces obesity (Strang and Evans, 1928; Newburgh and Johnston, 1930; Dabney, 1964). Several studies have compared the basal metabolic rate in obese children (Mossberg, 1948; Bruch, 1939) and in obese adults with that of comparable lean individuals (Bray et al., 1970; Boothby and Sandiford, 1922; Brozek and Grande, 1955; Strouse et al., 1924; Brown and Ohlson, 1946; Means, 1916; Nelson et al.,

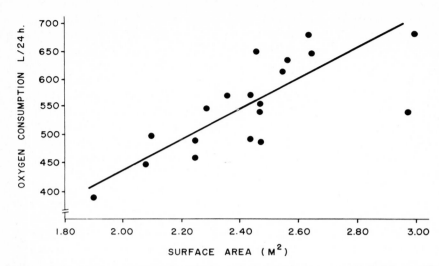

Figure 4–4. Oxygen consumption of obese patients. The oxygen needed for resting metabolism increased with the rise in surface area (M²). The slope of the line shows that 1100 kilocalories are required to support resting metabolism. (See Fig. 4–6 for calculation of the resting metabolism.) (From Bray et al.: Metabolism, *19*:418–420, 1970, reprinted with permission.)

1973). Oxygen requirements increase with body weight. This is shown in Figure 4–4 (Bray et al., 1970). The oxygen uptake or calorie expenditure had a linear relation to surface area. Had the data been plotted against body weight, the curve would have been similar over this range of body weights. In quantitative terms oxygen utilization ($\dot{V}_{O_2}$) and body weight can be related by the following equation (White and Alexander, 1965):

Oxygen consumption ($\dot{V}_{O_2}$) = 69 + 1.65 (body weight in kg)

Using this basis for comparison, the basal metabolic rate of obese subjects is usually the same as that of lean individuals. Boothby and Sandiford (1922) found that the BMR was within ± 10 percent of normal in 81 percent of the 94 obese patients whom they examined.

In a study of 82 obese individuals, Nelson et al. (1973) found that 53 (65 percent) were within ± 10 percent of normal and that only 7 (8.5 percent) were more than 20 percent above or below normal. To re-emphasize, however, this does not mean that obese patients require no more energy than lean ones, but rather that the energy requirements expressed in relation to surface area do not differ (Table 4–5). The absolute requirement for energy as measured by oxygen consumption increases in obese patients as the body weight rises (Fig. 4–4 and Table 4–3). The larger the surface area or body weight, the larger the metabolic expenditure. Oxygen uptake (energy expenditure) is lower when expressed per kilogram but not in terms of surface area (Table 4–2).

TABLE 4–5. *Metabolic Rate of Obese and Lean Subjects**

	Sex	No. Patients	Body Weight kg	Surface Area m^2	Oxygen Consumption ($\dot{V}_{O_2}$) ml/min	$\dfrac{\dot{V}_{O_2}}{kg}$	$\dfrac{\dot{V}_{O_2}}{m^2}$
Normal	M	35	70	1.83	269	3.84	147
	F	35	62	1.72	226	3.65	131
Obese	M	39	143	2.48	348	2.43	140
	F	125	124	2.23	274	2.21	122

*Adapted from Dobeln (1956) and White and Alexander: Acta Physiol. Scand., 37:(Suppl. 126) 1–79, 1956, and J. Appl. Physiol., 20:197–201, 1965, with permission.

Comparing obese and lean subjects by any method creates problems of interpretation (Schmidt-Nielsen, 1970; Durnin, 1959; Dobeln, 1956). Since the major difference between these groups is in body weight, attempts have been made to relate basal energy expenditure to lean body components rather than body weight or surface area. Johnston and Bernstein (1955) studied 17 females whose weight ranged from 39.8 to 186.4 kg. They found that oxygen consumption was correlated with surface area (r = .91), with lean body mass (r = .94) and with cell mass (r = .92). Miller and Blyth (1952) found a good correlation between oxygen consumption and the excretion of creatinine, but that has not been confirmed in another study (Bray et al., 1970). In studies on 19 grossly obese patients, Bray et al. found that oxygen consumption had the best correlation with surface area, body water and body fat. Thus for all its theoretical and technical limitations surface area appears to provide the most useful base for comparing metabolic differences between obese and lean people.

Nutritional status also affects metabolic rate. With caloric restriction basal metabolism declines in both lean (Grande et al., 1958) and obese subjects (Bray, 1969b). After two weeks of caloric restriction, basal metabolic rate can be reduced by as much as 20 percent or more (Fig. 4–5). The decline begins within 24 to 48 hours after decreasing caloric intake and continues to fall slowly over a number of weeks. With refeeding metabolic rate rapidly returns to normal.

Thermic Effects

A reduced or absent thermic effect of food (SDA) might also provide an important metabolic difference between lean and obese patients (Wang et al., 1924).

The thermic effect of food is clearly demonstrated in Figure 4–6. In this figure the resting oxygen consumption is shown throughout the day. After each meal there is a clear increase in energy utilization. The

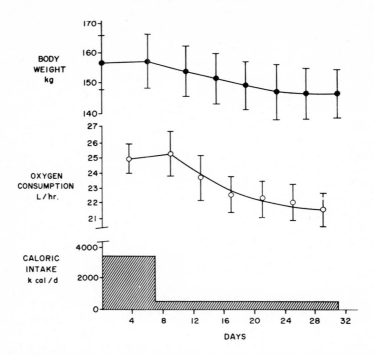

Figure 4–5. Effect of caloric restriction on oxygen consumption of 6 obese patients. After 1 week on a diet of 3500 kcal/day caloric intake was reduced to 450 kcal/day. Body weight declined but the drop in oxygen uptake was proportionally faster, representing a fall of 15 percent by the end of 2 weeks. (From Bray, G. A.: Lancet, 2:397–398, 1969b, reprinted with permission.)

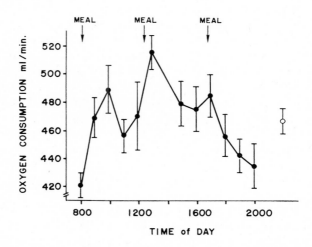

Figure 4–6. Oxygen consumption in one obese patient throughout the day on 7 consecutive days. The rise in oxygen consumption after each of the meals is evident. This rise was smallest after the evening meal. The open circle on the right is the mean figure for resting metabolism of this patient. (From Bray et al.: Metabolism, 19:418–429, 1970, reprinted with permission.)

basal metabolism in the morning was about 10 percent lower than the average value for the rest of the day.

Quantitative data on the thermic effect of food are limited in number. Strang and McClugage (1931) carefully examined caloric expenditure following a test meal fed to obese (18 to 60 percent overweight), normal (± 15 percent from ideal weight), and thin subjects. Measurements were obtained on 25 occasions on 18 subjects, but only 18 of these measurements met the exacting criteria for inclusion in this study. The standard meal produced an average increase of 57 calories in all three groups of patients. These authors conclude that no differences exist between lean and obese patients in the dissipation of calories following ingestion of a meal.

Differences do exist, however, in the response to environmental temperature. A low environmental temperature stimulates oxygen uptake in lean subjects, but has less effect in some obese subjects (Quaade, 1973). For these studies oxygen uptake of lean and obese subjects was measured before and during the last 10 minutes of a 30 minute interval of cooling under a thermal blanket. In the 10 lean subjects the oxygen uptake rose by 33 percent. The average for the 16 obese patients was only 11 percent. In the 4 obese subjects who admitted overeating there was a rise of 37 percent, but in the ones who denied overeating the rise was only 2.5 percent. Among 8 lean subjects who claimed to eat large quantities of food, exposure to the cold increased oxygen uptake by 41 percent, but in 5 lean subjects who ate limited quantities of food the rise was only 10 percent. This difference in the metabolic response to cooling, along with differences in spontaneous (self-paced) activities between big eaters and those who eat small amounts of food, may be important in the ease with which some people develop obesity.

The central issue in the development of obesity is a positive caloric balance. Yet there are only a few studies on the metabolic effects of overeating in man. In contrast there is a large literature on the effects of caloric restriction (see Chapter 7). The possibility that obese patients might differ from lean ones in the way in which they metabolize foods has been the subject of debate for over 50 years. Neumann (1902) measured his food intake and body weight for 3 years. His weight remained essentially constant over this time, while his daily caloric intake was 1766 the first year, 2199 the second and 2403 calories during the third year. Gulick (1922) performed a similar year long self-study where body weight remained constant but caloric intake varied from 1974 to 4113 kCal/day. The term "luxuskonsumption" was coined to describe the dissipation of excess calories which appeared to occur in each of these studies.

Animal data also support the concept of luxuskonsumption. Grafe (see Lusk, 1928, p. 388) presented data from dogs on the rise in oxygen consumption that followed periods of starvation. The fall in metabolic rate associated with starvation is rapidly reversed by refeeding. Grafe suggested that normal man might maintain a constant weight almost without regard to energy intake by dissipating excess calories ("burning them off"). This postulated ability to "burn off excess calories" is what is meant by luxuskonsumption. Inability to activate such a mechanism could clearly produce obesity.

A scheme showing the relationship of "luxuskonsumption" to BMR, physical activity and the thermic effects of food is shown in Figure 4–7 (Miller and Mumford, 1973). Over the range of energy intake from high (H) to low (L) the BMR and activity do not change. The thermic effect of food (SDA or dietary induced thermogenesis) rises with the intake of food, and above the SDA is "luxuskonsumption," which is necessary if energy homeostasis is to be maintained.

The experimental literature on whether "luxuskonsumption" exists is confused (Newburgh, 1931; 1944). Miller and Payne (1962) fed baby pigs a diet that was either high or low in protein. The pigs on the low (2 percent) protein diet ate 5 times as many calories as the pigs eating the high protein diet, yet the body weights were the same. They claimed that differences in carcass composition or activity could not have been enough to account for the stability of body weight in the face of these large differences in caloric intake. However, data from other laboratories show that a reduction in protein in the diet in-

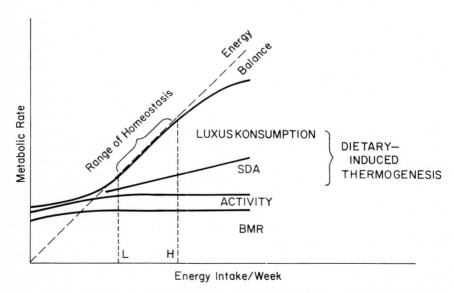

Figure 4–7. Distribution of calories between various metabolic compartments. Luxuskonsumption, if it exists, would be a form of dietary-induced thermogenesis which could not be related to specific dynamic action (SDA) of food. (From Miller and Mumford: Regulation de L'Equilibre, Paris, Masson et Cie, 1973, reprinted with permission.)

creases body fat (Blaxter, 1975). In pigs weighing 70 kg, those on a low protein diet of 13.5 percent had 23.4 percent body fat, and those eating 22.1 percent protein had only 17.1 percent body fat.

From these and other experimental studies Blaxter concluded: (1) that a reduction in caloric intake reduces the rate of fat deposition more than the deposition of protein; (2) that decreased protein intake which impairs protein synthesis leads to accumulation of fat; (3) that fat content increases markedly as body weight approaches maturity; and (4) that reaching a new equilibrium after increasing food intake may take many months or even years.

The evaluation of metabolic response to overeating in human subjects has been even more difficult. One of the earliest studies was by Mann et al. (1955) who increased the food intake of 3 medical students from 3000 to 6000 kCal/day. Exercise was simultaneously increased but was insufficient to prevent body weight from rising. Miller and Mumford (1967, 1973) examined the effects of feeding extra calories to normal subjects either as high or low protein diets, or by giving them one or many meals each day. In all of these experiments the weight gain was less than that expected from the number of extra calories which were ingested.

Several explanations were offered to account for the discrepancy between the amount of weight which was gained and the number of extra calories which were ingested. By using pedometers Miller and Mumford showed that there was no increase in activity during the period of overeating. Similarly there was no decrease in the absorption of calories from the gastrointestinal tract. Since extra calories did not appear in the stools, we can assume that the food which was fed was digested and absorbed.

From these studies Miller and Mumford (1973) suggested that there is a change in the thermic response to food and exercise when comparing subjects before and after periods of overeating. The thermic response to a meal increased with the size of the meal. When exercise was performed after a meal there was a greater thermic effect when exercising than when not exercising. They proposed that, during overeating, the thermic effect of the food plus that from exercise could account for the dissipation of some of the excess calories.

Stirling and Stock (1968) proposed a second mechanism for dissipation of calories. They noted that during cold exposure and after treatment with thyroid hormones the enzymes of the glycerophosphate cycle are increased (see Chapter 3). This cycle bypasses one step in the generation of ATP (Bray, 1969b), and to the extent that the activity of the cycle is increased the efficiency of biological oxidations is reduced. Such a mechanism provides one theoretical possibility for regulating the "efficiency" of metabolism. Bray showed that the activity of the glycerophosphate cycle was reduced with calorie restriction, and Galton and Bray found reduced activity of this cycle in adipose tissue from obese subjects. Whether the glycerophosphate cycle plays an important role in regulating metabolic efficiency is not presently known, and this mechanism is thus mainly of theoretical interest (Gordon, 1968) (see Chapter 3).

The metabolic response to overfeeding of normal human subjects has been extensively investigated by Sims and his collaborators (1968, 1973; Goldman et al., 1975) and others (Munro, 1950; Passmore, 1967, 1971). They found that the number of calories stored as fat in normal healthy men during several months of overeating was substantially less than the number of calories ingested. This has been confirmed by Bray et al. (1974) and the data on one of our subjects is shown in Figure 4–8. In this individual a supplement of 4000 calories was given each day for 28 days. No more than 71 percent of the ingested calories were stored during this period (assuming 7000 kCal/kg of weight gain).

Sims et al. (1973) have also shown that the number of calories needed to maintain body weight increases substantially after an acute weight gain by overeating. Before the period of overeating, the normal men required 1800 kCal/m² and had a surface area of 1.8 m². At the end of the experiment body weight had risen by 20 percent and the surface area by 10 percent to 2 m², but the caloric requirement to maintain this weight had increased to 700kCal/m² (see Fig. 4–7). Measurements of the efficiency with which metabolic processes were coupled to working muscles was measured by having the subjects ride a bicycle before

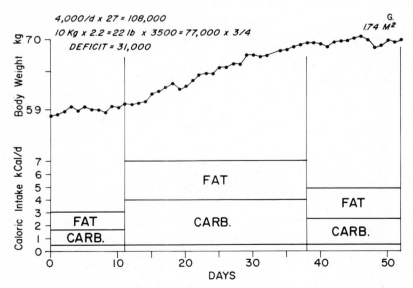

Figure 4–8. Weight gain during overfeeding. A 4000 kcal supplement was fed for 4 weeks to a normal male who had never been overweight. About 71 percent of the extra calories were estimated to have been stored. (From Bray, G. A., Campfield, L. A., and Whipp, B. J.: Studies during weight gain in normal volunteers. Submitted for publication.)

and after weight gain (Hanson, 1973; Whipp, 1975; Bray et al., 1974).

The effects of eating a meal on the energy expenditure during work on the bicycle were tested to examine the hypothesis proposed by Miller and Mumford (1973). The efficiency with which energy was generated on the bicycle before and after weight gain was unchanged (Bray, Whipp and Koyal, 1974). Under these rigorous conditions we were not able to provide experimental support for the proposal made by Miller and Mumford (1973).

A change in the basal or resting metabolic rate is a final mechanism for dissipating calories. Apfelbaum et al. (1971) found that BMR went up by about 15 percent after overfeeding normal subjects. Goldman (1975) has obtained similar data. Whether obese subjects who are overfed show any such changes in BMR is not known.

From this discussion, it should be clear that "luxuskonsumption" has little solid experimental support other than a small change in BMR which occurs with overfeeding. The "balance sheet" obtained during overfeeding is different from the one obtained during weight loss (see Chapter 8). There is always less energy during growth than the quantity of energy which is ingested. Blaxter (1971) has estimated the efficiency with which fat, carbohydrate and protein in the diet can be used by different species during weight gain. For carbohydrates this is about 75 percent, for proteins about 65 percent, and for fat about 85 percent. Thus on a mixed diet one would not expect the normal human being to use more than 75 percent of the ingested calories for storage in fat depots. These figures are only a little above the estimates obtained from the weight gain studies, and lead to serious doubt about the existence of "luxuskonsumption." Indeed in two careful studies on human subjects who were overfed, all of the extra calories could be accounted for (Passmore et al. 1955a,b; Wiley and Newburgh, 1933).

Physical Activity

Obesity limits both spontaneous physical activity and the maximal amount of work that can be performed. Keys et al. (1970) have shown the relation between obesity and inactivity (Figure 4–9). The percentage of men from each participating group in 7 countries who had sedentary occupations is plotted against the percentage of these men who were obese. The relationship is clear. One of the important factors in the high incidence of obesity among the American railwaymen who participated in this study is their sedentary and inactive occupations. Mayer et al. (1956) have reached similar conclusions from a study of 200 adult workers in a mill in West Bengal. These men were subdivided into five classes depending on the level of physical activity associated with their jobs. Body weight was inversely proportional to the level of activity on the job. Food intake was higher among men with the most sedentary occupations than in those with the high-

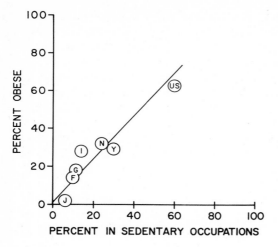

Figure 4-9. Obesity and sedentary occupations. As the percentage of men in sedentary occupations rose the percentage of obese men in the sample also rose. (Each circle represents a country: J=Japan; F=Finland; G=Greece; I=Italy; N=Netherlands; Y = Yugoslavia; US = United States.) (Adapted from Keys, A.: Circulation, *41*(1):1–211, 1970, with permission.)

est activity. The conclusion to be reached is that sedentary occupations are frequently associated with obesity.

The low level of physical activity in obesity has also been studied experimentally (Greenfield and Fellner, 1969). Rose and Mayer (1968) examined a group of 31 infants during the first six months of life. Caloric intake was measured along with triceps skinfold thickness, and the activity of the infants was recorded on an "actometer." The most striking conclusion from their observations was that the extremely thin infants were more active and ate more food than the fat infants who moved less and ate less. These observations suggest that the tendency to spontaneous inactivity is present at the earliest stages in the development of the overweight child.

Additional support for the concept that inactivity is an important factor in the genesis of obesity has come from other studies in children (Mayer, 1965). Bruch (1939) has observed that obese children tend to be inactive. Johnson et al. (1956) provided a more quantitative picture of this degree of inactivity in adolescents by studying 28 matched pairs of normal and obese youths. The obese girls had a lower caloric intake than the lean girls and also showed a significantly lower level of participation in school athletic programs. Stefanik et al. (1959) provided parallel data for adolescent boys. They studied the dietary and activity patterns in obese and lean boys during the school year by dietary history, and during a summer camp by dietary history and direct observation. During the school year there was no difference in the degree of activity, but during the camp experience the lean boys were somewhat more active. The data on the boys were not as clear cut as those from the girls, but nonetheless suggested that inactivity was more important than increased food intake in the genesis of obesity in adolescents.

Among adolescents the clearest demonstration of diminished activity are the studies with time-lapse photography at summer camp (Bullen et al., 1964). With this technique, it is possible to quantify the percentage of the picture frames involved in various degrees of activity. Bullen et al. have observed volleyball, swimming and tennis (Fig. 4–10) at two summer camps for girls. They found that the obese girls almost uniformly spent a smaller fraction of time in positions of activity than did the lean girls. In swimming, for example, the obese girls tended to spend their time floating in the shallow end of the pool. The lean girls, on the other hand, spent more of their time in the deep end where swimming is essential to stay afloat. Similar observations have been obtained in studies of lean and obese adolescent males. Thus in the adolescent it appears that obesity results as much from inactivity as from overeating.

Obese adults also tend to be inactive. Bloom and Eidex (1967) found that obese subjects spent more time in activities that required little energy than did lean subjects. The obese tended to spend more time in bed, and when out of bed, to spend more time sitting than did lean people. Curtis and Bradfield (1971) studied the energy expenditure of 6 obese women in detail. The mean energy expenditure in 4 of these subjects ranged from 2000 to 2600 kCal/day, values which are those to be expected for normal weight women and somewhat lower than expected for overweight women. When the activity of these obese women was compared with the activity of normal weight women published by Durnin et al. (1957), it was found that the obese

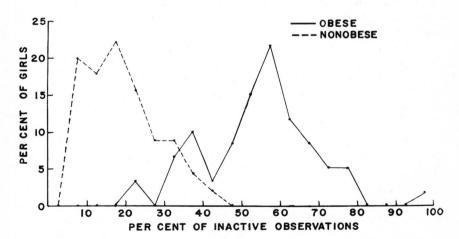

Figure 4-10. Activity of obese and lean girls playing tennis. Pictures taken with time lapse photography were analyzed for the percentages of inactive frames. Obese girls had nearly 60 percent inactive frames on average while the average for the lean girls was only 15 to 20 percent. (From Bullen et al.: Am. J. Clin. Nutr., *14*:211, 1964, reprinted with permission.)

women spent 5 percent less time in moderate activities and 5 percent more time sitting than the lean women.

In still another study, Chirico and Stunkard (1960) used pedometers to measure the distance walked by normal and obese men and women. An obese and lean individual of the same age and occupation were each given a pedometer to wear and the differences in readings were used to compare the distance walked for each pair of subjects. The lean woman walked further than the overweight woman in all but one pair. Among the men, however, there were several pairs in which the overweight man out-walked his lean partner. As a group, however, there was still a significant difference, with the lean men on average walking farther than the obese.

In addition to the reduced spontaneous activity of obese patients, excess body weight limits the performance of physical work. In the first place, the obese individual has more work to do every time he moves his body. This is shown in Table 4–6 (Passmore and Durnin, 1955). As body weight doubles, caloric requirements to move the extra mass almost double as well. Thus the sheer mass of the body significantly increases the work required to move it.

The performance of work by obese and lean subjects has been carefully examined using both the treadmill and the bicycle ergometer. Mocellin and Rutenfranz (1971) found that the maximal work output of children declined as they became more overweight. At 70 percent overweight, the maximum work under standard conditions was reduced by nearly 50 percent.

The efficiency with which the obese exercise under controlled conditions is probably not different from that observed in normal people. Astrand et al. (1960) studied 8 obese women and 4 obese men whose physical work was measured while riding a bicycle ergometer.

TABLE 4–6. *Effect of Body Weight and Speed of Walking on Energy Expenditure (kcal/min)**

BODY WEIGHT		SPEED OF WALKING MPH		
lb	kg	2.0	3.0	4.0
80	36.4	1.9†	2.7	3.5
100	45.5	2.2	3.1	4.1
120	54.6	2.6	3.6	4.7
140	63.7	2.9	4.0	5.2
160	72.8	3.2	4.4	5.8
180	81.9	3.5	4.8	6.4
200	91.0	3.8	5.3	7.0

*Adapted from Passmore and Durnin: Physiol. Rev., 35:801–840, 1955, with permission.
†kcal/min.

They found that the obese subjects showed little difference from the lean in mechanical efficiency. We have reevaluated this problem by taking into account the amount of energy which is expended in moving the legs alone to pedal the bicycle (Whipp et al., unpublished observations). In the very obese subject, moving the legs where the thigh diameter was over 70 cm requires a substantial expenditure of energy. If obese and lean subjects are compared under conditions in which leg movement is controlled, the efficiency of substrate utilization for riding the bicycle is not different for lean and grossly obese subjects. For both groups this is just over 30 percent.

Maximal oxygen uptake in 5 obese and 5 lean women was investigated by Moody et al. (1969) using 4 different methods. The maximal uptakes of oxygen were higher per kg of body weight in the obese women, but when expressed in terms of fat free body weight, they were similar (43.5 cc/kg for the lean and 43.4 cc/kg for the obese). This confirms the previous suggestions that maximal oxygen uptake should be related to fat free body weight (Buskirk and Taylor, 1957; Welch et al., 1958).

To explore further the relation between physical work and obesity, we have studied 10 healthy males weighing on average 72.8 kg with a group of moderately overweight men weighing 103.3 kg (Whipp, Wasserman, Koyal and Bray, 1975). Careful assessment of their pulmonary function showed that the obese men had a significantly smaller expiratory reserve volume in their lungs than the normal men (see Chapter 6). Arterial oxygen saturation was also significantly lower in the overweight men. Two forms of exercise were used. On the bicycle ergometer, three work rates were selected. Oxygen uptake was higher for the obese men at all three work rates. Thus at comparable work rates doing supported work, the obese men required consistently more oxygen than the normal weight men. This means that it took more energy for the overweight men to move their legs and the flywheel than it did for the normal weight men.

Of equal importance was the observation that the blood pressure of the obese men was consistently elevated during moderate and heavy exercise. When walking on the treadmill in these studies, the speed and grade were adjusted to provide oxygen uptakes which were similar to those obtained on the bicycle. This grade on the treadmill was much less for the overweight men than for the normal weight men. The amount of work performed on the treadmill at comparable oxygen uptakes was significantly lower for the overweight men than for the normal weight controls. The reduced level of work capacity for overweight men doing submaximal work might well limit the kinds of occupations for which overweight men are suitable. In particular, it might limit them in obtaining employment where physical requirements are substantial.

REFERENCES

Altman, P. L. and Dittmer, D. S. (eds.): Metabolism. Federation of American Societies of Experimental Biology, Bethesda, Maryland, 1968, p. 345.

Apfelbaum, M., Bostsarron, J. and Lacatis, D.: Effect of caloric restriction and excessive caloric intake on energy expenditure. Am. J. Clin. Nutr., 24:1405–1409, 1971.

Astrand, I., Astrand, P. O. and Stunkard, A. J.: Oxygen intake of obese individuals during work on a bicycle ergometer. Acta Physiol. Scand. 50:294–299, 1960

Astrand, P. O. and Rodahl, K.: Textbook of Work Physiology. New York, McGraw-Hill, 1970.

Atwater, W. P. and Benedict, F. G.: A respiration calorimeter with appliances for the direct determination of oxygen. Carnegie Institution of Washington, publ. 42, 1905, p. 193.

Atwater, W. O. and Benedict, F. G.: Experiments on the metabolism of matter and energy in the human body. Bull. U.S. Dept. Agric. 69, 1899, p. 112.

Aub, J. C. and DuBois, E. F.: Clinical Calorimetry. Arch. Int. Med., 19:823–831, 1917.

Banerjee, S. and Bhattacharjee, R. C.: Interrelations of the basal metabolic rate and body composition in adult male and female medical students. Indian J. Med. Res., 55:451–458, 1967.

Behnke, A. R.: The relation of lean body weight to metabolism and some consequent systematizations. Ann. N.Y. Acad. Sci., 56:1095–1142, 1953.

Blaxter, K. L.: Methods of measuring the energy metabolism of animals and interpretation of results obtained. Fed. Proc., 30:1436–1443, 1971.

Blaxter, K. L., Brockway, J. M. and Boyne, A. W.: A new method for estimating the heat production of animals. Quart. J. Exp. Physiol., 57:60–72, 1972.

Blaxter, K. L.: Energy utilization and obesity in domesticated animals. In: Obesity in Perspective. Fogarty International Center Series on Preventive Medicine, Vol. II, Part 2 (Bray, G. A. ed.), Washington, D.C., U.S. Government Printing Office, 1976.

Bloom, W. L. and Eidex, M. F.: Inactivity as a major factor in adult obesity. Metabolism, 16:679–684, 1967.

Boothby, W. M. and Sandiford, I.: Summary of the basal metabolism data on 8614 subjects with special reference to the normal standards for estimation of the basal metabolic rate. J. Biol. Chem., 54:783–803, 1922.

Boothby, W. M., Berkson, J. and Dunn, H. L.: Studies on energy metabolism of normal individuals: A standard for basal metabolism with a nomogram for clinical application. Am. J. Physiol., 116:468–484, 1936.

Booyens, J. and Hervey, G. R.: The pulse rate as a means of measuring metabolic rate. Can. J. Biochem, 38:1301–1309, 1960.

Bradfield, R. B.: A technique for determination of usual daily energy expenditure in the field. Am. J. Clin. Nutr., 24:1148–1154, 1971.

Bradfield, R. B., Curtis, D. E. and Margen, S.: Effect of activity on caloric response of obese women. Am. J. Clin. Nutr., 21:1208–1210, 1968.

Bray, G. A.: Calorigenic effect of human growth hormone in obesity. J. Clin. Endocrinol. Metab., 29:119–122, 1969a.

Bray, G. A.: Effect of caloric restriction on energy expenditure in obese patients. Lancet, 2:397–398, 1969b.

Bray, G. A., Whipp, B. J. and Koyal, S. N.: The acute effects of food intake on energy expenditure during cycle-ergometry. Am. J. Cliin. Nutr., 27:254–259, 1974.

Bray, G. A., Schwartz, M., Rozin, R. and Lister, J.: Relationships between oxygen consumption and body composition of obese patients. Metabolism, 19:418–429, 1970.

Brown, E. G. and Ohlson, M. A.: Weight reduction of obese women of college age. I. Clinical results and basal metabolism. J. Am. Diet. Assoc., 22:849–857, 1946.

Brozek, J. and Grande, F.: Body composition and basal metabolism in man: Correlation analysis versus physiological approach. Hum. Biol., 27:22–31, 1955.

Bruch, H.: Obesity in childhood. II. Basal metabolism and serum cholesterol of obese children. Am. J. Dis. Child., 58:1001–1022, 1939.

Bullen, B. A., Reed, R. B. and Mayer, J.: Physical activity of obese and non-obese adolescent girls, appraised by motion picture sampling. Am. J. Clin. Nutr., 14:211–223, 1964.

Buskirk, E. R., Iampietro, P. F. and Welch, B. E.: Variations in resting metabolism with changes in food, exercise and climate. Metabolism, 6:144–153, 1957.

Buskirk, E. and Taylor, H. L.: Maximal oxygen intake and its relation to body composition, with special reference to chronic physical activity and obesity. J. Appl. Physiol., 11:72–78, 1957.

Chirico, A. M. and Stunkard, A. J.: Physical activity and human obesity. N. Engl. J. Med., 263:935–940, 1960.

Consolazio, C. F., Johnson, R. E. and Pecora, L. J.: Physiological measurements of metabolism functions in man. New York, McGraw-Hill, 1963.

Consolazio, C. F. and Johnson, H. L.: Measurement of energy cost in humans. Fed. Proc., 30:1444–1453, 1971.

Curtis, D. E. and Bradfield, R. B.: Long-term energy intake and expenditure of obese housewives. Am. J. Clin. Nutr., 24:1410–1417, 1971.

Dabney, J. M.: Energy balance and obesity. Ann. Intern. Med., 60:689–699, 1964.

Dobelin, Von W.: Human standard and maximal metabolic rate in relation to fat free body mass. Acta Physiol. Scand., 37:(Suppl 126) 1–79, 1956.

DuBois, E. F.: Basal metabolism in health and disease. Philadelphia, Lea and Febiger, 1936.

Durnin, J. V. G. A.: The use of surface area and of body weight as standards of reference in studies on human energy expenditure. Br. J. Nutr., 13:68–71, 1959.

Durnin, J. V. G. A., Blake, E. C. and Allan, M. K.: The food intake and energy expenditure of some elderly men working in heavy and light engineering. Br. J. Nutr., 15:587–591, 1961a.

Durnin, J. V. G. A., Blake, E. C., Brockway, J. M., and Drury, E. A.: The food intake and energy expenditure of elderly women living alone. Br. J. Nutr., 15:499–506, 1961b.

Durnin, J. V. G. A., Blake, E. C. and Brockway, J. M.: The energy expenditure and food intake of middle-aged Glasgow housewives and their adult daughters. Br. J. Nutr., 11:85–93, 1957.

Durnin, J. V. G. A. and Brockway, J. M.: Determination of the total daily energy expenditure in man by indirect calorimetry: Assessment of the accuracy of a modern technique, Br. J. Nutr., 14:41–53, 1959.

Edelman, I. S. and Ismail-Beigi, F.: Thyroid thermogenesis and active sodium transport. Recent Prog. Horm. Res., 30:235–257, 1974.

Evans, E. S., Simpson, M. E. and Evans, H. M.: The role of growth hormone in calorigenesis and thyroid function. Endocrinology, 63:836–852, 1958.

Garrow, J. S. and Hawes, S. F.: The role of amino acid oxidation in causing "specific dynamic action" in man. Br. J. Nutr., 27:211–219, 1972.

Givoni, B. and Goldman, R. F.: Predicting metabolic energy cost. J. Appl. Physiol., 30:429–433, 1971.

Goldman, R. F.: Bioenergetics and the response to overfeeding. In: Obesity in Perspective. Fogarty International Center Series on Preventive Medicine, Vol. II, Part 1 and Part 2, (Bray, G. A. ed.), Washington, D.C., U.S. Government Printing Office, 1976.

Gordon, E. S.: Efficiency of energy metabolism in obesity. Am. J. Clin. Nutr., 21:1480–1485, 1968.

Grande, F., Anderson, J. T. and Keys, A.: Changes of basal metabolic rate in man in semistarvation and refeeding. J. Appl. Physiol., 12:230–238, 1958.

Greenfield, N. S. and Fellner, C. H.: Resting level of physical activity in obese females. (Guest editorial) Am. J. Clin. Nutr., 22:1418–1419, 1969.

Gulick, A.: A study of weight regulation in the adult human body during over-nutrition. Am. J. Physiol., 60:371–395, 1922.

Halmagyi, D. F., Broell, J., Gump, F. E. and Kinney, J. M.: Hypermetabolism in sepsis: correlation with fever and tachycardia. Surgery, 75:763–770, 1974.

Hanson, J. S.: Exercise responses following production of experimental obesity. J. Appl. Physiol., 35:587–591, 1973.

Henneman, P. H., Forbes, A. P., Moldawerm, M., Dempsey, E. F. and Carroll, E. L.: Effects of human growth hormone in man. J. Clin. Invest., 39:1223–1238, 1960.

Himms-Hagen, J.: Sympathetic regulation of metabolism. Pharmacol. Rev., 19:367–461, 1967.

Johnson, M. L., Burke, B. S. and Mayer, J.: Relative importance of inactivity and overeating in the energy balance of obese high school girls. Am. J. Clin. Nutr., 4:37–44, 1956.

Johnston, L. C. and Bernstein, L. M.: Body composition and oxygen consumption of overweight, normal, and underweight women. J. Lab. Clin. Med., 45:109–118, 1955.

Johnston, M. W. and Newburgh, L. H.: Calculation of heat production from insensible loss of weight. J. Clin. Invest., 21:357–363, 1942.

Keys, A.: Coronary heart disease in seven countries. Circulation, 41:(Suppl 1) 1–211, 1970.

Keys, A., Taylor, H. L. and Grande, F.: Basal metabolism and age of adult man. Metabolism, 22:579–587, 1973.

Krieger, I.: The energy metabolism in infants with growth failure due to maternal deprivation, undernutrition, or causes unknown. Pediatrics, 38:63–76, 1966.

Lusk, G.: The Elements of the Science of Nutrition. 4th ed. Philadelphia, W.B. Saunders Company, 1928.

Lusk, G.: Editorial review: The specific dynamic action. J. Nutr., 3:519–530, 1931.

Magnus-Levy, A.: Basal metabolism in the same person after an interval of fifty years. J.A.M.A., 118:1369, 1942.

Mann, G. V., Teel, K., Hayes, O., McNally, A. and Bruno, D.: Exercise in the disposition of dietary calories. N. Eng. J. Med., 253:349–355, 1955.

Matson, J. R. and Hitchcock, F. A.: Basal metabolism in old age. Am. J. Physiol., 110:329–341, 1934.

Mayer, J., Roy, P. and Mitra, K. P.: Relation between caloric intake, body weight and physical work: Studies in an industrial male population in West Bengal. Am. J. Clin. Nutr., 4:169–175, 1956.

Mayer, J.: Inactivity as a major factor in adolescent obesity. Ann. N.Y. Acad. Sci., 131:502–506, 1965.

Mayfield, M. E.: The indirect measurement of energy expenditure in industrial situations. Am. J. Clin. Nutr., 24:1126–1138, 1971.

Means, J. H.: The basal metabolism in obesity. Arch. Int. Med., 17:704–710, 1916.

Melville, P. H. and Mezey, A. G.: Emotional state and energy expenditure. Lancet, 1:273–274, 1959.

Miller, A. T. and Blyth, C. S.: Estimation of lean body mass and body fat from basal oxygen consumption and creatinine excretion. J. Appl. Physiol., 5:73–78, 1952.

Miller, D. S. and Mumford, P.: Gluttony. I. An experimental study of overeating on low or high protein diets. Am. J. Clin. Nutr., 20:1212–1222, 1967.

Miller, D. S. and Mumford, P.: Luxuskonsumption. In: Energy balance in man. (M. Apfelbaum, ed.) Paris, Masson et Cie., 1973, pp. 195–207.

Miller, D. S. and Mumford, P.: Obesity: Physical activity and nutrition. Proc. Nutr. Soc., 25:100–107, 1966.

Miller, D. S., Mumford, P. and Stock, M. J.: Gluttony: II. Thermogenesis in overeating man. Am. J. Clin. Nutr., 20:1223–1229, 1967.

Miller, D. S. and Payne, P. R.: Weight maintenance and food intake. J. Nutr., 78:255–262, 1962.

Mocellin, R. and Rutenfranz, J.: Investigations of the physical working capacity of obese children. Acta Paed. Scand. (Suppl.) 217:77–79, 1971.

Moody, D. L., Kollias, J. and Buskirk, E. R.: Evaluation of aerobic capacity in lean and obese women with 4 test procedures. J. Sports Med., 9:1–9, 1969.

Mossberg, H. O.: Obesity in children. A clinical-prognostical investigation. Acta Paediatr. Scand. (Suppl II), 35:1–122, 1948.

Munro, H. N.: The energy metabolism of man during overfeeding. Br. J. Nutr., 4:316–323, 1950.

Nelson, R. A., Anderson, L. F., Gastineau, C. F., Hayles, A. B. and Stamnes, C. L.: Physiology and natural history of obesity. J.A.M.A., 223:627–630, 1973.

Neumann, R. O.: Experimentelle Beiträge zur Lehre von dem täglichen Nahrungsbedarf des Menschen unter besonderer Berücksichtigung der notwendigen Eiweifsmenge. Arch. für Hygiene, 45:1–87, 1902.

Newburgh, L. H.: Obesity: 1. Energy metabolism. Physiol. Rev., 24:18–31, 1944.

Newburgh, L. H.: The cause of obesity. J.A.M.A., 97:1659–1661, 1931.

Newburgh, L. H. and Johnston, M. W.: The nature of obesity. J. Clin. Invest., 8:197, 1930.

Passmore, R.: Energy balances in man. Proc. Nutr. Soc., 26:97–101, 1967.

Passmore, R.: The regulation of body weight in man. Proc. Nutr. Soc., 30:122–127, 1971.

Passmore, R. and Durnin, J. V. G. A.: Human energy expenditure. Physiol. Rev., 35:801–840, 1955.

Passmore, R., Meiklejohn, A. P. and Dewar, A. D.: An analysis of the gain in weight of overfed thin young men. Brit. J. Nutr., 9:27–37, 1955b.

Passmore, R., Meiklejohn, A. P. and Dewar, A. D.: Energy utilization in overfed thin men. Brit. J. Nutr., 9:20–26, 1955a.

Pitt-Rivers, R. and Tata, J. R.: The thyroid hormone. (Callow, R. K., Campbell, P. N., Datta, S. P., and Engel, L. L., eds.) London, Pergamon Press, 1959.

Quaade, F.: Insulation as a creative and maintaining factor in leanness and obesity. In.: Energy balance in man. (M. Apfelbaum, ed.) Paris, Masson et Cie, 1973, pp. 135–140.

Recommended Dietary Allowances. National Academy of Sciences. Washington, D.C., 8th revised edition, 1974.

Rose, G. A. and Williams, R. T.: Metabolic studies on large and small eaters. Br. J. Nutr., 15:1–9, 1961.

Rose, H. E. and Mayer, J.: Activity, caloric intake, fat storage, and energy balance of infants. Pediatrics, 41:18–29, 1968.

Schmidt-Nielsen, K.: Energy metabolism, body size, and problems of scaling. Fed. Proc., 29:1524–1532, 1970.

Sims, E. A. H., Goldman, R. F., Gluck, C. M., Horton, E. S., Kelleher, P. S. and Rowe, D. W.: Experimental obesity in man. Trans. Assoc. Am. Physicians, 81:153–170, 1968.

Sims, E. A. H., Danforth, E., Jr., Horton, E. S., Bray, G. A., Glennon, J. A. and Salans, L. B.: Endocrine and metabolic effects of experimental obesity in man. Rec. Prog. Horm. Res., 29:457–487, 1973.

Southgate, D. A. T. and Durnin, J. V. G. A.: Calorie conversion factors. An experimental reassessment of the factors used in the calculation of the energy value of human diets. Brit. J. Nutr., 24:517–535, 1970.

Stefanik, P. A., Heald, F. P. and Mayer, J.: Calorie intake in relation to energy output of obese and non-obese adolescent boys. Am. J. Clin. Nutr., 7:55–62, 1959.

Stirling, J. L. and Stock, M. J.: Metabolic origins of thermogenesis induced by diet. Nature (Lond), 220:801–802, 1968.

Strang, J. M. and Evans, F. A.: The energy exchange in obesity. J. Clin. Invest., 6:277–289, 1928.

Strang, J. M. and McClugage, H. B.: The specific dynamic action of food in abnormal states of nutrition. Am. J. Med. Sci., 182:49–81, 1931.

Strouse, S., Wang, C. C. and Dye, M.: Studies on the metabolism of obesity. II. Basal metabolism. Arch. Intern. Med., 34:275–281, 1924.

Swanson, H. E.: The effect of temperature on the potentiation of adrenalin by thyroxine in the albino rat. Endocrinol., 60:205–213, 1957.

Wang, C. C., Strouse, S. and Saunders, A. D.: Studies on the metabolism of obesity. III. The specific dynamic action of food. Arch. Intern. Med., 34:573–583, 1924.

Welch, B. E., Riendeau, R. P., Crisp, C. E. and Isenstein, R. S.: Relationship of maximal oxygen consumption to various components of body composition. J. Appl. Physiol., 12:395–398, 1958.

Whipp, B. J.: The physiological and energetic basis of work efficiency. In: Obesity in Perspective. Fogarty International Center Series on Preventive Medicine, Vol. II, Part 2. (Bray, G. A. ed.) Washington, D.C., U.S. Government Printing Office. 1976.

Whipp, B. J., Bray, G. A. and Koyal, S. N.: Exercise energetics in normal man following acute weight gain. Am. J. Clin. Nutr., 26:1284–1286, 1973.

Whipp, B. J., Bray, G. A., Koyal, S. N. and Wasserman, K.: Exercise energetics and respiratory control in man following acute and chronic elevation of caloric intake. In: Obesity in Perspective. Fogarty International Center Series on Preventive Medicine, Vol. II, Part 2. (Bray, G. A. ed.) Washington, D.C., U.S. Government Printing Office. 1976.

White, R. I. and Alexander, J. K.: Body oxygen consumption and pulmonary ventilation in obese subjects. J. Appl. Physiol., 20:197–201, 1965.

Wiley, F. H. and Newburgh, L. H.: The doubtful nature of luxuskonsumption. J. Clin. Invest., 10:733–744, 1933.

World Health Organization. Energy and protein requirements. Technical Report series No. 522, 1973.

CHAPTER 5

EXPERIMENTAL AND CLINICAL FORMS OF OBESITY

Obesity, like high blood pressure and anemia, is a symptom, not a disease (Bray, Davidson and Drenich, 1972). It represents a visible consequence of ingesting more calories than are being utilized. This statement summarizes in the simplest terms the essence of obesity; however, it does not provide an adequate understanding of the basic etiologic factors or of the natural history of obesity. In the present chapter we will review the normal growth of fat in experimental animals and man, and follow this by an examination of the excessive or abnormal growth of fat. Finally, we will discuss several attempts to classify obesity into different etiologic types and look at factors underlying the development of obesity, stressing both genetic and environmental components (Conn, 1944).

NORMAL GROWTH OF BODY FAT

Experimental Animals

In most animals, body fat content is only a small fraction of total body weight at birth. The increase of fat during postnatal growth has been studied in experimental animals by Widdowson and McCance (1960), who compared rats which grow rapidly with slow growing rats (see also Zucker and Zucker, 1961). In both animals there is an increase of fat from approximately 3 percent of body weight in the slow growing rats to as much as 15 percent in the fast growing rats by the 14th day of life. Following weaning from maternal milk, there is a drop in body fat; it falls to 2 percent of body weight in the slow growing rats and to 7 percent in the fast growing animals. Thereafter body fat gradually increases to approximately 13 percent of body weight by 160 days in the slow growing animals and to 22 percent at the same age in the fast growing rats. Thereafter body fat increases slowly throughout the remainder of life. In addition to the effects of age, there are important differences in body fat content of male and female rats, with males having considerably more fat in adult life than females (see Chapter 1).

Human Beings

In human beings body fat begins to accumulate in the last trimester of pregnancy. At birth body fat represents approximately 12 percent of body weight. Body fat continues to increase during the first 6 to 12 months of life, reaching approximately 30 percent of body weight by one year of age (see Fig. 1–6). From this peak at the end of 12 months of life, the percentage of body fat gradually declines in normal boys and girls to between 12 and 14 percent of total weight, at which level it remains until the onset of puberty. When the pubertal growth spurt begins in girls, body fat content usually increases so that by the end of puberty (age 16) it represents approximately 24 percent of body weight (the 90th percentile of body fat for girls of this age is 28.7 percent (Cheek, 1968). For boys body fat rises from 12 percent at age 5 to approximately 17 percent by age 10. With puberty the percentage of body fat declines to 11 percent by age 16 (the 90th percentile for body fat in boys at age 16 is 18.3 percent; Cheek, 1968). At the end of puberty, therefore, body fat content is significantly lower for boys than for girls. The mean with two standard deviations for body weight and body fat in males and females is shown in Fig. 5–1 (from Cheek, 1968). A body fat content above 20 percent of body weight for males and 30 percent for females at age 18 represents obesity.

The remainder of adult life is usually associated with a steadily increasing percentage of body fat (see Chapter 5, 1 and 2, and Fig. 2–1). From age 20 to 60 there is a rise in body fat from 18 percent to 36 percent in males and from 25 percent to approximately 40 percent in females. For the average person there is a small rise in total body weight during the same period. There is a corresponding decline in lean body mass.

METHODS OF CLASSIFICATION

Obesity has been classified in a number of ways, several of which are summarized in Table 5–1. These approaches to classification can be divided into a number of subgroups: descriptive (Noorden, 1900; Bauer, 1945; Zondek, 1926; Jarlov, 1932; Rony, 1940; Vague et al., 1974); anatomic (Hirsch and Knittle, 1970); functional (Kemp,

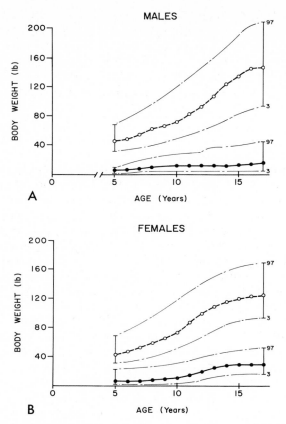

Figure 5–1. Body weight and body fat of males and females during growth. The mean body weight and body fat with the range from the 3rd to the 97th percentiles are plotted for males (A) and females (B) age 5 to 17 years. (Adapted from Cheek, D. B.: Human growth: Body composition, cell growth energy and intelligence. Philadelphia, Lea and Febiger, 1968.)

1972); and etiologic or mechanistic (Mayer, 1960; Bray, 1974a; Bray et al., 1974b; Bray, 1975). One of the most widely used classifications is that of von Noorden, who popularized the terms "exogenous" and "endogenous" obesity. The exogenous obese are those who are fat because they eat too much. Endogenous obesity, on the other hand, includes the various endocrinopathies associated with corpulence. Bauer and Zondek extended the approach of Noorden by adding localized fat deposits (lipomatoses).

The classification used by Jarlov (1932) further expands the observations of von Noorden by dividing endogenous and exogenous obesity into 13 categories (only 3 of which are shown) plus two categories of localized fat deposits (lipomatoid and lipodystrophic). Rony (1940) simplified these older classifications by categorizing

TABLE 5–1. *Chronolgy of Classification of Excessive Fat Accumulations*

STUDY	YEAR	CLASSES
Noorden	1900	1. Exogenous 2. Endogenous
Bauer	1923	1. 'Rubens' type 2. 'Breeches' type 3. Fat over upper half of body 4. Fat over lower half of body
Zondek	1926	1. Alimentary (gluttony) 2. Endocrine (thyroid, pituitary, genital, pineal, pancreatic) 3. Localized (lipomatosis)
Jarlov	1932	1. Hypertrophic — diffuse 2. Plethoric 3. Myxematoid 4. Lipomatoid
Rony	1940	1. Specific forms (hypothalamic, pituitary, adrenal thyroid) 2. Essential 3. Mixed
Vague	1956	1. Gynoid 2. Android
Mayer	1960	1. Metabolic 2. Regulatory
Kemp	1966	1. Childhood 2. Early adult life 3. Pregnancy 4. Middle life
Hirsch and Knittle	1970	1. Hypercellular 2. Normocellular
Bray and York	1971	1. Genetic 2. Hypothalamic 3. Dietary 4. Physical inactivity 5. Endocrine

obesities into those for which a specific cause could be identified and those he called "essential" obesity, for which no specific cause was present.

The other classifications in Table 5–1 utilize information from experimental animals (Mayer, 1953, 1960; Bray and York, 1971), from cellularity of adipose tissue (Hirsch and Knittle, 1970), from age of onset (Kemp, 1972), and from anthropomorphic measurements (Vague, 1974). We will discuss 3 of these in more detail: (1) an anatomic classification based on the number of adipocytes and their localization; (2) an etiologic classification in which specific factors are identified where possible; and (3) a developmental classification based on the age of onset of obesity.

ANATOMIC CLASSIFICATION

Obesity can be classified by the part or parts of the anatomy which it affects. Generalized or diffuse obesity involves all parts of the body, while localized obesity affects only certain areas. Generalized obesity can be further subdivided into two groups; that which occurs in subjects with a normal number of fat cells and that which occurs in subjects with an increased number of fat cells. In Chapter 3, we noted that the accumulation of body fat can occur in one of two ways; by storing excess triglyceride in adipocytes which already exist (hypertrophy), or by increasing the number of adipocytes (hyperplasia). It is conceivable that increased caloric intake acts as a stimulus to evoke the appearance of new fat cells, resulting in augmentation of their total number.

This classification can be applied to both man and animals. Among the rodents three recessively inherited forms of obesity have an increased number of fat cells (Johnson and Hirsch, 1972; Johnson et al., 1971). An increased number of fat cells is also observed in the perirenal fat deposits of mice fed a high fat diet (Lemonnier, 1972). Other deposits in the inguinal region however, do not have an increased number of cells. These animals, therefore, represent a "mixed" form. Three other experimental models of obesity have a normal number of fat cells. These include the yellow mouse ($A^y a$) with dominantly inherited obesity, the Psammomys obesus and rats with hypothalamic obesity.

Several studies have shown that obese patients can be subdivided on the basis of the number of fat cells. In one study Bjurlf examined this question by measuring the size, thickness and number of fat cells in the abdominal adipose tissue obtained at autopsy from 60 males. The size of the fat cells was correlated with body weight, reflecting differences in nutrition. The number of fat cells, on the other hand, was related to the thickness of the subcutaneous fat. Bjurlf concluded that the genetic factors in obesity (see below) were reflected, at least in part, in determining the number of fat cells.

This basic concept of normal (normocellular) or increased numbers of fat cells (hypercellular obesity) has been confirmed and amplified by the use of more elegant techniques developed by Hirsch and Gallian (1968) and by Sjostrom et al. (1971), and Bray (1970) (see Chapter 3). These investigators have clearly shown that all fat people have enlarged adipocytes and that all obesity is "hypertrophic" from the anatomic viewpoint (Bjorntorp, 1974). Most patients with juvenile onset obesity have, in addition, an increased number of fat cells (Table 5–2) (Hirsch and Knittle, 1970; Knittle, 1972; Brook, 1970; Brook et al., 1972; Bjorntorp and Sjostrom, 1971). Knittle (1974) has measured the number of fat cells for normal and obese children (more than 20 percent overweight). In Figure 5–2 the upper panel shows the number of fat cells for the obese and the lower panel for the lean. Although an overlap is obvious, the progressive rise in number of fat

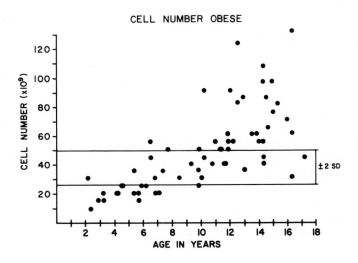

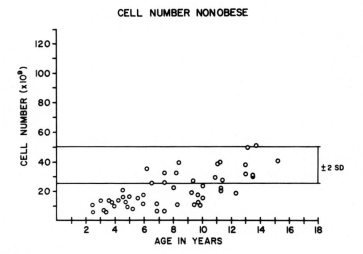

Figure 5–2.   Number of fat cells in obese and nonobese children. (Reprinted from Knittle, J. L.: Triangle, *13*:57–62, 1974.)

cells in the obese children between ages 4 and 12 indicates the importance of this period of life for multiplication of fat cells (see discussion on the age of onset below). Thus two groups are defined: those with a normal number of fat cells, and a second group with an increased total number of fat cells.

Localized accumulations of fat are also of several kinds. Lipomas are localized accumulations of fat which may be single or multiple. The solitary lesions are usually 1 to 2 cm in diameter and soft, but on occasion they can grow to over 15 cm in diameter. The histology reveals an encapsulated accumulation of fat which has all of the characteristics of normal fat tissue. These tumors can be found in almost every organ in the body (Das Gupta, 1970). Studies on the formation of fat by these lipomas have yielded interesting results. Gellhorn and Marks (1961) found that the lipomatous tissue incorporated acetate into fatty acids more rapidly than the adjacent normal adipose tissue.

Atkinson et al. (1974) have extended these observations to the study of extracts of lipomatous tissue. Normally the conversion of the carbons from glucose 6-phosphate into glyceride-glycerol can be inhibited by adding citrate to the extract of adipose tissue. With an extract from a lipoma, on the other hand, there was no inhibition when citrate was added. Extending these observations further, they showed that the enzyme phosphofructokinase from normal adipose tissue is usually inhibited by citrate, but that enzyme from lipomatous tissue of 4 obese patients was not. The appearance of lipomas may thus result from a change in the chemical properties of phosphofructokinase, which is one of the regulatory enzymes concerned with controlling fatty acid synthesis. In lipomatous tissue, formation of triglyceride continues when it would have been inhibited in normal fat.

Multiple lipomas are unquestionably inherited as a simple dominant trait (Das Gupta, 1970). The number of individual tumors may vary from 2 to 3 to as many as 500 in one patient. In individuals with von Recklinghausen's disease lipomas may be encountered along with neurofibromas. Lipomatosis of discrete parts of the skeletal muscle has been described in Maffucci's syndrome. Madelung's disease consists of lipomatosis of the neck and axillae which does not involve the lymph nodes. There are as yet no biochemical studies on the lipomatous tissue in these individuals.

Liposarcomas are relatively rare, in comparison with lipomas. In one series the ratio was 120:1. Males are affected more frequently than females. These tumors have a predilection for the lower extremities, with nearly 60 percent being found there (Das Gupta, 1970). Histologically they can be subdivided into 4 types. (1) The well differentiated myxoid type, which is found mainly in adults. These are unlikely to metastasize. (2) The poorly differentiated myxoid type is a malignant tumor which is difficult to remove and may metastasize. (3) The round cell or adenoid type contains large round cells and usually metastasizes. (4) The mixed type is usually very malignant with a survival varying from 1 month to 4 years (Sharp et al., 1969).

There are four types of idiopathic localized accumulations of fat. Adiposis dolorosa (also called Dercum's disease) was originally described in 1888. Our one patient with this syndrome was typical of the group, for the onset of her disease occurred during the menopausal years. The disease is manifested in obese women by painful nodules in the subcutaneous fat on the arms, thighs and abdomen. The hands and face are not usually involved. The nodules do not become inflamed and have the histologic appearance of normal fat. The clinical course is benign and there is no known treatment for this disease.

Weber-Christian disease differs in several respects from Dercum's disease (MacDonald and Feiwel, 1968). First, it is a relapsing disease with a febrile course. Second, it occurs in women who are 20 to 40 years old. There have been only 11 deaths in more than 120 reported cases. The nodules in the subcutaneous tissue may be single or multiple, and may be tender or painless. Degeneration of the nodules with liquefication occurs in some patients, while other patients show only plaques. The patients may have fever and generalized symptoms. The 20 year old woman who was presented to Harbor General Hospital with this illness subsequently developed mild joint symptoms, but this is distinctly unusual.

ETIOLOGIC CLASSIFICATION

GENETIC FACTORS

This classification has been modified from an etiologic classification proposed for experimental animals (Table 5–2) (Bray and York, 1971). The groups have been rearranged to emphasize the relative importance of genetic and environmental factors.

EXPERIMENTAL STUDIES. The importance of genetic factors in the development of corpulence can be shown for experimental animals and for man. In experimental animals obesity or the susceptibility to develop obesity can be transmitted genetically (Bray and York, 1971). Mayer (1960) noted that genetically obese (ob/ob) mice differed in a number of ways from mice with obesity resulting from treatment with gold thioglucose. He referred to the genetically obese mouse as an example of "metabolic" obesity. Hypothalamic obesity was considered to be a "regulatory" obesity (Table 5–1).

Among experimental animals a number of forms of obesity are genetically transmitted. A summary of these is presented in Table 5–3. These genetically transmitted forms of obesity have a number of characteristics in common (Bray and York, 1971; Bray et al., 1974a, b;

TABLE 5–2. *A Classification of Obesity Based on Genetic and Environmental Factors*

ETIOLOGY	EXPERIMENTAL ANIMALS	MAN
Predominantly genetic	Dominant Recessive Polygenic	Hypercellular Laurence-Moon-Bardet-Biedl syndrome Morgagni's syndrome Growth hormone deficiency
Nutritional	High fat diet Desert rodents fed a chow diet	Infant feeding
Inactivity	Restriction	Inactivity
Endocrine	Insulin injections Hypophysectomy	Cushing's syndrome Insulinoma Hypogonadism Acquired hypopituitarism
Hypothalamic	Electrolytic or chemical injury	Tumors Inflammation
Drugs	—	Phenothiazines Corticosteroids
Social and economic factors	—	Ethnic origin Social class Psychological predisposition

TABLE 5–3. *Genetically Transmitted Obesity in Rodents*

Single gene
   Dominant inheritance
     Yellow mouse (A^y; A^{vy}; A^{iy})
   Recessive inheritance
     Obese mouse (ob/ob)
     Diabetes mouse (db/db)*
     Fatty rat (fa/fa)
     Obese hypertensive rat. (f/f)
   Sex-linked inheritance (Tfm/Y-males)
Inbred strains
   Obese strain of Chickens (OS) (Wick. et al., 1974)
   New Zealand obese mouse (NZO)
   Japanese KK mouse
Hybrid strains
   C_3FI F_1 (Wellesley mouse)
   LAF_1

*Adipose mouse (ad/ad) described by Falconer and Isaacson (1959) is an allele of (or identical with) the diabetes gene.

Renold et al., 1975). All the animals are hyperphagic, that is, they all eat more food than lean controls. Food intake may be only slightly elevated, but in some instances it may increase more than twofold. The fat animal is usually inactive compared to his lean litter mate. Hyperglycemia of varying degrees is present in most of the mice, but is not routinely found in the fatty rat (Bray et al., 1974a). All animals, however, are hyperinsulinemic, with values in some strains reaching very high levels. Insulin resistance (i.e., a diminished response to the administration of exogenous insulin) is present in many of these forms of obesity. However, this resistance can be reversed in one of two ways; by decreasing body weight (Batt and Miahle, 1966) or by damaging the pancreatic islets with alloxan or streptozotocin (Mahler and Szabo, 1971) (see Chapter 7).

The so-called yellow mouse was originally described in detail by Danforth in 1927. It inherits obesity as a dominant trait which is lethal in the homozygous form (Weitze, 1960; Bray and York, 1971). The obesity in these mice begins at puberty and progresses during most of the animal's life. They have enlarged fat cells, but the total number of fat cells is not increased. The gene for this trait is carried on chromosome 2, but the biochemical defect is not known.

There are 3 rodents which inherit obesity as an autosomal recessive Mendelian trait. These are the diabetes mouse (Coleman and Hummel, 1975) (gene symbol, db), the obese mouse (Ingalls et al., 1950) (gene symbol, ob), and the fatty rat (Zucker and Zucker, 1961) (gene symbol, fa). The adipose mouse (gene symbol ad) was originally described by Falconer and Isaacson (1959) and is an allele of or identical with db (Coleman and Hummel, 1975). The ob gene is located on chromosome 4, while chromosome 6 carries the db gene (Coleman and Hummel, 1975). When the ob and db genes are on the same genetic stock, the syndrome in the homozygous (ob/ob or db/db) animals is phenotypically identical. When this background is the C57B1/6J strain, the ob or db trait manifests itself as gross obesity with hyperphagia, hypometabolism, hyperinsulinemia and hyperglycemia. When the genetic trait is contained on the C57B1/Ks background, the homozygous animals develop a ketotic form of diabetes and eventually die of ketoacidosis.

The islets of Langerhans in the pancreas of the C57B1/Ks db/db mouse do not enlarge and insulin secretion is inadequate. The only current way to differentiate between mice carrying the ob/ob and db/db gene is in experiments with parabiosed mice. (Coleman, 1973). When db/db mice are attached to lean animals, the lean mice reduce their food intake and die. Mice with ob/ob gene do not show this effect when parabiosed to lean animals. On the basis of these experiments, Coleman has suggested that db/db mice may produce a "satiety factor" to which they cannot respond, whereas the ob/ob animals can respond to "satiety factor" but cannot produce it (Coleman and Hummel, 1975).

The fatty rat described by Zucker and Zucker (1961) is the only rat in which obesity is inherited as an autosomal recessive trait. The "fatty" rat and the obese (ob/ob) mouse have an increased number of adipose cells. Whether this is a reflection of the genetic defect or the overeating observed in early life is not presently known. The biochemical basis for the obesity in these animals is also unknown. The hypothalamus, the adipose tissue, and the pancreas have been the principal organs to be incriminated, but definitive evidence is not available (Bray and York, 1971; Renold et al., 1975). The obese hypertensive rat has recently been described (Koletsky, 1975). This animal has a recessively inherited form of obesity with hypertension hyperlipidemia. The shortened life span in these animals is due to renal and vascular disease.

CLINICAL STUDIES.   Genetic factors in human obesity manifest themselves in two ways. First, there are a group of rare diseases in which the evidence suggests that genetic factors are of major importance. There are, in addition, the "genetic factors" which under appropriate environmental conditions lead to the development of obesity. We will deal first with the forms of obesity in which genetic factors are of prime importance, and then examine the genetic factors in obesity as elucidated from studies of twins, of adopted children and from family studies.

Genetic forms of obesity in man are less well defined than in experimental animals. It is the author's belief that the hypercellular form of obesity may be genetically inherited. This form of corpulence is discussed below under the general heading of childhood onset progressive juvenile obesity, although most accurately it is one of the varieties of "essential obesity." Five other types of human obesity may be genetically transmitted. These are the Laurence-Moon-Bardet-Biedl (LMBB) syndrome, the Alström-Hallgren syndrome, the Prader-Willi syndrome, the syndrome of hyperostosis frontalis interna (Morgagni-Stewart-Morel), and triglyceride storage disease.

The Laurence-Moon-Bardet-Biedl Syndrome (LMBB)

The Laurence-Moon-Bardet-Biedl syndrome includes five cardinal features: retinal degeneration, obesity, mental deficiency, polydactyly and hypogenitalism (Table 5–4). Laurence and Moon (1866) described four patients with this syndrome. Bardet noted the polydactyly (1920) and Biedl demonstrated its familial occurrence (1922). In addition to these major features, clinical findings of congenital heart disease, strabismus and nephropathy may be detected.

In a review of the syndrome in 1958, Bell collected 368 pedigrees from the literature and found parental consanguinity in 23.4 percent.

TABLE 5–4. *Clinical Features of the Laurence-Moon Bardet-Biedl Syndrome (LMBB)**

	MEN		WOMEN	
	No.	Percent	No.	Percent
Pigmentary retinopathy	152	95	103	91.2
Obesity	142	88.8	106	93.8
Mental retardation	139	86.9	99	87.6
Polydactyly	120	75.0	81	71.1
Hypogenitalism	119	74.4	60	53.1

*Adapted from Bell: *In* The Treasure of Human Inheritance. (L. S. Penrose, ed.) Vol. 5, Part 3, London, Cambridge University Press, 1958, pp. 51–96.

Among 26 pedigrees (38 sibships) in Switzerland, Klein and Ammann (1969) found consanguinity in 52.6 percent. In Israel consanguinity was present in 50 percent (Ehrenfeld et al., 1970). Decreased visual acuity at school age is frequently the first sign of this disease, but it may be preceded by nightblindness. The pigmentary retinopathy is typical in only 18.7 percent of the Swiss cases. Whether typical or atypical, vision steadily deteriorates, with most being blind by age 30.

Hypogenitalism is more common in men than in women. There are reports of women with the LMBB syndrome having children, but no reports of men being fathers (Bell, 1958). Small testes, feminine hair distribution, and occasionally gynecomastia have been described in the males. Polydactylism is usually manifested as an extra digit on the hypothenar (cubital) side. It may occur on any extremity and all 4 were involved in 26.3 percent (Klein and Ammann, 1969). Syndactyly is less frequent. The fifth cardinal feature is mental retardation which is present in over 70 percent. It is generally a mild feeble mindedness. The obesity usually appears in childhood and is progressive. It was present in 88.8 percent of the men and 93.8 percent of the women reviewed by Bell (1958). In well over half of the patients, body weight was more than 3 standard deviations above normal, and in one patient body weight was over 200 kg (440 lbs) (Klein and Ammann, 1969).

The Alström Syndrome

In 1959 Alström and his colleagues described 3 patients who had obesity, blindness in childhood, nerve deafness and diabetes mellitus. Although retinal degeneration and obesity were present (suggesting the LMBB syndrome), the absence of polydactyly and mental retardation, and the presence of nerve deafness and diabetes mellitus led them to suggest this as a separate syndrome.

Ten patients have now been reported with this syndrome (Goldstein and Fialkow, 1973). Table 5–5 compares the features of the LMBB syndrome with those of Alström's syndrome. The earliest sign in the latter syndrome is blindness, which usually begins in the first

TABLE 5–5. *Features of the Laurence-Moon-Bardet-Biedl Syndrome (LMBB) and Alström's Syndrome**

Characteristic	LMBB Syndrome Percent	Alström's Syndrome Percent
Retinal degeneration	90	100
Obesity	95	100
Mental retardation	85	0
Polydactylism	80	0
Nerve deafness	4	100
Diabetes mellitus	6	90
Nephropathy	7	90

*Adapted from Goldstein and Fialkow (1973), with permission from the Williams and Wilkins Co.

two years of life. It is due to a diffuse retinitis. The obesity usually begins between ages 2 and 10. Body weight ranges between 116 and 230 percent of "ideal." As adults, however, obesity had subsided in 3 of the 10 patients. Nerve deafness was a constant feature and was usually detected by age 7. Diabetes mellitus and renal disease appear later. Acanthosis nigricans, baldness and hypogonadism may also be features. The hypogonadism is not present in females, and is less severe in males than it is in the LMBB syndrome.

The Prader-Willi Syndrome

The Prader-Willi syndrome is characterized by hypotonia, mental retardation, obesity, short stature and hypogenitalism, and these features were present in the five patients studied at the Harbor General Hospital. This syndrome was originally described in 1956 (Prader et al., 1956), and 14 cases were reviewed by the authors seven years later (Prader and Willi, 1963). Since that time more than 200 cases have been described in the literature (Dunn, 1968; Medical Staff Conference, 1970; Hall and Smith, 1972).

In contrast with the two syndromes discussed above, a clear demonstration of the genetic inheritance in the Prader-Willi syndrome has not yet been provided. Most of the parents are healthy, and there are only two instances of consanguinity (Brissenden and Levy, 1973). Monozygotic twins with the Prader-Willi syndrome were reported by Ikeda et al. (1973) and by Brissenden and Levy (1973) who also noted 3 pairs of dizygotic twins with this defect. These observations strengthen the likelihood that it is a genetically transmitted disease. The parents are usually not obese, but 6 siblings with the same problem have occurred in families. Chromosomal studies have usually been normal, although Dunn (1968) observed three instances with defects, two with a long Y chromosome and the other with an extra Y

(XYY). Five other reports of chromosomal defects have been noted (Brissenden and Levy, 1973) but there is no constant clinical picture associated with these chromosomal changes.

The clinical features in 32 patients with the PW syndrome are listed in Table 5–6. Pregnancy is usually unremarkable but the mother may note a reduction in intrauterine fetal activity. Breech presentation is more common. Birth weights are generally normal or low. Hypotonia may be observed at or before birth. All of the children have small hands and feet and a characteristically pleasant face. The dermatoglyphics (finger prints) on the hypothenar area may show an open loop pattern. Motor development is slow, and during the first year of life the patients are frequently below average for both height and weight. Treatment with growth hormone does not increase the rate of growth (Raiti et al., 1973). Bone age may be delayed. Dentition is frequently retarded and the enamel may be of poor quality.

The onset of obesity, which is a uniform part of this syndrome, is usually delayed until the second or third years of life, but after that it is progressive. Indeed the pattern of growth in the first year of life shows relative underweight compared with the obesity which develops between ages 3 and 5. The testes have usually not descended at birth and the scrotum is small. Hypogonadism is another characteristic of the syndrome. During the first two years of life there is also a decline in intelligence, which in one series averaged 55, (Hall and Smith, 1972). With the development of obesity, there are often temper tantrums and problems with emotional adjustment.

Laboratory investigation reveals a delayed bone age in the males. Skull x-rays, electroencephalogram (EEG), and electromyogram are

TABLE 5–6. *Features of the Prader-Willi Syndrome**

FEATURE	PERCENTAGE
Breech presentation	40
Non-term delivery	43
Birth Weight <5 lbs. (<2268 g)	21
Hypotonia	100
Feeding problems	100
Delayed milestones	100
Mental deficiency	97
Personality problems	71
Obesity	100
Short stature	94
Small hands and feet	79
Cryptorchidism (males)	84
Hypogenitalism (males)	100
Delayed bone age	50
Strabismus	40
Abnormal glucose tolerance	30

*Adapted from Hall and Smith: J. Pediatr., *81*:286–293, 1972.

usually normal. Muscle biopsies are also usually normal. Protein-bound iodine (PBI) and thyroxine have generally been within normal limits (Tolis et al., 1974; Morgner et al., 1974). The rise in thyrotropin (TSH) following an injection of thyrotropin-releasing hormone (200 μg TRH) was normal (Morgner et al., 1974; Bolaños et al., 1973), and so was the rise in prolactin (Tolis et al., 1974). Gonadotropins (FSH and LH) in the serum are low (Ikeda et al., 1973; Morgner et al., 1974; Zarate et al., 1974) and show a variable or diminished response to luteinizing releasing hormone (LRH) (Tolis et al., 1974).

In one study prolonged treatment with clomiphene resulted in a rise in serum gonadotropins and early signs of testicular maturation in one patient (Hamilton et al., 1972), but was without effect in another study (Tolis et al., 1974). Other studies, however, indicate failure of maturation of the pituitary control of testicular or ovarian function. One formulation of this syndrome is the concept of hypothalamic disease, which produces hypogonadism, hyperphagia and mental retardation. The release of insulin and the impaired output of growth hormone are similar to those functions in other obese children (Parra et al., 1973), although some children with the PW syndrome will release growth hormone (Tolis et al., 1974).

A syndrome of growth resistance, obesity and mental retardation with precocious puberty may be a clinical variant of the Prader-Willi syndrome. The three published cases (MacMillan, Kim and Weisskopf, 1972; Parkin, 1973) are in girls. They resemble patients with typical Prader-Willi syndrome except for the precocious puberty. A second variant (or alternatively a new syndrome) with obesity, hypotonia and mental deficiency was described by Cohen et al. (1973). Two of the 3 cases were in siblings. There was no consanguinity and the onset of obesity was in midchildhood, in distinction to the Prader-Willi syndrome. The tapered extremities, cubitus valgus, genu valgum and hyperextensibility of the wrists were distinctive features. The addition of anomalies of the face, mouth and the limbs leads the authors to think this is a distinctive syndrome.

Hyperostosis Frontalis Interna (Morgagni-Stewart-Morel Syndrome)

This syndrome is characterized by virilism, obesity and hyperostosis of the frontal bones, and occurs almost exclusively in older women (Henschen, 1949; Julkunen et al., 1971). Although it may begin at any age, the majority of cases occur in the third to the sixth decades. In addition to the characteristics described above, a variety of neurological and neuropsychiatric symptoms such as headache, dizziness, irritability, disturbances of equilibrium, impairment of memory, mental slowness and occasional seizures may be present. About 50 percent of the patients have pronounced obesity. X-rays of the skull show a diffuse or spotted thickening of the squamus portion of the orbital plate. This radiologic picture results from thickening of the inner table of the skull with new very dense bone. The outer table is never involved. One clue to the obesity is provided by the pathologic study of the brain in 4 patients (Morel; see Rony, 1940). In the wall of the third ventricle he observed lesions consisting of excess pigment and fatty degeneration. Ritter (1938), however, found no similar lesions in his morphologic study of the hypothalamus from different types of obesity (see Rony, 1940). This syndrome is rare and I have seen no patients with it.

Triglyceride Storage Disease

By analogy with the many metabolic defects in the liver which lead to the accumulation of glycogen, Galton et al. (1974) and Gilbert et al., (1973) have presented four patients who may have abnormalities in the adipose tissue which hinder the mobilization of triglyceride and produce a triglyceride storage disease. The first patient was an infant with the accumulation of fat on the dorsum of the hands. The fat from the periphery showed a smaller stimulation of adenyl cyclase by norepinephrine than the abdominal fat (see Chapter 3), suggesting a defect in activation of adenyl cyclase.

In the other 3 cases from one family there appeared to be an abnormality in the formation of the hormone sensitive lipase in the fat cells. Generalized obesity was present in most members of this kindred. The stimulation of lipolysis by adding isoproterenol to adipose tissue was reduced, but the activation of adenyl cyclase was normal (Atkinson et al., 1974). On the basis of these two families, Galton et al. (1974) proposed three types of triglyceride storage disease. Type I results from a defect in the activation of the adenyl cyclase complex in adipose tissue and the consequent low levels of cyclic AMP. Type II results from a failure of cyclic AMP to activate normally the hormone sensitive lipase. Type III triglyceride storage disease, known also as primary familial xanthomatosis, results from a defect of an acid lipase. In this condition there is accumulation of foam cells throughout the viscera. The concept encompassed by triglyceride storage diseases is attractive and may provide important new methods for examining the function of adipose tissue.

FAMILIAL FACTORS IN OBESITY

Additional insight into the genetic factors in obesity have come from studies of twins and from studies on familial patterns of body weight (Astwood, 1962). The most important studies on body weight in identical and fraternal twins have been published by Newman et al. (1937), by Von Verscheuer (1927) and Shields (1962). Each study examined many parameters in identical twins and found that body weight was the most variable. Newman et al. found that among the 50 pairs of identical twins reared together, the mean difference in body weight averaged 4.1 lb, with only one pair showing a difference in body weight of more than 12 pounds.

Among 19 pairs of identical twins reared separately, however, the mean deviation in body weight was 9.9 lbs, more than twice that for twins reared in the same family. Five of these 19 pairs had a more than 12 pound difference in body weight, indicating that environmental factors may play an important role in the appearance of obesity in selected individuals. In 52 pairs of fraternal (dizygotic) twins, deviation in body weight was 10.0 lbs, which was almost identical with that of the identical twins separated in early life. In 18 (35 percent) of these dizygotic (fraternal) twins, the body weights deviated by more than 12 pounds. In siblings of the same sex, the deviation in body weight was similar to that for fraternal twins.

The importance of environmental factors on the body weight of identical twins was also shown in the studies of Von Verscheuer (1927), who studied 57 pairs of identical twins aged 3 to 51. Eight pairs were lean and 4 pairs obese. The average percentage deviation in body weight was greater than for any other measurement. For all twins in this study it was 2.58 percent, compared with a percentage difference of 1.27 percent for the circumference of the neck, 0.62 percent for height and 1.18 percent for the difference in the size of the waist. When those twins reared in the same environment (i.e., having the same birth weight, growing up together and living in the same town) were compared with those twins in whom one or more of these features did not hold, the deviation in body weight was 1.39 percent for those with the same environment and 3.60 percent for those with differences in their environment.

The data of Shields (1962) compares the weight and height in 44 monozygotic twins reared in the same home with 44 pairs of identical twins reared in separate homes. The height of the monozygotic twins reared together was only slightly less than that of the twins reared apart. In contrast to the other studies, the body weights were the same. This may have been skewed by differences of 31 and 62 pounds found in two pairs of "separated" twins. However, differences of 29 and 31 pounds were also observed in twins reared in the same home. In twins reared together, 43 percent differed in weight by less than 7 pounds, the same percentage as in twins reared separately. Thus the Shields study shows that large differences in body weight can occur in identical twins whether they are reared in the same or in different environments.

Rony (1940) extended these observations further by examining the deviation in body weight of 10 pairs of "lean" identical twins and eight pairs of "obese" twins which had been published in the literature. The body weight deviated by less than 3 percent in 8 of the 10 lean pairs, but in only one of the eight obese pairs was the difference in body weight that small. The greatest reported difference in body weight between identical (monozygotic) twins is 50 kg (110 lbs) (Ruedi, 1971). This pair of twins had 27 identical blood groups strongly supporting their identity. Thus environmental factors would appear to be more important in determining body weight than in determining height, intelligence quotients or other parameters of physiology.

Another analysis of the relationsip between genetic and environmental factors has come from the study of adopted children. Withers (1964) used this approach in a study of 142 individuals. The correlations between body weight of a father or mother and their adopted child were very low ($r = .113$ and $r = .157$), but there was a higher correlation between the weight of a father and his natural child ($r = .592$) or a mother and her natural child ($r = .34$). Although a role for genetic factors emerges from these studies, they also demonstrate the importance of environment, since there is a relatively low correlation between the body weights of parents and their natural children.

Genetic factors have also been examined by family studies comparing the obesity in parents with the weight of the children. The data from some of these studies are summarized in Table 5–7. Although various criteria were used for determining the presence of obesity or overweight in these subjects and their relatives, the high incidence of obesity in parents is obvious. More than 60 percent of the obese patients had one or both parents who were obese. Mothers were more frequently obese than fathers (Angel, 1949). Gurney (1936) examined the progeny in various families in relation to the weight classification

TABLE 5–7. *Frequency of Obesity in Parents of Obese Children*

Year	Author	Number of Obese Subjects	One or Both Parents Obese *Percent*	Mother Only *Percent*	Father Only *Percent*	Both Parents *Percent*
1931	Dunlop	523	69	39	12	18
1934	Ellis	50	44	26	12	6
1936	Gurney	61	83	43	15	25
1940	Rony	250	69	—	—	—
1945	Bauer	275	73	—	—	—
1948	Mossberg	270	80	36	12	32
1949	Angel	116	78	36	15	25
1953	Iverson	40	77	25	20	32
1964	Withers	100	84	28	13	43
1973	Craddock	78	63	—	—	—
1976	Bray*	239	69	33	11	25

*Present report

of the parents. When both parents were stout, 73 percent of the off-spring were stout (65/89), whereas only 9.1 percent were stout when both parents were lean (16/176). When one parent was stout and the other lean, 41.2 percent of the offspring were stout.

Davenport (1923) made a detailed analysis of the weight status of offspring in relation to the weight of the parents. He defines his sub-groups by use of the body mass index (BMI $=$ wt/ht^2). When the parents were both in the overweight group, the body weight of the offspring was twice as variable as when the parents were from the slender or very slender groups. In addition, the progeny of overweight parents were more likely to have body weight in the middle of the weight range than the progeny of slender parents. These findings suggested to Davenport that obese persons frequently carry genes for both obesity and leanness, whereas the lean person is more likely to be "homozygous" with respect to the traits which determine body weight. His findings also indicated that two and sometimes three unit characteristics may be involved in determining body weight, and that in matings of slender and obese parents, the genes for fatness tend to predominate.

Withers (1964) has also analyzed the nature of the inheritance of traits for fatness in an industrial factory and in a group of British school children. There was a notable association of body type among parents and siblings. In his analysis of both populations, it appeared that fathers transmitted somatotypic traits for mesomorphy to their sons and daughters. In both populations the mother transmitted both en-domorphy (roundness) and ectomorphy (leanness) to both sons and daughters. This is depicted in Figure 5–3.

In summary, it is clear that single and polygenic inheritance are involved in the transmission of obesity in man and in animals. From the practical point of view, however, it is clear that in susceptible individuals (those who are genetically predisposed) environmental factors may play a role of overriding importance.

NUTRITIONAL FACTORS

EXPERIMENTAL STUDIES.   Manipulation of the diet can produce obesity in one of two ways; by changing the frequency of eating or by changing the composition of the diet. The first technique involves manipulating eating patterns. If rats which normally eat 6 to 8 meals a day are trained to eat only one or two times a day, they will become fatter (Tepperman and Tepperman, 1970; Fabry and Tepperman, 1970; Leveille, 1970; Cohn et al., 1965). The best example of this is shown by the studies of tube-fed rats reported by Cohn et al. (1965). If rats in one group are allowed to eat ad libitum, and rats in the second group are fed an identical quantity of food by stomach tube twice a

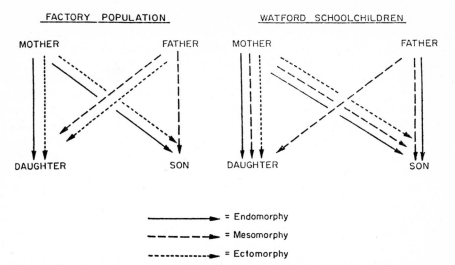

Figure 5–3. The transmission of body type in two populations. Note that the endomorphy was transmitted from mother to daughter and son and that the father transmitted mainly mesomorphy. (Reprinted from Withers, R. F. J.: Eugen. Rev., 58:81–90, 1964.)

day, the content of body fat in the tube-fed rats will be up to twice as high as in the animals which fed ad libitum.

The amount of body fat in tube-fed rats is influenced by a number of factors. One of these is the composition of the diet (Cohn et al., 1965). As the percentage of fat in the diet was increased, the body fat of the tube-fed rats increased more rapidly than in the rats which fed ad libitum. The protein content of the diet was also important. With a protein-free diet, the body fat in the tube-fed animals was only 15 percent higher than in rats feeding ad lib. Body fat rose to 35 percent when the diet contained 18.5 percent protein and showed a further rise to 52 percent when the diet had 67 percent protein. By manipulating the temporal sequence in which protein, fat and carbohydrate are fed, Cohn observed that the greatest accumulation of fat occurs when protein intake is separated from the intake of carbohydrate and fat. Nitrogen excretion is enhanced in the tube-fed rats, which implies that the carbon skeletons for fat synthesis come from the dietary amino acids.

In summary, dietary composition has a profound effect on the quantity of calories stored during tube-feeding of experimental animals. The greatest quantities of excess calories are stored when the intake has a low carbohydrate and high fat ratio and is much lower when there is a high carbohydrate content. Dietary alterations markedly influence enzymatic adaptation. Most of the enzymatic changes occur when rats are adapted to nibbling a high carbohydrate diet. With a high fat diet, few if any adaptive changes are observed. Thus one can dissociate the adaptive lipogenic changes which appear to reflect the rate at which carbohydrate must be processed from the total lipogenic capacity, i.e., total caloric retention which seems to be greatest under conditions where the fat content in the diet is high.

Allowing animals to eat only two hours per day is another approach to the study of the periodicity of food intake. Under these circumstances, food intake is initially lower than when animals are allowed to eat ad libitum. After a few days of adaptation, however, food intake increases, but usually not to the level found in lean animals (an exception is the study by Hollifield and Parson, 1962). Because the quantity of food ingested at each meal is greater, the gastrointestinal tract enlarges and elongates. This hypertrophy is reflected in the increased rate at which food can be absorbed. In spite of this adaptation, however, the rise in blood glucose is less in the meal-fed rats than in the nibbling rats, whether the glucose is administered directly into the gastrointestinal tract or into the peritoneal cavity (Leveille, 1970). Thus the meal-eating rat has a greater capacity to dispose of glucose than the rat eating 4 to 6 smaller meals each day.

Studies on energy metabolism of animals adapted to unusual forms of food intake reveal that during the post-absorptive period (i.e., just after eating) metabolism is higher than normal, but that over the total 24 hour period total energy expenditure is less than in animals eating food in a normal fashion.

The enzymatic adaptations in both adipose tissue and liver of rats which are fed for only a 2 hour period have been studied extensively. For this discussion the enzymatic activities in liver and adipose tissue can be divided into three groups: (1) the glycolytic enzymes which convert glucose into glycogen and pyruvate; (2) the lipogenic enzymes which convert carbon from glucose and pyruvate to long chain fatty acids and which generate NADPH; and (3) the gluconeogenic enzymes which convert pyruvate or glycerol into glucose.

In the animal adapted to eat its food in a short period once a day (meal-fed), the adipose tissue, diaphragm and liver contain more glycogen than the corresponding tissue of animals which eat many small meals (nibblers). The enzymes involved in gluconeogenesis and in lipogenesis are increased. Among this group, the activity of citrate cleavage enzyme (citrate:ATP-lyase), of acetyl-coA carboxylase and of fatty acid synthetase is increased by more than 100 percent. The enzymes of the pentose-phosphate cycle which are involved in the generation of NADPH are also enhanced, as are pyruvate carboxylase and malic enzyme.

Most of the increase in enzymatic activity occurs between the sixth and eighth day following the initiation of a meal-feeding program. However, before the enzyme levels have changed, there was already a highly significant increase in the rate of fatty acid synthesis (lipogenesis from glucose or acetate). It would thus appear that the increased activity of the NADPH-generating enzymes is a consequence of the enhanced rate of substrate conversion to fatty acid rather than the converse. The mechanism by which the increased flow of substrate into fatty acids occurs in the first few days after beginning periodic ingestion of food is at present not clear (Baker and Huebotter, 1973).

Changing the composition of the diet is still another way to produce obesity in experimental animals. When rats which maintain a normal body weight eating laboratory chow are fed a high fat diet, they do not decrease food intake sufficiently to compensate for the high caloric density of the diet and they become obese (Schemmel et al., 1970). The extra weight of such rats is almost entirely fat. As might be anticipated, there is an important genetic component in this response. Most strains of rats become grossly obese when fed the high fat diet but one strain does not. The biochemical basis for this difference is unclear.

Another example of the interaction of genetic and environmental factors is seen in the exaggerated obesity of mice fed a high fat diet (Fenton and Chase, 1951). The yellow mouse usually becomes obese after puberty. The magnitude of this obesity is greatly exaggerated if the animals are fed a high fat diet. Another example of the effect of dietary composition is the appearance of obesity in the sand rat (Psammomys obesus) and spiny mouse (Acomys cahirinus) when their diet is changed to laboratory chow from the leafy foods in their natural habitat in the arid deserts of Egypt and Israel. If the intake of laboratory chow is limited, however, the animals do not become obese (Hackel et al., 1966). Since all of the abnormalities in metabolism which result when Psammomys obesus is fed laboratory chow are prevented by restricting caloric intake, the disorder probably lies in the "caloristat" or ponderostat which regulates caloric storage (see Chapter 2).

HUMAN STUDIES.   Overfeeding may be of particular importance in the onset of childhood obesity (Cochrane, 1965; Fomon, 1971). The incidence of "obesity" among preschool and school age children appears to be rising. In 1951 12 percent of the adolescents and 9 percent of the 6 year olds in a suburban school system were overweight (ht/wt ratio) or obese (skinfolds), and by 1971 these figures had increased to 20 percent for adolescents and 15 percent for the younger age group (Mayer, personal communication). Experimental studies by Knittle and Hirsch (1970) (see Chapter 3) have shown that the total number of adipocytes in rats can be modified by infant nutrition (1968). Eid (1970) found that the infants who gained excessive amounts of weight during the first six weeks of life had a significantly greater likelihood of being obese later in childhood. Huenemann (1974) has recently sustained this finding. The children who grew most rapidly during the first six months were most likely to be obese.

Mellbin and Vuille (1973), however, were unable to use the early growth rate as a predictor of body weight in later childhood. Thus although exceptions exist, the weight of evidence suggest that body weights early in life may be predictive of future obesity. Taitz (1971) pursued this concept further by examining the feeding patterns of infants and found that the ones fed an artificial formula were significantly heavier than expected from height and weight tables. Breast-fed infants showed a less dramatic weight gain. In a similar fashion Fomon et al. (1971) compared the weight gain and milk intake of infants during the first 112 days of life. The bottle-fed infants at the 10th percentile for birth weight were similar in weight at all ages up to 112 days. Infants at the 90th percentile for birth weight who were fed by bottle, however, were heavier and longer at 112 days of age than those who were breast-fed.

Fomon et al. (1969) went further and fed infants with one of two formulas. One contained 67 kCal/100 ml and the other provided 133 kCal/100 ml. The infants receiving the more concentrated food (133 kCal/100 ml) drank less than the other group. Of particular interest was the gain in body weight. During the first 6 weeks the infants receiving the more concentrated formula ingested more calories each day and gained more weight. It is this same period of life which some authors think is predictive of obesity in children at age 6 (Eid, 1970). Huenemann (1974a,b), however, could find no relation between the rate of weight gain in children and whether as infants they received early nutrition from a bottle or from the breast.

In summary, the available data suggest that those infants who grow more rapidly in the early weeks of life may be the fattest in later childhood. Although there are differences of opinion, current evidence suggests that both the quantity and quality of the food available during the first weeks of life may be a major environmental factor in the etiology of childhood obesity. The early introduction of solid foods may also hasten the appearance of obesity (Jelliffe, 1973).

The relation of the frequency of eating to the development of human obesity remains an unsettled question. It has been observed clinically that obese individuals frequently eat fewer meals than normal weight people but this is a difficult point to document. Huenemann et al. (1966a) noted a reduction in the number of breakfasts eaten by the obese boys and girls. More direct evidence on the relation of obesity to the frequency of food intake was obtained by Fabry et al. (1964) in a survey of 379 men aged 60 to 64. The men who ate 1 or 2 meals per day were heavier, had thicker skinfolds, had higher levels of cholesterol, and frequently had impaired glucose tolerance than men who ate three or more meals per day. Fabry extended this finding in a study of school children (Fabry et al., 1966). Children who were fed only 3 meals per day tended to gain more weight than children eating 5 or 7 meals per day.

The frequency of eating also changes the metabolism of glucose and the concentration of cholesterol. Cohn (1964) found that when normal volunteers ate several small meals a day, they had lower concentrations of cholesterol than when the same total intake was eaten in a few large meals. This reduction of cholesterol with frequent ingestion of small meals has been confirmed in several other studies (Gwinup et al., 1963; Jagannathan et al., 1964; Irwin and Feeley, 1967; Young et al., 1972). Glucose tolerance curves are also improved when eating three or more meals as compared with one or two large meals (Fabry et al., 1964; Gwinup et al., 1963; Young et al., 1972).

In one laboratory study six grossly obese patients were fed a 5000 calorie diet for 8 weeks. During one four week period the calories were divided into 20 small meals and during the other 4 weeks they ate one large meal. The period with one large meal was associated with more rapid formation of fat as measured by the glucose incorporation of carbon into fatty acids in adipose tissue (Bray, 1972). Of the enzymatic changes which were studied, the only one which showed a significant alteration during the rapid food ingestion was the cycloplasmic glycerol-3-phosphate dehydrogenase. This contrasts with the numerous enzymatic changes which have been observed in the adipose tissue of rats (Leveille, 1970).

RESTRICTED ACTIVITY

EXPERIMENTAL STUDIES.   Restriction of physical activity to produce obesity in the experimental animal was used by Ingle (1943) to study this problem. In his experiment body weights of over 800 g were produced by housing rats in small cages with access to a palatable diet. This contrasted with weights of less than 500 g in the control animals. Mayer et al. (1954) have graphically demonstrated this phenomenon (Fig. 5–4). In this study rats were exercised up to 8 hours per day. Food intake was proportional to energy expenditure when activity ranged between 1 and 5.5 hours per day. When activity was less than 1 hour per day, however, food intake compensated inappropriately. At higher levels of work, food intake could not match energy needs and the animals lost weight. At very low levels of energy output, both food intake and body weight increased.

This is a fascinating observation that requires additional experimental study. It suggests that at low levels of physical activity, food intake may paradoxically increase. These adaptations, however, do not occur with female rats (Oscai et al., 1974). Moreover, patterns of activity are dictated largely by environmental considerations. In animals living in the wild, there is an important relation between body fat content and total body weight. Small animals have a smaller percentage of body fat than large ones. This ranges between 3 percent of fat

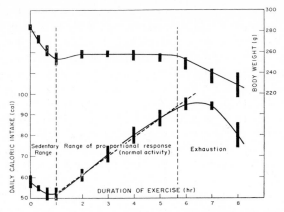

Figure 5–4.   Daily calorie intake of rats exercised for varying periods of time each day. Body weight is given in the upper section. Bars denote the standard deviation. In the "sedentary range" body weight tended to rise as did the food intake. (Reprinted from Mayer et al.: Am. J. Physiol., *177*:544–548, 1954.)

for the mouse to over 30 percent for the whales living in the ocean (Pitts and Bullard, 1968). With captivity, the percentage of body fat of many mammalian species increases. Thus the transition from life in the "wild" to the captive or domestic state may be accompanied by an increase in body fat content.

HUMAN STUDIES.   An effect of physical activity on food intake has also been suggested in man. The observations of Mayer et al. (1956) showed that with sedentary occupations, food intake and body weight tend to be higher than with moderate degrees of activity. In a clinical study Greene (1939) observed that the onset of obesity was associated with inactivity in 67.5 percent of his patients (104/154). The epidemiologic studies of Keys et al. (1970) also show the importance of inactivity as a factor in the prevalence of obesity (see Chapter 4, Fig. 4–9). The highest frequency of overweight men was found in the groups with sedentary occupations. These observations suggest the importance of shifting patterns of physical activity in the regulatory systems controlling the storage, distribution and utilization of calories which ultimately are responsible for obesity. Since such patterns of activity and inactivity are largely environmentally determined, they represent an important and potentially approachable area for modification during treatment (see Chapter 8).

ENDOCRINE ASPECTS

EXPERIMENTAL STUDIES.   There are several endocrine abnormalities which can induce mild or moderate degrees of obesity in the experimental animal (Bray, 1974c). These include administration of insulin (Hoebel and Teitelbaum, 1966), administration of glucocorticoids (Hollifield, 1968), castration (Wade, 1972) and hypophysectomy.

Insulin injections will produce gross obesity (McKay et al., 1940). When preparations of protamine zinc insulin are injected daily for several weeks, body weight may double. When the insulin injections are discontinued, body weight returns to control levels (Hoebel and Teitelbaum, 1966). There are at least two possible mechanisms for this effect. The first hypothesis suggests that insulin produces hyperphagia indirectly by lowering blood sugar. The second hypothesis is that insulin acts directly on the brain to increase feeding activity (for details see Chapter 2).

Administration of glucocorticoids to rats (Hollifield, 1968) or the engrafting of ACTH-producing tumors onto mice can increase body fat (Mayer, 1960). In the rat steroid administration modifies the metabolism of adipose tissue toward increased fat storage, but total body weight does not increase. In the mouse with an ACTH-producing tumor, however, body fat increases, and this model has been used as an example of "metabolic obesity."

Female rats weigh less than male rats. Moreover, the female rat has a cyclic variation of food intake, running activity and body weight which correlates with the estrus cycle. On the day of proestrus and during estrus, running increases sharply and there is a corresponding fall in food intake and a drop in body weight. In the days between estrus, running is reduced, food intake increases and body weight rises (Wade, 1972). After castration this cyclic pattern is abolished and there is a rise in body weight to a new plateau. If estrogen is injected, there is a decrease in food intake. If estrogen is given to castrated female rats in a cyclic fashion, the running activity, food intake and body weight of the normally cycling female animal can be reproduced (see Chapter 2).

Hypophysectomy may be accompanied by obesity and it can be prevented by treatment with growth hormone. In the experimental animal, the administration of growth hormone will reduce body fat content. Thus growth hormone plays a role in the distribution of calories between fat stores and nonfat stores and enhances the conversion of fat stores into utilizable energy for protein deposition and body growth.

Diabetes Mellitus and Obesity

In the adult-onset form of diabetes, weight gain frequently precedes or is associated with the onset of the disease (Drash, 1973). If the excess weight is lost, the impairment of glucose tolerance reverts toward normal and the symptoms diminish (see Chapter 7). In one estimate, approximately 25 percent of the patients who attended an obesity clinic were diabetic, and approximately 70 percent of the diabetics were obese (Baird quoted by Keen, 1975). Joslin, Dublin and Marks (1935) noted that a third or more of the diabetics were more than 20 percent overweight, and that more than 60 percent of the diabetics were above desirable weight.

Pyke and Please (1957) studied the relation between diabetes and obesity in 946 patients and noted that the frequency of obesity was lowest in the diabetics under 30 and highest in the diabetics between 30 and 60. In those over 60 the frequency of obesity was intermediate. This distinction on the basis of body weight between juvenile and adult onset diabetes can be seen in Table 5–8, which compares the body mass index, height and weight of 20 patients whose diabetes began before age twenty with 20 patients who were older than twenty when their diabetes began. None of the juvenile-onset diabetics was overweight but 60 percent of the adult onset group were. Keen (1975) has also observed an increase in body mass index (i.e., overweight) among civil servants who developed diabetes mellitus as compared with those who were known diabetics. The relation of the diabetes and obesity has also been examined in epidemiologic studies. West and Kalbfleisch (1971) have compared the incidence of diabetes and obesity with the index of relative body weight in several countries (Fig. 5–5). As relative weight increased from country to country, the prevalence of diabetes also increased.

However, not all obese patients develop diabetes. Experimental evidence suggests that obesity increases the demands on the pancreas to produce insulin (see Chapter 7). When the pancreas is unable to meet these demands because it has been injured by chemical, viral or genetic factors, then the demands of obesity may lead to failure of the pancreas (see Fig. 7–9). Support for this concept has come from studies on body weight and the frequency of diabetes among siblings of diabetics. When the propositus (i.e., the first member of the family with diabetes to be seen) was obese, the frequency of diabetes among the other siblings was lower than if the propositus were not obese.

When obesity was present in the siblings of diabetic propositi,

TABLE 5–8. *Body Weight Among Adult and Juvenile Diabetics†*

Age at Onset	Number	Age Years	Duration Years	Weight		Height		BMI* KG/M²
				LB	KG	IN	CM	
Adult	20	50.6 ±2.37°	8.2 ±1.83	171.6 ±1.94	77.8 ±0.88	64.7 ±0.17	164.3 ±0.43	28.97 ±1.55
Juvenile	21	16.6 ±1.77	6.6 ±1.39	112.6 ±8.04	51.1 3.65	61.4 ±1.44	156.0 3.65	20.42 .75

†Consecutive patients seen at Harbor General Hospital.
*BMI = Body Mass Index
°Standard error of the mean (SEM)

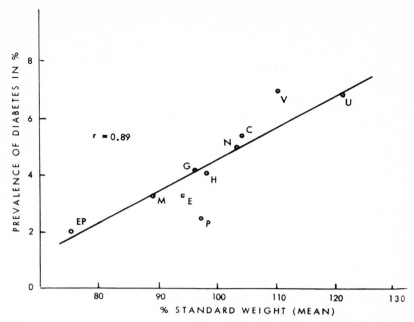

Figure 5–5. Prevalence of diabetes mellitus in relation to body weight. Standard weights for samples from 10 countries were compared with the prevalence of diabetes mellitus in the same groups. The population with the higher standard weight showed a higher prevalence of diabetes. (U=Uruguay; V=Venezuela; C=Costa Rica; N=Nicaragua; G=Guatemala; H=Honduras; E=El Salvador; P=Panama; M=Malaya; EP=East Pakistan.) (Reprinted from West and Kalbfleisch: Diabetes, 20:99–108, 1971.)

however, the frequency of diabetes was higher in those who were obese (10.8 percent and 27.3 percent) than when the siblings were not obese (4.8 percent and 7.3 percent). Thus obesity had placed an extra burden on the pancreas of these diabetics and had precipitated diabetes. These data and the experiments with animals would implicate obesity as a source of environmental "stress" which can precipitate failure of the pancreas and diabetes if the pancreas is already diseased. However, an entirely normal pancreas can apparently meet the demands for extra insulin production imposed by obesity.

Insulin and Insulinomas

Hyperinsulinism, whether from endogenous production or exogenous injection, may also be associated with obesity. Insulinomas are tumors of the pancreas which secrete insulin (Kavlie and White, 1972). In patients with these tumors, an associated weight gain is seen in less than one half of the patients (see Chapter 7). The injection of insulin 5 to 15 u/day into lean subjects can increase body weight (see Rony, 1940 review of early literature).

Cushing's Disease

Cushing's disease is probably the form of endocrine disease most often associated with obesity (Soffer et al., 1961; Burke and Beardwell, 1973). This illness is associated with weight gain, hypertension, glucose intolerance, hirsutism, amenorrhea, plethora and fullness of the face. It can result from hyperplasia of the adrenal glands when they are stimulated by excess ACTH from the pituitary, from a tumor or from injections. Excess corticosteroids may be produced by an adenoma or carcinoma of the adrenal glands, or may be given as treatment for other diseases.

The pattern of weight gain in Cushing's syndrome is characteristic. Fat is accumulated on the trunk, in the supraclavicular fossa and over the dorsal posterior cervical region. The arms and legs are usually spared. The development of obesity as a manifestation of Cushing's disease is most striking in children. In this age group linear growth stops and fat accumulates rapidly (Chen, Kenny and Drash, 1969). In one obese boy with adrenal hyperplasia who was operated on at the Harbor General Hospital, removal of the adrenals was followed by return of body weight to normal. Because Cushing's disease is a curable form of obesity, its differential diagnosis requires careful attention (see Chapter 7).

Polycystic Ovaries

The syndrome of polycystic ovaries described by Stein and Leventhal (Goldzieher and Green, 1962) may be a combination of hypothalamic and endocrine obesity. The complex consists of reduced or absent menses and of moderate hirsutism and weight gain which usually develops in young women shortly after menarche. These women are often infertile. It is of interest that menstruation and fertility can frequently be restored by wedge resection of the ovary. Studies on these women have failed to provide a clear understanding of the mechanism for the abnormalities in the ovary. Hypersecretion of the adrenal, which is often observed in these patients, is also unexplained and may well be caused by several factors. However, the complex of hyperphagia, hypofunction of the gonads and hyperfunctioning of the pituitary-adrenal system is reminiscent of some of the defects observed in experimental animals with obesity, particularly the yellow obese mouse in which obesity, mild hyperglycemia and enlarged adrenal glands develop at or just after puberty.

HYPOTHALAMIC OBESITY

EXPERIMENTAL ANIMALS.   Hypothalamic injuries that induce obesity can be produced with at least three different approaches (see

Chapter 2). The experimental picture produced in animals with these lesions depends upon the extent and location of the injury. Following an electrolytic injury to the ventromedial nucleus, the estrus cycle may become irregular and unpredictable. Food intake increases sharply and may rise twofold (Stevenson, 1969). The increased food intake and decreased physical activity lead to a "dynamic phase" with progressive weight gain. Metabolic rate is normal or slightly diminished. After a period of increased food intake, body weight reaches a new plateau or "static phase." Food intake is only slightly increased or may return to normal.

If the obese rat with a hypothalamic lesion is fasted, it loses weight; as soon as it again has access to food, however, the animal regains weight to the same or a slightly higher level than the one at which fasting began (Kennedy, 1953). Thus the introduction of a hypothalamic lesion has altered the point at which body weight can be regulated. Weight gain after hypothalamic injury is an example of hypertrophic obesity; that is, in these animals there is an enlargement of individual adipocytes with no increase in the total number of fat cells (Hirsch and Han, 1969) (see Chapter 3).

Studies of the endocrine and metabolic alterations in animals with hypothalamic obesity have revealed several interesting facts. First, the glucose concentration in plasma is unaltered in the obese animal. Second, there is an increase in the quantity of unsaturated acids and a decrease in unsaturated fatty acids (Haessler and Crawford, 1967). Third, the obese animals are hyperinsulinemic (Hales and Kennedy, 1964). This was originally suggested by finding hypertrophy of the beta cells in the islets of Langerhans (Kennedy and Parker, 1963) and has been confirmed by direct measurements of plasma insulin (Frohman and Bernardis, 1968; Frohman et al., 1969; Han, 1968). The hyperinsulinemia occurs promptly after injury to the hypothalamus if food intake is allowed but does not occur if all food is removed (Slaunwhite et al., 1972).

The stimulus of food intake leads to an exaggerated output of insulin from the pancreatic beta cells of rats with hypothalamic injury. In spite of hyperinsulinemia, rats with hypothalamic obesity do not become hypoglycemic but rather maintain a normal or elevated blood sugar. This could occur either because peripheral clearance of glucose was reduced or because glucose production was increased. The removal of glucose has been measured and is normal or increased (Frohman et al., 1972a, b). Moreover, the muscle and adipose tissues of rats with hypothalamic obesity respond normally to insulin. It thus appears that in hypothalamic obesity glucose production must be enhanced, but the mechanism for this is unclear.

A pathogenetic sequence for this syndrome in animals is present in Figure 5–6. Injury to the ventromedial nucleus releases the vagus from tonic inhibition (Ridley and Brooks, 1965; Powley and Opsahl,

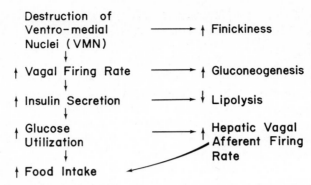

Figure 5–6. A model of hypothalamic obesity. (Reprinted from Bray and Gallagher: Medicine, in press 1975, with permission of The Williams and Wilkins Co.)

1974a, b). The increased vagal firing rate would sensitize the islets of Langerhans in the pancreas to release more insulin when nutrients are absorbed. The increased insulin increases glucose utilization in peripheral tissues and possibly in the hypothalamus (Bray, 1974c; York and Bray, 1972). The increased utilization may, in turn, account for the hyperphagia which provides the calories to develop obesity.

HYPOTHALAMIC OBESITY IN MAN. A syndrome of obesity accompanying injury to the ventromedial hypothalamus occurs in all species which have been investigated, including man. Table 5–9 is a list of the various diseases which have been reported to produce obesity after injury to the hypothalamus in man. Tumors are by far the most frequent. Of these the craniopharyngioma, a congenital tumor developing from cells originating in the anlage of Rathke's pouch, accounts for over 75 percent.

The original description of hypothalamic obesity has been attributed to Mohr in 1840. However, the classical clinical descriptions are

TABLE 5–9. *Hypothalamic Diseases Associated with Obesity*

DISEASE	NUMBER OF CASES
Malignancy	
Solid Tumors	
Craniopharyngioma	253
Others	32
Leukemia	15
Inflammatory disease	
Postencephalitic	10
Sarcoidosis	6
Tuberculosis	4
Trauma	15
Vascular	1

usually attributed to Babinski (1900) and Fröhlich (1901) (Bruch, 1939c). Each described a patient in whom a hypothalamic tumor was associated with the development of obesity and, in the case of Fröhlich's patient, delayed puberty. Over the ensuing years, many other cases with and without delayed puberty have been described (Erdheim, 1904; Heldenberg et al., 1972; Svolos, 1969; Bray and Gallagher, 1975).

We have had the chance to study 10 patients with hypothalamic obesity. Table 5–10 lists the etiologic factors in our patients. It is obvious that tumors were the major cause in our series, as in others. Patient No. 2 developed her obesity at 6 months of age in association with a dermoid cyst of the third ventricle. When brought to us, she was already obese. Her weight rose sharply after the initial operation and remained consistently above the 97th percentile. Her weight has continued to rise and at her last visit at age 14 she weighed in excess of 250 pounds (114 kg) (Fig. 5–7).

Patient No. 6 was found to have a chordoma at the base of the clivus. Chordomas are tumors arising from the embryologic notochord (Mabrey, 1935). In the adult the residuum of this tissue is found in the nucleus pulposis of the intervertebral disc. Occasionally chordomas become malignant. Most such tumors are observed in the region of the coccyx, but about one third of them are intracranial. Usually the symptoms are those of intracranial tumor; our patient is the only reported case with obesity, but it should be noted that this only developed after neurosurgical intervention.

Patient No. 7 had a lipoma of the interpeduncular fossa, and patient No. 8 had a craniopharyngioma. This tumor, developing from the embryologic remnants along the stalk of the hypophyseal duct, is the commonest cause of hypothalamic obesity in man (Bray and Gallagher, 1975a). In our series, however, there was only one patient with this problem. One man (No. 9) in our series had a ruptured aneurysm

TABLE 5–10. *Etiologic Factors in Hypothalamic Obesity*

PATIENT	AGE (YEARS)	SEX	HEIGHT CM	WEIGHT KG	WEIGHT GAIN KG	DIAGNOSIS
1.	4½	F	104	30	—	Trauma
2.	15	F	137	126	60	Tumor
3.	18	F	—	105	55	Inflammation
4.	22	M	186	143	61	Tumor plus surgery
5.	22	F	176	95	32	Tumor
6.	25	F	169	115	62	Tumor plus surgery
7.	30	M	169	119	45	Tumor plus surgery
8.	40	F	161	107	37	Tumor
9.	41	M	173	109	34	Aneurysm
10.	55	F	152	97	26	Tumor

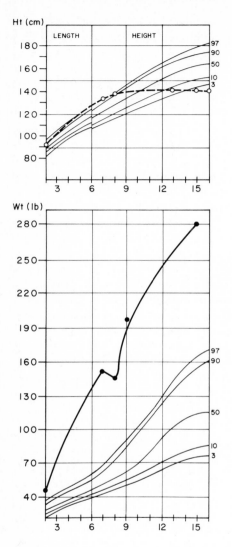

Figure 5–7. Weight gain in a 14 year old girl. The solid line in the lower panel and the broken line in the upper panel show weight and height against the normal grid. (Reprinted from Bray and Gallagher: Medicine, in press 1975.)

of the internal carotid artery. The aneurysm had been clipped and his obesity developed following relief of internal hydrocephalus with a ventriculo-jugular shunt. Prior to that time, his weight had been constant at less than 160 pounds, but following this second operation he gained 100 pounds in 6 months. The other two men had a glioma of the optic nerve (No. 5) and a pituitary tumor which extended above the sella (No. 4). Patient No. 10 had a meningioma of the right optic nerve, and another patient had a large pituitary tumor. Patient No. 3 had a granulomatous disease of the hypothalamus (Fig. 5–8). This figure shows the sequence of involvement in many regions of the hypothalamus prior to increased food intake.

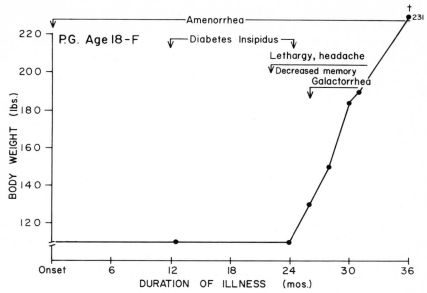

Figure 5–8. Hypothalamic syndrome in an 18 year old girl with granulomatous disease. (Reprinted from Bray and Gallagher: Medicine, in press 1975.)

Patients with hypothalamic obesity are rare. In reviewing many large series of patients with craniopharyngioma, the frequency of obesity varied from 0 to 40 percent (Bray and Gallagher, 1975). In a review of 108 cases, Svolos (1969) noted that 31 were obese and 5 were emaciated. The degree of obesity in these 31 patients was highly variable with 13 being 5 to 10 kg overweight; 8 others between 10 and 15 kg overweight; and only 11 patients being more than 15 kg overweight. Thus only 10 percent of this group exceeded their expected weight by more than 15 kg, and in only one was it greater than 25 kg. This individual had gained more than 50 kg during her illness.

In addition to our patients, we have found 68 cases of hypothalamic obesity reported in the literature where enough data is shown to be able to analyze weight gain. Most patients with hypothalamic obesity developed their problem before age 40, and only 9 of the 68 were over 40 years old. Craniopharyngioma was the major source of pathology in these patients, with other lesions being much less common. In our patients the evidence suggests that most of the obesity occurred by hypertrophy of the fat cells, although, in one patient, it was possible that hyperplasia had occurred as well. The distribution of body weight among these patients showed the following pattern. Over half of the patients gained less than 20 kg. In our series of 10 patients, they all gained more than 20 kg. None of the patients in the literature except those in the present series have gained more than 100 kg.

Such an increment in body weight represents a two and one half to threefold increase in total body fat. Indeed, there were only two other reported patients with weights between 125 and 140 kg. It is thus clear that in patients weighing over 120 kg, the obesity is rarely due to hypothalamic injury. In addition to the relatively limited total body weight, none of the patients gained more than 125 kg. Thus gross obesity of the generalized hypercellular kind which develops in early life is unlikely to be the result of a primary hypothalamic lesion.

The location of the tumors which produce obesity by impinging on the hypothalamus are such that additional symptoms are almost invariably present. Headache, diminished vision, and abnormalities of the reproductive system (amenorrhea in women and loss of libido in men) are the most frequent associated symptoms. Polyuria, polydipsia, diabetes insipidus, somnolence and behavioral disorders occurred with a considerably lower frequency. Thus hypothalamic obesity in man is invariably associated with other manifestations of intracranial disorders.

In general the metabolic characteristics of these ten patients with hypothalamic obesity were similar to the findings in patients with spontaneous or "essential" obesity. Unless endocrine function had been altered by damage to the pituitary from the tumor or at surgery, the responses of thyroid, adrenal and pituitary glands were similar to that expected of obese individuals (see Chapter 7). Serum levels of insulin however, were higher during fasting in patients with hypothalamic obesity than in individuals with essential obesity. The explanation for this phenomenon appears to be related to the way in which the hypothalamus controls insulin secretion.

A working model of this concept is presented in Figure 5–6. In man, as in animals, destruction of the ventromedial hypothalamus releases vagal inhibition and the increased firing of the vagus leads to increased insulin secretion. This in turn leads to increased glucose utilization and glucose output with an increased tendency to eat. We can summarize by saying that hypothalamic obesity in man is a hypertrophic form of the obesity associated with increased food intake, weight gain, and hyperinsulinemia.

PHARMACOLOGIC AGENTS

Some drugs can also lead to an increase in body weight. Cyproheptadine (Periactin) has been shown to increase food intake without an alteration in metabolism in human subjects. This drug and the phenothiazines are probably the major drugs which increase body fat. One study found that, on admission to a mental institution, men averaged 5 pounds less than "desirable" for their height, only to gain 7 pounds during the average stay of 35 months (Waltzkin, 1969). The frequent use of phenothiazines may play an important role in this weight gain (Klett and Caffey, 1960). Although estrogens alone or in birth control pills have been reported to produce weight gain, this is largely the result of fluid retention and probably not the result of increased fat accumulation.

Smoking is another pharmacologic factor affecting body weight. There is a large body of apocryphal data about weight gain, increased food intake and hunger following cessation of cigarette smoking. In one study of a population of Welsh miners (Khosala and Lowe, 1972), nonsmokers were found to weigh about 15 pounds more than smokers at most ages. Ex-smokers approached the body weight of the nonsmokers. That is, they tended to regain the 15 pounds of body weight by which the smoking and nonsmoking groups differed (see Chapter 1).

SOCIAL AND ECONOMIC FACTORS

Obesity in the United States and in Britain is more prevalent in the lower socioeconomic groups (Goldblatt et al., 1965; Moore et al., 1962; Silverstone and Stunkard, 1968; Stunkard et al., 1972) (see Chapter 1). Using a scale of 12 to divide socioeconomic groups, Goldblatt et al. found that among the highest group (i.e., most educated and affluent) only 4 percent were overweight, whereas in the lowest socioeconomic groups 36 percent were overweight. These effects are most prominent in women (Chapter 1, Fig. 1–10, 1–11).

Similar conclusions have been drawn from the Ten State Nutrition Survey (1972). There was significantly more obesity as assessed by skinfold thickness in the lower socioeconomic groups. Ethnic differences were also present. Black males were consistently less obese than white males. Black women, on the other hand, showed a consistently higher prevalence of obesity at all ages than white women. Both black and white males in the lower income levels had a higher prevalence of obesity than black or white males in the higher income levels. The effects of income levels in women produced a more complex picture. Among older women both black and white, lower income was associated with a lower prevalence of obesity. For younger women, the relationship was not clear cut. In some age groups, obesity was more prevalent in women from the lower income groups, but not in all.

The importance of social factors can also be seen in children. Stunkard et al. (1972) found that overweight children were present among first graders from the lower socioeconomic groups, but that no overweight children from the highest socioeconomic groups could be identified by this age. When overweight did appear, it was less prevalent in the children from the higher social classes than from the lower classes.

Additional social factors are related to the duration of residence in the United States. Fourth generation Americans of comparable economic and social levels show a lower incidence of obesity than do recent immigrants. The cohort analysis from Framingham also indicates important social factors. That is, women born later in this century weigh less at the same age than women born earlier in this century (see Chapter 1). The reverse is true for men. That is, men born later in the century are heavier than those born earlier when compared at the same age. Thus while women seem to be getting lighter, men seem to be getting heavier.

PSYCHOLOGICAL FACTORS

Psychological factors in the development of obesity are widely recognized, but attempts to define a specific personality type in association with obesity have proven difficult (Stunkard, 1959). Much of the early work on the psychological factors of obesity came from studies of single patients who had undergone intensive psychiatric analysis. Formulations based on these cases were tantalizing and tended to focus on the oral features of the obese patient as important in the development of this syndrome.

A review of psychological factors in obesity indicates several different approaches to the problem. One of these comes from the extensive studies of Bruch (1957, 1973). She identifies two types of obesity. The first is called reactive obesity and results from ingestion of excess food as an emotional reaction to situations in the environment. According to Bruch (1973), this type of abnormality is a reflection of inappropriate responses to the feeding situation during growth and development of the child. The second type of obesity which she identifies is called developmental. In these individuals, emotional problems are minimal.

Hamburger (1958) formed a classification based on his study of 18 patients. Group 1 consisted of those individuals who overate in response to emotional tensions. The second group were the individuals who overate as a substitute gratification for other emotional needs. The third group were those individuals who overate as a symptom of underlying emotional illness. In the final group he defined overeating in the individual in whom there was an addiction to food (Swanson and Dinello, 1970).

Still a third approach to classifying the emotional problems of obese patients was used by Darling and Summerskill (1953) and by Sucsek (1954). They grouped obese individuals into those who are reasonably well adjusted psychologically, and those who are maladjusted. In a study of 100 obese patients, Sucsek found that there were many different personality types. Only 30 percent of those patients were sufficiently anxious to be comparable to the group of patients seeking psychiatric help for anxiety. From an analysis of the profiles on the Minnesota Multiphasic Personality Inventory (MMPI) and the Thematic Apperception Test (TAT), certain features stood out. The obese as a group tended to be more strong, dominating and independent than individuals with psychosomatic illnesses such as peptic ulcer or ulcerative colitis. Sucsek was impressed with the relative infrequency with which obese patients needed psychiatric help, and we have had the same experience.

The unitary concept of a specific personality constellation in the obese patient was dealt a death blow by the studies of Weinberg, Mendelson and Stunkard (1961), who measured several personality features of obese and nonobese men. The hypotheses which they tested were: (1) that obese men are more anxious than normal weight men; (2) that obese men are more dominant, more conscious of their status and more self accepting; (3) that obese men tend to be more verbal; (4) that they tend to be more intellectually conforming; (5) that they tend to describe their mothers as stronger than their fathers; and (6) that they are more feminine.

Using a variety of psychological tests, Weinberg et al. (1961) could find no support for any of these differences between obese and normal weight men. Lefley (1971) also tested the hypothesis that obesity is a denial of the feminine role. In her study of 30 obese and 30 matched control subjects, however, the obese individuals showed a significantly higher femininity score than did the lean controls.

The psychological features of massively obese patients have also been evaluated. Atkinson and Ringuette (1967) reported on 21 obese patients who averaged 127 percent above their desirable weight. Psychiatric diagnoses were made in 19 cases, but clinical findings varied considerably. Significant depressive symptoms were present in only two patients. From studies with the MMPI (Minnesota Multiphasic Personality Inventory) a diversity of personality types was observed. There was a moderate degree of anxiety and a mild to moderate degree of depression by this test.

In another study at Harbor General Hospital a group of 12 massively obese women had been examined psychologically before and after intestinal bypass surgery. None of these patients had had serious psychiatric illness, but most showed moderate personality disturbances with passive aggressiveness as the predominant trait. Depression was common but not severe. Ingestion of food had frequently been used to reduce the feelings of emotional deprivation which had been present since early childhood and were historically associated with unstable marriages in the family of many of these patients. Such characteristics as stubbornness, defiance, the need for autonomy and wariness of entangling relationships, as well as conflicts over exhibitionism, were prominent features in the personality structures of these patients. These characteristics contribute to the traditional reputation of the obese as "difficult" patients.

The personality characteristics of children with obesity have also been examined (Bruch, 1941). Werkman and Greenberg (1967) studied 42 normal weight girls and 88 obese adolescents at two summer camps. Several different tests of personality were used. The obese girls showed considerably more anxiety and some degree of immaturity and depression. The single finding that cut across all of the test results, however, was the attempt by the obese girls to present themselves as "hypernormal." Similar findings led Monello and Mayer (1963) to suggest that the adolescent with obesity behaves as a minority.

The most consistent and important differentiation between juvenile and adult onset types of obesity may live in the perception of body image. Stunkard and Mendelson (1967) and Stunkard and Burt (1967) examined the relationship of body image and onset of obesity. Distortion of body image is almost entirely limited to individuals whose obesity is begun in childhood or adolescence. Individuals whose obesity began in adult life show little change in body image. This concept has been extended by Cappon and Banks (1968) and by Bailey et al. (1970). This phenomenon has been of interest because of the diversions observed with diet induced weight reduction (see Chapter 8).

A DEVELOPMENTAL CLASSIFICATION
BASED ON THE AGE OF ONSET

The third feature of the classification of obesity is based on the age at onset. This has been broadly divided into two groups; childhood, meaning from birth to age 18, and adult onset (see Table 5–11). In general the onset of obesity in the early years of life is more likely to be associated with genetic factors than its onset later in life. Of the cases of obesity identified by various surveys of the population, approximately one third of the cases have their onset in the childhood years, and the remaining two thirds in the adult years. One important reason for this distinction is that obesity beginning in childhood may be accompanied by an increased number of adipocytes. In contrast, a normal number of fat cells characterizes the adipose tissue when obesity begins in adult life (Hirsch and Knittle, 1970; Bjorntorp, 1974).

OBESITY BEGINNING IN CHILDHOOD

Childhood obesity can be subdivided into several etiologic groups as listed in Table 5–11. Many of these etiologic subgroups have

TABLE 5–11. *Classification of Obesity by Age at Onset*

AGE AT ONSET	ETIOLOGIC FACTORS	ANATOMIC CLASSIFICATION
Childhood	Genetic	?
(0 to 18 years)	Infant feeding	?
	Endocrine	Normocellular
	Hypothalamic	Normocellular
	Unknown	
	Progressive	Hypercellular
	Infantile	?
	Drugs	?
Adulthood	Feeding patterns	Normocellular
(over 18 years)	Inactivity	"
	Endocrine	"
	Pregnancy	"
	Hypothalamic	"
	Drugs	"

already been discussed. We will focus the present discussion on two forms of "essential childhood obesity." The first of these has its onset in infancy and is more benign than the progressive form which has its onset later in childhood.

OBESITY BEGINNING IN INFANCY. Can the potentially obese child be identified at birth by an increased weight? The data on this point are conflicting. Bornhardt (1936) and Gordon (1937) found that 20 to 30 percent of the birth weights in their group of obese children exceeded 4 kg (see Mossberg, 1948). Bruch (1939a) reported that birth weights of 90 obese children were not significantly different from the birth weights of children who did not become obese in childhood. Heald and Hollander (1965) likewise found no difference in birth weights between 158 obese females and 94 nonobese controls (7.004 ± 1.2 vs 7.188 ± 0.9 pounds).

In a retrospective analysis of birth weights from 98 obese children, Wolff (1955) found an identical distribution for birth weights of the obese and normal children from the same hospital (Fig. 5–9). From his data, it is not possible to determine which children would become obese later in life on the basis of body weight at birth. On the other hand, Mossberg (1948) found that 56.5 percent of the 504 obese children in Sweden had birth weights which were more than 3 standard deviations above normal. Quaade (1955) also found that birth weights were significantly higher in his obese children, and Shukla et al. (1972) have recently reported similar findings.

The basis for the discrepancies between various authors is unclear. They may reflect the particular population under study. McKeown and Record (1957b) noted that the mean birth weight of an infant increases with the height and the weight of the mother. Thus if one author were examining the offspring from heavier mothers, these

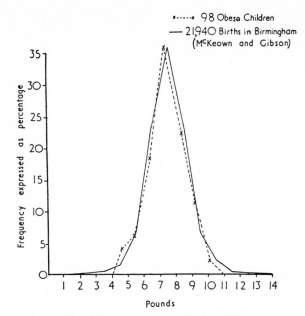

Figure 5–9. Birth weight of lean and obese children. The frequency of each birth weight is compared for 21,940 infants born in Birmingham, England. The birth weights of 98 obese children are superimposed. (Reprinted from Wolff, 1955, with permission of the Oxford University Press.)

infants might be significantly heavier than infants from mothers of normal weight. Whatever the interpretation, it would seem fair to conclude that normal birth weight has little prognostic significance. However, an increased birth weight, particularly if the child has obese parents or a familial tendency towards obesity, may indicate a child who will become overweight.

In the analysis of the age of onset in 504 cases of childhood obesity, Mossberg (1948) observed two periods of peak incidence in the prepubertal years. The first of these occurred in the first two years of life. If obesity were present in more than one relative in the family, the onset of obesity occurred in the first three years in 59 percent. In families where none, or at most one relative, was "obese," only 31 percent of children had the onset of their obesity before 3 years of age.

Some of the features of obesity beginning in infancy have recently been clarified by Court and Dunlop (1974) (Table 5–12). The pattern of growth in the group of 20 children with obesity beginning before age two followed the normal growth curves, although their weights remained more than 3 standard deviations above average. In addition to the normal growth pattern, these children tended to do well at school and were described as "active" by their parents. They were emotionally stable and had normal indices of lipolysis (i.e., the concentrations of glycerol and free fatty acids in plasma were normal).

TABLE 5–12. *Two Forms of Juvenile Obesity**

	ONSET IN INFANCY	ONSET IN CHILDHOOD
Age (years)	2	2 to 12
Growth pattern	Follows upper limit of normal	Deviates progressively from normal
Performance in school	Succeeds	Fails
Activity	Active	Inactive
Emotionality	Stable	Unstable
Triglycerides	Normal	High
Lipolysis (FFA-glycerol)	Normal	Reduced

*Adapted from Court and Dunlop: *In* Proceedings of First International Congress on Obesity. London, Newman Publishing Ltd., 1975.

Children whose obesity started between 2 and 12 years of age showed a number of contrasts. They deviated from the normal lines for growth. These children tended to do poorly at school and were described as "inactive" by their parents. They were subject to emotional outbursts and had lower levels of glycerol and fatty acids than the group whose obesity began in infancy. This latter group might be termed "benign" obesity, whereas the group beginning in middle childhood appears to be more "malignant."

One variety of malignant obesity is labelled "progressive" to distinguish it from grossly obese patients whose weight is stable. Progressive obesity is a particularly ominous form of weight gain. It usually begins in childhood and continues throughout life. These individuals have at least two characteristics in common. The incremental weight gain for each individual is nearly the same year after year. Among patients who reach 140 kg (300 lb) or more by age 30, this increment has ranged from 4.5 to more than 10 kg/year. The constancy of incremental weight gain means that this increment can be used to predict future weight gain. The relationship between age and body weight (in lb) for a group of 20 grossly obese patients who were admitted to the Tufts New England Medical Center between 1966 and 1969 is shown in Fig. 5–10. Note that there is a positive correlation between body weight and age with a slope of 4.5 kg/year.

The second common characteristic of this group of patients is that they must be "hyperphagic;" that is, they must be continually eating more than their body requires. As noted in Chapter 4, the metabolic or energy requirements increase with body weight. Any patient who continues to gain weight year after year requires ever increasing intake of food to maintain the higher energy requirements. To allow for extra weight gain an extra increment is required. These relationships are illustrated further by a patient seen on several occasions at the UCLA Medical Center over a period of 15 years. When I saw him, he was 32 years old and weighed 545 lb. (247 kg); he had gained an average of 17 lb/year (7.7 kg/year). On his initial visit at age 17, his weight was 295 lb. We would have predicted 289 lb (17 × 17) (131 kg). He was seen again at age 24 weighing 390 lb (177 kg). We would have predicted 408 lb (185 kg). He was thus progressively gaining weight at close to 17 lb (7.7 kg) per year with no apparent end in sight and with an ever increasing food intake to maintain present weight and allow for continuing weight gain.

CHILDHOOD ONSET OBESITY.   The second critical period for development of obesity was between the ages of 2 and 11 years. Table 5–13 summarizes the frequency of childhood obesity originating in each of these two age groups. Obese children tend to be taller than age-matched contemporaries. Bruch (1939a) compared the height of 102 boys and girls against chronologic standards. With few exceptions the obese children were above average height. Mossberg (1948) showed clearly that skeletal age was advanced by approximately one year over the chronologic age, but that it had a good correlation with height age. Wolff (1955) found that obese children were 0.3 inches taller than age-matched controls, but this difference was not statistically significant. Quaade (1955) likewise found no difference in height in 50 obese children. Although growth in childhood may be accelerated, the adult height of obese children may be less than normal (Lloyd et al., 1961).

Prevalence

Most of the published studies do not allow a distinction between obesity which begins in infancy and that which begins in later childhood or adolescence. For this reason, we have discussed childhood onset obesity in the following paragraphs as though it were a "single" entity. This, however, is clearly not true (Trygstad, 1972). The prevalence of obesity (or overweight) in childhood depends on the criteria

TABLE 5–13.   *Frequency with which Obesity Begins at Various Ages in Children*

AUTHOR	YEAR	NO. OF PATIENTS	AGE OF ONSET OF OBESITY (PER CENT)		
			0 to 4	5 to 11	11 to 18
Rony	1932	50	64	34	2
Ellis	1934	50	26	68	6
Gordon	1937	50	30	70	
Bruch	1939	83	82	18	
Mossberg	1948	493	77	23	
Salans	1972	62	37	47	16

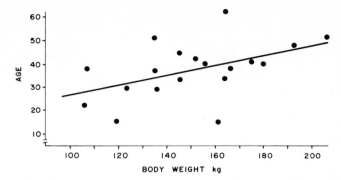

Figure 5–10. Relation between body weight and age in patients with progressive obesity. There was a positive correlation between the age and body weight of these 20 patients who were studied at the Clinical Study Center at Tufts New England Medical Center. The weight gain in this group of patients averaged 4.5 kg/year (10 lb/year).

used for measurement (Hammond, 1955; Stuart and Sobel, 1946; Tanner and Whitehouse, 1962; Tanner et al., 1966).

Using the Wetzel grid, Johnson, Burke and Mayer (1956) observed that 10 percent of the boys and girls in a school in Boston could be classified as obese (Mayer, 1965-1966). In studies of other sections in the United States, the incidence ranges from 15 percent in 9 year old girls to 45 percent for 16 year old girls in Iowa. Using overweight as a criterion 32 percent of the 14 year olds and 39 percent of the 16 year olds in Oregon were overweight (Morgan, 1959). In the longitudinal studies of the school children in Berkeley, California (Huenemann et al., 1966a), obesity was assessed by a formula involving the sum of 11 circumferences and 6 to 8 bony diameters from which body fat and lean body mass could be calculated (see Chapter 1). For this study mild obesity in boys was defined as 20 percent of body weight as fat; marked obesity was a body fat of 25 percent or more of body weight. For girls mild obesity was 25 percent body fat and marked obesity, 30 percent fat. With these figures the prevalence of marked obesity between the 9th and 12th grades stayed nearly constant for boys at 6, 7 and 5 percent respectively. For girls there was a rise in prevalence from 3 to 7 percent between 9th and 11th grades.

In a more recent study by Dwyer et al. (1967), obesity was estimated from the thickness of the triceps skinfold. A measurement of greater than 26 mm was called obesity. With this criterion 15 percent of the 446 girls in their study were obese. When obesity was defined as a ponderal index of 12.4 or less, 23.3 percent of the high school girls were obese (Canning and Mayer, 1966). The prevalence of obesity had been estimated by Hampton et al. (1961) at 14 percent for a population in high school, but the criteria were different from those of Dwyer et al. (1967).

Using a triceps skinfold of greater than 28 mm gave a prevalence for obesity of 39 percent among high school population in Berkeley, California. Christakis et al. (1966), using criteria of height and weight compared to the Baldwin-Wood table, found the prevalence of obesity to be 23 percent in a New York high school. These estimates of prevalence of obesity in the United States are considerably higher than the 2 to 3 percent reported by Lloyd (1972) for English children. The figures from Sweden (Borjeson, 1962) also show a much lower prevalence of obesity than in the United States. In Canada, however, nearly 9 percent of 5549 school children were obese using triceps and subscapular skinfolds (Boileau and Lizotte, 1973). Obesity thus appears to be more prevalent in North American children than in European children.

Food Intake

Estimates of food intake in adolescents have been obtained in several studies (Bruch, 1940a). Johnson, Burke and Mayer (1956) compared the food intake of 28 obese high school girls with 28 girls who were matched for height, age and grade in school. The mean caloric intake for the obese girls was 1965 calories per day and for the lean controls 2,706 calories per day. Stefanik, Heald and Mayer (1959) examined the food intake of 14 obese boys at a summer camp and compared them with 14 boys of normal weight. The body weights of the overweight boys were 138.5 pounds compared with 118 pounds for the normal weight ones. That these differences in weight reflected differences in obesity was indicated by the increased skinfold thickness over the arm and abdomen observed in the obese adolescent boys.

Caloric intake was estimated under two conditions. The first was the average daily food intake obtained during the school year as reported in careful nutritional histories obtained at the beginning of the camp season. These estimates gave a value of 3476 calories per day for the nonobese group and 3011 calories per day for the obese group. During the course of the camp season, the boys were observed and a second dietary history obtained at the end of the camp season. Estimated caloric intake during camp season was 4628 calories for the nonobese and 3430 calories per day for the obese group. As might be expected, the duration of time spent in sedentary activities tended to be higher for the obese boys than for the lean ones. Caloric intake was also assessed by Huenemann et al. (1966b). The mean caloric intake per kg of body weight declined with increasing obesity, and this decline was particularly prominent when examining data from the most obese group. In these studies Huenemann et al. (1966b) also observed that the adequacy of the diet tended to be inversely related to the body weight (Hampton et al., 1967).

Growth and Development

Bruch (1939a) reviewed earlier literature on this question and showed in her patients that menarche occurred on average at 11½ to 12 years in the obese girls and at 13 to 13½ in control populations. Wolff (1955) found that signs of puberty occurred 1 to 2 years earlier in 47 obese girls than in the control group of normal weight girls. Mossberg (1948) observed an average age of 13 years for menarche in the obese girls as contrasted with 14.4 years for the controls. Hammar et al. (1972) also found an early menarche in obese girls. However, Heald and Hollander (1965) failed to detect any difference in age of menarche in their study (12.2 years for the obese vs 12.3 years for the controls). Mossberg and Bruch both found that puberty in obese males occurred on average at an earlier age than in normal boys. Wolff confirmed this and he concluded that puberty was advanced by about one year. Thus both obese males and females develop sexually at an earlier age.

Metabolic and Endocrine Changes

Measurements of metabolic expenditure indicate that the obese adolescent has a normal basal oxygen requirement and a decreased expenditure for physical activity (Heald, 1966, 1972). Measurements of basal oxygen uptake have indicated that the total caloric requirement of obese children and adolescents is higher than for corresponding normal weight children of the same height (Mossberg, 1948; Bruch, 1939b; Nelson et al., 1973). These three groups have observed that if the oxygen consumption is corrected for differences in surface area, there is no difference in basal energy requirements between lean and obese subjects (Bruch, 1940b). Physical activity on the part of obese individuals, however, is clearly reduced (Stunkard and Pestka, 1962) (see Chapter 4). The most striking studies are those of Bullen et al. (1964) who used time lapse motion pictures taken during sessions at a summer camp to quantify the activity of obese and lean children. From these studies it appears that the degree of activity expended in tennis, volleyball and swimming was less for the obese girls than for corresponding lean ones (see Chapter 4). Abnormal glucose tolerance and hyperinsulinemia may also be found in obese children (Court et al. 1971; Parra, et al., 1971; Grant, 1967; Heald et al. 1965; Schultz and Parra, 1970).

Psychological Features

Several studies have focused on the attitudes of the adolescent toward food and body weight (Iverson, 1953). Huenemann et al.

(1966a, b) noted that "teenagers had a high degree of interest in their body conformation which was sustained from the 9th through the 12th grades. Many were generally dissatisfied with their size and shape. Boys desired mainly to gain weight and size, girls to lose weight and reduce certain dimensions."

Dwyer et al. (1967) have examined 446 high school girls for their degree of obesity and for their attitudes toward dieting. Of this group, 15 percent were obese as assessed by the thickness of the triceps skinfold. There was a positive relationship between degree of obesity and the percentage of this group of girls who had dieted. In the obese group 97 percent of the girls had dieted, while only 27 percent of those in the lean group had dieted. In addition, there was a discrepancy between the weight actually reported and the desired weight which increased with the degree of obesity. The body weight desired by the obese girls was 9 to 10 pounds more than what the girls who were below average weight wanted to weigh. Thus the awareness of actual body weight was lower in the obese girls than in their lean contemporaries.

Similar alterations in awareness of external factors have been observed in studies of body image. Monello and Mayer (1963) administered a word association test, a sentence completion test and a schematic appreciation test to 100 obese and 65 nonobese subjects. The obese subjects used words such as calories, diets, reducing, fattening, fat, heavy and overweight with much greater frequency than did the nonobese subject.

In the sentence completion test, the obese subjects behaved in a passive fashion while the nonobese subjects tended to respond in an "active" manner. For example, the obese subjects often described a picture with a child and a cookie jar in it as a situation in which the child was receiving cookies from his mother, while the nonobese tended to view the same picture as the child taking cookies from the jar. In addition to passivity on these tests, the obese subjects tended to withdraw and show isolation and rejection. Monello and Mayer suggested that obese individuals view their surroundings in the same way that the other minorities do and that many of their psychological attitudes reflect this view.

Prognosis

The prognosis of childhood obesity is, in general, poor (Bryans, 1967). Haase and Hosenfeld (1956) noted that 80 percent of the obese children remained obese as adults. A poor prognosis has also been observed by Mullins (1958). Among 373 consecutive admissions to an outpatient department in London, 44 percent of the women and 26 percent of the men were more than 20 percent overweight, and approximately one third of them had the onset of obesity in childhood.

The most convincing studies, however, were published by Abraham and Nordsieck (1960). They compared the body weight of adults with childhood weight documented from school records. The school records on height and weight of all children in Hagerstown, Maryland who were ages 10 to 13 in 1937 to 1939 were examined, and 50 of the heaviest of each sex were selected for comparison with 50 of each sex who had average body weights as children. Of these 200 only 120 could be located for re-examination. The average age was 31, providing an interval of 20 years after these first weights.

The results are summarized in Table 5–14. Of those who were overweight as children, over 80 percent remained overweight as adults. However, a significant percentage of those with average weights in childhood became overweight in adult life. The outlook for the most overweight was even worse. More than 90 percent of those who were 20 percent or more overweight as children remained moderately or markedly overweight as adults. Of the moderately overweight girls (10 to 20 percent), 50 percent were less than average weight as adults compared with only 8 percent for those who were more than 20 percent overweight.

Mossberg (1948) has re-evaluated in later life 328 obese children from his series. The prognosis for infantile obesity was good and few of them were obese later in life. In children with diffuse obesity, however, the prognosis was worse, particularly among the more obese girls. However, it was not bad for the obese boys. These data which include long term evaluation indicate a need for caution in interpreting prognosis from body weights obtained in infancy. Although there is no doubt of the high frequency with which fat children become fat adults, not all types of fatness in childhood have the same prognosis.

OBESITY BEGINNING IN ADULT LIFE

WOMEN.   There are several events in the life of a woman which may be associated with weight gain. These include: marriage, the initiation of treatment with oral contraceptives, pregnancy and the menopause. Lowe and Gibson (1955) observed that at the same ages

TABLE 5–14.   *Prognosis of Childhood Obesity**

| | CHILDHOOD WEIGHT STATUS (PERCENT) | |
OVERWEIGHT ADULTS	*Average*	*Overweight*
Males	42	86
Females	18	80

*Adapted from Abraham and Nordsieck: Public Health Reports, 75:263-273, 1960.

married women without children are heavier than single women. The explanation for the effect of marital status independent of pregnancy has not been explained. The results are not due to oral contraceptives, since these data were collected before such medications were available.

Administration of oral contraceptives has frequently been associated with weight gain. The nature of the extra weight, however, is not entirely settled. Most of the data suggest that the gain in weight results from retention of fluid and that little or no extra fat is added. However, some women have great difficulty in losing weight after stopping these medications, and it is possible that the effect of these agents might be similar to the effects of pregnancy.

Pregnancy increases the weight gain of many women. (Gurney, 1936) Sheldon (1949) has reported a series of women who experienced large weight gains during pregnancy. In this review he described weight gain varying from 28 pounds (12.7 kg) to 110 pounds (50 kg). This study was done on a small group of women who gained weight in pregnancy and there is no way to extrapolate these findings to larger groups of women. To provide this missing data, McKeown and Record (1957a, b, c) re-examined the change in body weight of women who delivered babies between April, 1949 and March, 1950. Maternal weights were obtained early in pregnancy and corrected to the 124th day of gestation. Subsequent weights were obtained at 3, 6, 9, 12 and 24 months postpartum. The changes in weight between the first measurement and two years after delivery varied from a loss of 31 pounds to a gain of 38 pounds. The lone exception was a woman who gained 54 pounds. It was thus apparent that substantial weight gain (over 50 pounds) in pregnancy occurred in less than 1 percent of the sample.

When the data were examined by subdividing the women into groups based on the number of pregnancies they had had and the age at the time of pregnancy, several trends became obvious. First, there was an increase in weight with increasing age regardless of the number of pregnancies, a fact which has been noted previously (Chapter 1). The change in weight from three months after delivery to the end of the year after delivery showed that older women gained more weight (or lost less weight) than the younger women. Finally, during the time from the initial weighing until three months after delivery the weight gain was greater in the women with more previous pregnancies. For example, a woman going through her first pregnancy gained on average 1.7 pounds. With the second pregnancy, 3.9 pounds, and for a woman with three or more pregnancies the gain was 4.4 pounds. Those who gained most during pregnancy tended to lose more in the period from 3 to 12 months postpartum. These data can also be broken down by the number of pregnancies. On average, a woman would be 4.0 pounds heavier two years after her first pregnancy than if she had not become pregnant. The expected weight gain after the second pregnancy would be 5.9 pounds and after three or more it would be 6.2 pounds.

In a further analysis McKeown and Record (1957c) showed that at any given height the amount of weight added increases as the initial weight increases. Thus women who are obese at the start tend to gain more than those who are lean. This effect of pregnancy on weight gain is most pronounced in short women. The patients were arbitrarily divided into those below and above 64 inches (162.2 cm). There was no effect of initial weight status on the weight gain during pregnancy of the taller women. However, there was a pronounced effect of pregnancy on weight gain of shorter women. Weight gain was least in those who were 5 to 15 percent below expected weight and rose progressively as relative weight increased. Thus initial weight status in short women, the number of previous pregnancies and age all play a role in the weight gain during pregnancy, but a weight gain of more than 50 pounds (22 kg) is very uncommon.

Weight gain might also be associated with menopause. The data from the Framingham study, however, found no association with changes in weight and menopause (Kannel and Gordon, 1974). Indeed, the weight gain of women who had surgical menopause was greater than those who underwent menopause naturally. Since the maximum weight in women is achieved in the early forties and shows little change thereafter through age 60, it would appear that the endocrine changes associated with the menopause do not play a significant role in obesity. Summers et al. (1971) believe that the coexistence of obesity with hypertension and fibromyomas in the uterus constitutes a distinct syndrome in women.

MEN.   There are no critical periods for men as there are for women, but the decade from age 20 to age 30 appears to be associated with the greatest change in body weight. This may result from changes in life style which are associated with these years. In Western societies men leave school at the end of the teenage years and during the next decade gradually settle into a pattern of living which will be with them all of their lives. This reduction in physical activity which is associated with these changes may be the most important factor in this process. Although there are no critical periods, the detrimental medical consequences of excess weight may be more significant in men. These consequences are reviewed in Chapter 6.

REFERENCES

Abraham, S. and Nordsieck, M.: The relationship of excess weight on children and adults. Public Health Reports, 75:263–273, 1960.

Alström, C. H., Hallgren, B., Nilsson, L. B. and Asander, H.: Retinal degeneration combined with obesity, diabetes mellitus and neurogenous deafness. Acta Psychiatr. Scand., 34 (Suppl 129): 1–35, 1959.

Angel, J. L.: Constitution in female obesity. Am. J. Phys. Anthrop., 7:433–471, 1949.

Astwood, E. B.: The heritage of corpulence. Endocrinol., 71:337–341, 1962.

Atkinson, J. N. C., Galton, D. J. and Gilbert, C.: Regulatory defect of glycolysis in human lipoma. Br. Med. J., 1:101–102, 1974.

Atkinson, R. M. and Ringuette, E. L.: A survey of biographical and psychological features in extraordinary fatness. Psychosom. Med., 29:121–133, 1967.

Babinski, M. J.: Tumeur du corps pituitaire sans acromegalie et avec de developpement des organes genitaux. Rev. Neurol., 8:531–533, 1900.

Bailey, W. L., Shinedling, M. M. and Payne, I. R.: Obese individuals' perspective of body image. Percept. and Mot. Skills, 31:617–618, 1970.

Baker, N. and Heubotter, R. J.: Lipogenic activation after nibbling and gorging in mice. J. Lipid Res., 14:87-94, 1973.

Bardet, G.: Thése pour le doctor en medicine: sur syndrome d'obésite congénitale avec polydactylie et rétinite pigmentaire (Contribution a l'étude. des formes cliniques de l'obésité hyphosphysaire, Paris, 1920).

Batt, R. A. L. and Miahle, P.: Insulin resistance of the inherently obese mouse-obob. Nature, 212:289–290, 1966.

Bauer, J.: Constitution and disease. New York, 2nd edition, 1945.

Bell, J.: The Laurence-Moon syndrome. In: L. S. Penrose (ed.) The Treasury of Human Inheritance. Vol. 5, Part 3, London, Cambridge University Press, 1958, pp. 51–96.

Biedl, A.: Ein geschwisterpaar mit adiposogenitaler dystrophie, Deutsche Med Wschr 48:1630, 1922.

Bjorntörp, P. and Sjöström, L.: Number and size of adipose tissue fat cells in relation to metabolism in human obesity. Metabolism, 20:703–713, 1971.

Bjorntörp, P.: Effects of age, sex and clinical conditions on adipose tissue cellularity in man. Metabolism, 23:1091–1102, 1974.

Bjurulf, P.: Atherosclerosis and body-build with special reference to size and number of subcutaneous fat cells. Acta Med. Scand., 166:(Supp 349)1–99, 1959.

Boileau, J. G. and Lizotte, P.: Étude longitudinale d'une population d'enfants obèses en milieu scolaire. In: Regulation de l'equilibre energetique chez l'homme (Energy Balance in Man). (Apfelbaum, M., Miller, D. S. and Mumford, P., eds.) Paris, Masson et Cie, 1973, pp. 243–246.

Bolaños, F., Lopez-Amor, E., Vazquez, G. and Monato, R. L. T.: Study on the hypothalamic-pituitary-gonadal axis in the Prader-Willi Syndrome. (abs). Revista Invest. Clinica, 25:108–109, 1973.

Borjeson, M.: Overweight children. Acta Pediatr.(Upps)51(Suppl 132): 1–76, 1962.

Bornhardt, M.: Ueber Fettsucht im Kindesalter und ihre Prognose mit besonderer Berücksichtigung der Frage der Dystrophia adiposogenitalis. Monatschr. F. Kinderh., 67:270–272, 1936.

Bray, G. A. (ed.): Obesity in Perspective, Fogarty International Center Series on Preventive Medicine, Vol. II, Part I. Washington, D.C., U.S. Government Printing Office, 1975. pp. 13-18 DHEW Publ. No. (NIH) 75-708

Bray, G. A.: Measurement of subcutaneous fat cells from obese patients. Ann. Intern. Med., 73:565–569, 1970.

Bray, G. A., Davidson, M. B. and Drenick, E. J.: Obesity: A serious symptom. Ann. Intern. Med., 77:779–795, 1972.

Bray, G. A.: Lipogenesis in human adipose tissue: Some effects of nibbling and gorging. J. Clin. Invest., 51:537–548, 1972.

Bray, G. A.: The Varieties of Obesity. In: Treatment and Management of Obesity. (G. A. Bray, and J. E. Bethune, eds.) Chapter 5, Section II. Hagerstown, Harper and Row, 1974a pp. 61–76.

Bray, G. A., Luong, D. and York, D. A.: Regulation of Adipose Tissue Mass in Genetically Obese Rodents. In: The Regulation of the Adipose Tissue Mass. Proceedings of the IV International Meeting of Endocrinology, Marseilles, in Vague, J. and Boyer, J. eds.) Excerpt Medica, (Amsterdam) 1974b. pp. 111–121.

Bray, G. A. and Gallagher, T. F., Jr.: Manifestations of hypothalamic obesity in man: A comprehensive investigation of eight patients and a review of the literature. Medicine 54:301-330, 1975.

Bray, G. A.: Endocrine factors in the control of food intake. Fed. Proc. 33:1140–1145, 1974c.

Bray, G. A. and York, D. A.: Genetically transmitted obesity in rodents. Physiol. Rev., 51:598–646, 1971.

Bray, G. A.: The varieties of obesity: Some lessons from experimental medicine. *In*: Obesity, Burland, W. L., Samuel, P. and Yudkin, J., (eds.) Edinburgh, Churchill Livingstone, 1974, pp. 6-21.

Brissenden, J. E. and Levy, E. P.: Prader-Willi syndrome in infant monozygotic twins. Am. J. Dis. Child, *126*:110–112, 1973.

Brook, C. G. D.: Adipose cell size and number in obese children. Arch. Dis. Child, *45*:819, 1970. (Abs)

Brook, C. G. D., Lloyd, J. K. and Wolf, O. H.: Relation between age of onset of obesity and size and number of adipose cells. Br. Med. J., *2*:25–27, 1972.

Bruch, H.: Obesity in childhood; physical growth and development of obese children. Am. J. Dis. Child, *58*:457–484, 1939a.

Bruch, H.: Obesity in childhood; basal metabolism and serum cholesterol of obese children. Am. J. Dis. Child, *58*:1001–1022, 1939b.

Bruch, H.: Progress in Pediatrics. The Frohlich syndrome. Report of the original case. Am. J. Dis. Child, *58*:1282–1289, 1939c.

Bruch, H.: Obesity in childhood. III. Physiologic and psychologic aspects of the food intake of obese children. Am. J. Dis. Child, *59*:739–831, 1940a.

Bruch, H.: Obesity in childhood. IV. Energy expenditure of obese children. Am. J. Dis. Child, *60*:1082–1109, 1940b.

Bruch, H.: Obesity in childhood and personality development. Am. J. Orthopsychiatr., *2*:467–474, 1941.

Bruch, H.: Eating disorders; obesity, anorexia nervosa and the person within. New York, Basic Books, 1973.

Bruch, H.: The importance of overweight. New York, W. W. Norton Co., Inc., 1957.

Bryans, A. M.: Childhood obesity—prelude to adult obesity. Can. J. Public Health, *58*:486–490, 1967.

Bullen, B. A., Reed, R. B. and Mayer, J.: Physical activity of obese and nonobese adolescent girls appraised by motion picture sampling. Am. J. Clin. Nutr., *14*:211–223, 1964.

Burke, C. W. and Beardwell, C. G.: Cushing's syndrome. Q. J. Med., *42*:175–204, 1973.

Canning, H. and Mayer, J.: Obesity—its possible effect on college acceptance. N. Eng. J. Med., *275*:1172–1174, 1966.

Cappon, D. and Banks, R.: Distorted body perception in obesity. J. Nerv. Ment. Dis., *146*:465–467, 1968.

Cheek, D. B.: Human growth: Body composition, cell growth energy and intelligence. Philadelphia, Lea and Febiger, 1968.

Chen, R., Kenny, F. M. and Drash, A. L.: Cushing's disease in a boy: Serial steroid and growth hormone studies. Johns Hopkins Med. J., *125*:134–145, 1969.

Christakis, G., Sajecki, S., Hillman, R. W., Miller, E., Blumenthal, S. and Archer, M.: Effects of a combined nutrition education and physical fitness program on the weight status of obese high school boys. Fed. Proc., *25*:15–19, 1966.

Cochrane, W. A.: Overnutrition in prenatal and neonatal life: A problem. Can. Med. Assoc. J., *93*:893–899, 1965.

Cohen, M. M., Jr., Hall, B. D. and Smith, D. W., Graham, C. B. and Lampert, K. J.: A new syndrome of hypotonia, obesity, mental deficiency and facial, oral, ocular and limb anomalies. J. Pediatr., *83*:280–284, 1973.

Cohn, C.: Feeding patterns and some aspects of cholesterol metabolism. Fed. Proc., *23*:76–81, 1964.

Cohn, C., Joseph, D., Bell, L. and Allweiss, M. D.: Studies on the effects of feeding frequency and dietary composition on fat deposition. Ann. N.Y. Acad. Sci., *131*:507–518, 1965.

Coleman, D. L. and Hummel, K. P.: Obesity and diabetes-like syndromes in mice. *In*: Obesity in Perspective. Fogarty International Center Series on Preventive Medicine, Vol. II, Part II. (Bray, G. A., ed.) Washington, D.C., U.S. Government Printing Office, in press, 1976.

Coleman, D. L.: Effects of parabiosis of obese with diabetes and normal mice. Diabetologia, *9*:294–298, 1973.

Conn, J. W.: Obesity. II. Etiological aspects. Physiol. Rev., *24*:31–45, 1944.

Court, J. M. and Dunlop, M.: Obese from infancy: A clinical entity. In Howard, A. (ed.) Recent advances in Obesity Research: I Proc. 1st International Congress on obesity. International Congress on Obesity, London, Newman Publishing Ltd., 1975 pp 34-36.

Court, J. M., Dunlop, M., Leonard, I. and Leonard, R. F.: Five-hour oral glucose tolerance test in obese children. Arch. Dis. Child, 46:791–794, 1971.

Craddock, D.; Obesity and its Management. Edinburgh, Churchill Livingstone 1973
2nd ed.

Danforth, C. H.: Hereditary adiposity in mice. J. Hered., 18:153–162, 1927.

Darling, C. D. and Summerskill, J.: Emotional factors in obesity and weight reduction.
J. Am. Diet. Assoc., 29:1204–1207, 1953.

Das Gupta, T. K.: Tumors and tumor-like conditions of the adipose tissue. Curr. Probl.
Surg., 1–60, 1970.

Davenport, C. B.: Body build and its inheritance. Publication No. 329, Carnegie Institution, Washington, 1923.

Drash, A.: Relationship between diabetes mellitus and obesity in the child.
Metabolism, 22:337–344, 1973.

Dunlop, D. M., and Lyon, R. M. M.: A study of 523 Cases of Obesity. Edinburgh Med J.
38:561-577, 1931.

Dunn, H. G.: The Prader-Labhart-Willi syndrome: review of the literature and report of
nine cases. Acta Ped. Scand., (Suppl.)186:1–38, 1968.

Dwyer, J. T., Feldman, J. J. and Mayer, J.: Adolescent dieters: Who are they? Physical
characteristics, attitudes and dieting practices of adolescent girls. Am. J. Clin. Nutr.,
20:1045–1056, 1967.

Ehrenfeld, E. N., Rowe, H. and Auerbach, E.: Laurence-Moon-Bardet-Biedl syndrome
in Israel. Am. J. Ophthal., 70:524–532, 1970.

Eid, E. E.: Follow-up study of physical growth of children who had excessive weight
gain in first six months of life. Br. Med. J., 2:74–76, 1970.

Ellis, R. W. B. and Tallerman, K. M.: Obesity in childhood; A Study of 50 cases. Lancet,
2:615–620, 1934.

Erdheim, J.: Uber Hypophysenganggeschwulste und Hirncholesteatome. Sitzungsb.
Akad. Wissenschaften (Wien), 113:537–726, 1904.

Fabry, P., Fodor, J., Hejl, Z., Braun, T. and Zvolankova, K.: The frequency of meals: its
relationship to overweight, hypercholesterolemia, and decreased glucose tolerance.
Lancet 2:614–615, 1964.

Fabry, P., Hejda, S., Cerny, K., Osancova, K. and Pechar, J.: Effect of meal frequency in
school children. Changes in the weight-height proportion and skinfold thickness. Am.
J. Clin. Nutr., 18:358–361, 1966.

Fabry, P. and Tepperman, J.: Meal frequency — a possible factor in human pathology.
Am. J. Clin. Nutr., 23;1059–1068, 1970.

Falconer, D. S. and Isaacson, J. H.: Adipose, a new inherited obesity in the mouse. J.
Hered., 50:290–292, 1959.

Fenton, P. F. and Chase, H. B.: Effect of diet on obesity of yellow mice in inbred lines.
Proc. Soc. Exptl. Biol. Med. (N.Y.), 77:420–422, 1951.

Fomon, S. J.: A pediatrician looks at early nutrition. Bull. N.Y. Acad. Med., 47:569–578,
1971.

Fomon, S. J., Filer, L. J., Thomas, L. N., Rogers, R. R. and Proksh, A. M.: Relationship
between formula concentration and rate of growth in normal infants. J. Nutr.,
98:241–245, 1969.

Fomon, S. J., Thomas, L. N., Filer, L. J., Jr., Ziegler, E. E. and Leonard, M. T.: Food
consumption and growth of normal infants fed milk-based formulas. Acta Pediatr.
Scand.(Suppl)223:1–36, 1971.

Frohlich, A.: Ein Fall von Tumor der Hypophysis Cerebri ohne Akromegalie. Wiener.
Klin. Rdsch., 15:883–886, 1901.

Frohman, L. A. and Bernardis, L. L.: Growth hormone and insulin levels in weanling
rats with ventromedial hypothalamic lesions. Endocrinol., 82:1125–1132, 1968.

Frohman, L. A., Bernardis, L. L., Schnatz, J. D. and Burck, L.: Plasma insulin and
triglyceride levels after hypothalamus lesions in weanling rats. Am. J. Physiol.,
216:1496–1501, 1969.

Frohman, L. A., Goldman, J. K. and Bernardis, L. L.: Metabolism of intravenously
injected ^{14}C-glucose in weanling rats with hypothalamic obesity. Metabolism,
21:799–805, 1972a.

Frohman, L. A., Goldman, J. K. and Bernardis, L. L.: Studies of insulin sensitivity in
vivo in weanling rats with hypothalamic obesity. Metabolism, 21:1133–1142, 1972b.

Galton, D. J., Gilbert, C., Reekless, J. P. D. and Kaye, J.: Triglyceride storage disease. A group of inborn errors of triglyceride metabolism. Q. J. Med., 43:63–71, 1974.

Gellhorn, A. and Marks, P. A.: The composition and biosynthesis of lipids in human adipose tissue. J. Clin. Invest., 40:925–932, 1961.

Gilbert, C., Galton, D. J. and Kaye, J.: Triglyceride storage disease: A disorder of lipolysis in adipose tissue in two patients. Br. Med. J., 1:25–27, 1973.

Goldblatt, P. B., Moore, M. E. and Stunkard, A. J.: Social factors in obesity. J.A.M.A., 192:1039–1044, 1965.

Goldstein, J. L. and Fialkow, P. J.: The Alström Syndrome: Report of 3 cases with further delineation of the clinical, pathophysiological and genetic aspects of the disorder. Medicine, 52:53–71, 1973.

Goldzieher, J. W. and Green, J. A.: The polycystic ovary. I. Clinical and histologic features. J. Clin. Endocrinol. Metab., 22:325–338, 1962.

Gordon, M. B.: Endocrine obesity in children: Clinical and laboratory studies and results of treatment. J. Pediat., 10:204–220, 1937.

Grant, D. B.: Fasting serum insulin levels in childhood. Arch. Dis. Child, 42:375–378, 1967.

Greene, J. A.: A clinical study of the etiology of obesity. Ann. Intern. Med., 12:1797–1803, 1939.

Gurney, R.: Hereditary factor in obesity. Arch. Intern. Med., 57:557–561, 1936.

Gwinup, G., Byron, R. C., Roush, W., Kruger, F. and Hamwi, G. J.: Effect of nibbling versus gorging on glucose tolerance. Lancet 2:165–169, 1963.

Haase, K. E. and Hosenfeld, H.: Zur Fettsucht im Kindesalter. Zeitschrift fur Kinderheilkunde, 78:1–27, 1956.

Hackel, D. B., Frohman, L., Mikat, E., Lebovitz, H. E., Schmidt-Nielsen, K. and Kinney, T. D.: Effect of diet on the glucose tolerance and plasma insulin levels of the sand rat. Diabetes, 15:105–114, 1966.

Haessler, H. A. and Crawford, J. D.: Fatty acid composition and metabolic activity of depot fat in experimental obesity. Am. J. Physiol., 213:255–261, 1967.

Hales, C. N. and Kennedy, G. C.: Plasma glucose, nonesterified fatty acids and insulin concentrations in hypothalamic-hyperphagic rats. Biochem. J., 90:620–624, 1964.

Hall, B. D. and Smith, D. W.: Prader-Willi syndrome. J. Pediatr., 81:286–293, 1972.

Hamburger, W. W.: The psychology of weight reduction. J. Am. Diet. Assoc., 34:17–22, 1958.

Hamilton, C. R., Jr., Scully, R. E. and Kliman, B.: Hypogonadotropinism in Prader-Willi syndrome. Induction of puberty and spermatogenesis by clomiphene citrate. Am. J. Med., 52:322–329, 1972.

Hammar, S. L., Campbell, M. M., Campbell, V. A., Moores, N. L., Sareen, C., Gareis, F. J. and Lucas, B.: An interdisciplinary study of adolescent obesity. J. Pediatr., 80:373–383, 1972.

Hammond, W. H.: Measurement and interpretation of subcutaneous fat with norms for children and young adult males. Br. J. Prev. Soc. Med., 9:201–211, 1955.

Hampton, M. C., Huenemann, R. L., Shapiro, L. R. and Mitchell, B. W.: Caloric and nutrient intake of teenagers. J. Am. Diet. Assoc., 50:385, 1967.

Han, P. W.: Energy metabolism of tube-fed hypophysectomized rats bearing hypothalamic lesions. Am. J. Physiol., 215:1343–1350, 1968.

Heald, F. P.: The natural history of obesity. Adv. Psychosom. Med., 7:102–115, 1972.

Heald, F. P.: Natural history and physiological basis of adolescent obesity. Fed. Proc., 25:1–3, 1966.

Heald, F. P. and Hollander, R. J.: The relationship between obesity in adolescence and early growth. J. Pediatr., 67:35–38, 1965.

Heald, F. P., Muller, P. S. and Daugela, M. Z.: Glucose and free fatty acid metabolism in obese adolescents. Am. J. Clin. Nutr., 16:256–264, 1965.

Heldenberg, D., Tamir, I., Ashner, M. and Werbin, B.: Hyperphagia, obesity and diabetes insipidus due to a hypothalamic lesion in a girl. Helv. Paediat. Acta, 27:489–494, 1972.

Henschen, F. Morgagni's Syndrome: Hyperostosis Frontalis Interna, Virilismus, Obesitas. Edinburgh, Oliver and Boyd, 1949.

Hirsch, J. and Gallian, E.: Methods for the determination of adipose cell size in man and animals. J. Lipid Res., 9:110–119, 1968.

Hirsch, J. and Han, P. W.: Cellularity of rat adipose tissue: Effects of growth, starvation and obesity. J. Lipid Res., 10:77–82, 1969.

Hirsch, J. and Knittle, J. L.: Cellularity of obese and nonobese human adipose tissue. Fed. Proc., 29:1516–1521, 1970.

Hoebel, B. G. and Teitelbaum, P.: Weight regulation in normal and hypothalamic-hyperphagic rats. J. Comp. Physiol. Psychol., 61:189–192, 1966.

Hollifield, G.: Glucocorticoid-induced obesity–a model and a challenge. Am. J. Clin. Nutr., 21:1471–1474, 1968.

Hollifield, G. and Parson, W.: Metabolic adaptations to a "stuff and starve" feeding program. I. Studies of adipose tissue and liver glycogen in rats limited to a short daily feeding period. J. Clin. Invest., 41:245–249, 1962.

Huenemann, R. L., Hampton, M. C., Shapiro, L. R. and Behnke, A. R.: Adolescent food practices associated with obesity. Fed. Proc. 25:4–10, 1966a.

Huenemann, R. L., Shapiro, L. R., Hampton, M. C. and Mitchell, B. W.: A longitudinal study of gross body composition and body conformation and their association with food and activity in a teenage population. View of teenage subjects on body conformation, food and activity. Am. J. Clin. Nutr., 18:325–338, 1966b.

Huenemann, R. L.: Environmental factors associated with preschool obesity. I. Obesity in six month-old children. J. Am. Diet. Assoc., 64:480–487, 1974a.

Huenemann, R. L.: Environmental factors associated with preschool obesity. II. Obesity and food practices of children at successive age levels. J. Am. Diet. Assoc., 64:488–491, 1974.

Ikeda, K., Aska, A., Inouye, E. et al.: Monozygotic twins concordant for Prader-Willi syndrome. Jap. J. Human Gen., 18:220–225, 1973.

Ingalls, A. M., Dickie, M. M. and Snell, G. D.: Obese, new mutation in the mouse. J. Hered., 41:317–318, 1950.

Ingle, D. J.: A simple means of producing obesity in the rat. Proc. Soc. Expt. Bio. Med., 72:604–605, 1949.

Irwin, I. M. and Feeley, R. M.: Frequency and size of meals and serum lipids, nitrogen and mineral retention, fat digestibility and urinary thiamine and riboflavin in young women. Am. J. Clin. Nutr., 20:816–824, 1967.

Iverson, T.: Psychogenic obesity in children. Acta Ped., 42:8–19, 1953.

Jagannathan, S. N., Connell, W. F. and Beveridge, J. M. R.: Effects of gourmandizing and semicontinuous eating of equicaloric amounts of formula-type high fat diets on plasma cholesterol and triglyceride levels in human volunteer subjects. Am. J. Clin. Nutr., 15:90–93, 1964.

Jarlov, E.: The clinical types of abnormal obesity. Acta Med. Scand.(Suppl), 42:1–70, 1932.

Jelliffe, D. B.: Infantile overnutrition. (letter) Br. Med. J., 2:546, 1973.

Johnson, M. L., Burke, B. S. and Mayer, J.: The prevalence and incidence of obesity in a cross-section of elementary school children. Am. J. Clin. Nutr., 4:231–238, 1956.

Johnson, P. R. and Hirsch, J.: Cellularity of adipose depots in six strains of genetically obese mice. J. Lipid Res., 13:2–11, 1972.

Johnson, P., Zucker, L. M., Cruce, J. and Hirsch, J.: The cellularity of adipose depots in the genetically obese Zucker rat. J. Lipid Res., 12:706–714, 1971.

Joslin, E. P., Dublin, L. I. and Marks, H. H.: Studies in diabetes mellitus. III. Interpretations of the variations in diabetes incidence. Am. J. Med. Sci., 189:163–192, 1935.

Julkunen, H., Heinonen, O. P. and Pyorala, K.: Hyperostosis of the spine in an adult population. Its relation to hyperglycemia and obesity. Ann. Rheum. Dis., 30:605–612, 1971.

Kannel, W. B. and Gordon, T.: 3. Obesity and cardiovascular disease. The Framingham study. In: Obesity Symposium, December 4/5th, 1973. Servier Research Institute, Burland, W. L., Yudkin, J. and Samuel, P., eds.) London, 1974.

Kavlie, H. and White, T. T.: Pancreatic islet beta cell tumors and hyperplasia: Experience in 14 Seattle hospitals. Ann. Surg., 175:326–335, 1972.

Keen, H.: The Incomplete Story of obesity and diabetes. In Recent Advances in Obesity Research. (A. Howard, ed.): I. Proceedings of the first International Congress on Obesity. London, Newman Publishing Ltd., 1975, pp. 116-127.

Kemp, R.: The overall picture of obesity. Practitioner, 209:654–660, 1972.

Kennedy, G. C.: Role of depot fat in the hypothalamic control of food intake in rat. Proc. R. Soc. Lond. (Biol.); 140:578–592, 1953.

Kennedy, G. C. and Parker, R. A.: The islets of Langerhans in rats with hypothalamic obesity. Lancet 2:981–982, 1963.

Keys, A.: Coronary heart disease in seven countries. Circulation, 41(Suppl 1): 1–211, 1970.

Khosala, T. and Lowe, C. R.: Obesity and smoking habits by social class. Br. J. Prev. Soc. Med., 26:249–256, 1972.

Klein, O. and Ammann, F.: The syndrome of Laurence-Moon-Bardet-Biedl and allied diseases in Switzerland. J. Neurol. Sci., 9:479–513, 1969.

Klett, C. J. and Caffey, E. M., Jr.: Weight changes during treatment with phenothiazine derivatives. J. Neuropsychiat., 2:102-108, 1960.

Knittle, J. L.: Childhood obesity. Bull. N.Y. Acad. Med., 47:579–589, 1971.

Knittle, J. L.: Obesity in childhood: A problem in adipose tissue cellular development. J. Pediatr., 81:1048–1059, 19722.

Knittle, J. L.: Obesity and the cellularity of the adipose depot. Triangle, 13:57–62, 1974.

Knittle, J. L. and Hirsch, J.: Effect of early nutrition on the development of rat epididymal fat pads: cellularity and metabolism. J. Clin. Invest., 47:2091-2098, 1968.

Koletsky, S.: Pathologic findings and laboratory data in a new strain of obese hypertensive rats. Am. J. Pathol. 80:129-142, 1975.

Laurence, J. Z. and Moon, R. C.: Four cases of "retinitis pigmentosa," occurring in the same family, and accompanied by general imperfections of development. Ophthal. Rev., 2:32–41, 1866.

Lefley, H. P.: Masculinity-femininity in obese women. J. Consult. Clin. Psychol., 37:180–186, 1971.

Lemonnier, D.: Effect of age, sex and sites on the cellularity of the adipose tissue in mice and rats rendered obese by a high-fat diet. J. Clin. Invest., 51:2907-2915, 1972.

Leveille, G. A.: Adipose tissue metabolism: Influence of periodicity of eating and diet composition. Fed. Proc., 29:1294–1301, 1970.

Lloyd, J. K., Wolf, O. H. and Whalen, W. S.: Childhood obesity: A long-term study of height and weight. Br. Med. J., 2:145, 1961.

Lloyd, J. K.: Obesity in childhood. Adv. Psychosom. Dis., 7:110–115, 1972.

Lowe, C. R. and Gibson, J. R.: Changes in body weight associated with age and marital status. Br. Med. J., 2:1006–1008, 1955.

Mabrey, R. E.: Chordoma: A study of 150 cases. Am. J. Cancer., 25:501–517, 1935.

MacDonald, A. and Feiwel, M.: A review of the concept of Weber-Christian panniculitis with a report of five cases. Br. J. Dermatol., 80:355–361, 1968.

MacKay, E. M., Callaway, J. W. and Barnes, R. H.: Hyperalimentation in normal animals produced by protamine insulin. J. Nutr., 20:59–66, 1940.

MacMillan, D. R., Kim, C. B. and Weisskopf, B.: Syndrome of growth resistance, obesity and intellectual impairment with precocious puberty. Arch. Dis. Child., 47:119–121, 1972.

Mahler, R. J. and Szabo, O.: Amelioration of insulin resistance in obese mice. Am. J. Physiol., 221:980–983, 1971.

Mayer, J.: The obese hyperglycemia syndrome of mice as an example of metabolic obesity. Am. J. Clin. Nutr., 8:712–718, 1960.

Mayer, J.: Genetic, traumatic and environmental factors in the etiology of obesity. Physiol. Rev., 33:472–508, 1953.

Mayer, J.: Obesity in adolescence. Med. Clin. North Am. 49:421–432, 1965.

Mayer, J.: Physical activity and anthropometric measurements of obese adolescents. Fed. Proc., 25:11–14, 1966.

Mayer, J., Marshall, N. B., Vitale, J. J., Christensen, J. H., Moshagekhi, M. B. and Stare, F. J.: Exercise, food intake and body weight in normal rats and genetically obese adult mice. Am. J. Physiol., 177:544–548, 1954.

Mayer, J., Roy, P. and Mitra, R. P.: Relation between caloric intake, body weight and physical work.: Studies in an industrial male population in West Bengal. Am. J. Clin. Nutr., 4:169–175, 1956.

McKeown, T. and Record, R. G.: The influence of reproduction on body weight in women. J. Endocrinol., 15:393–409, 1957a.

McKeown, T. and Record, R. G.: The influence of body weight on reproductive function in women. J. Endocrinol., 15:410–422, 1957b.

McKeown, T. and Record, R. G.: The influence of weight and height on weight changes associated with pregnancy in women. J. Endocrinol., 15:423–429, 1957c.

Medical Staff Conference. The Prader-Willi syndrome. Calif. Med., 112:65–73, 1970.

Mellbin, T. and Vuille, J. C.: Physical development at 7 years in relation to velocity of weight gain in infancy with special reference to incidence overweight. Br. J. Prev. Soc. Med., 27:225–235, 1973.

Monello, L. F. and Mayer, J.: Obese adolescent girls. An unrecognized "minority" group? Am. J. Clin. Nutr., 13:35–39, 1963.

Moore, M. E., Stunkard, A. J. and Srole, L.: Obesity, social class and mental illness. J.A.M.A., 181:962–966, 1962.

Morgan, A. F. (ed.): Nutritional Status U.S.A. California Agricultural Experiment Station Bulletin, No. 769, 1959.

Morgner, K. D., Geisthövel, W., Niedergerke, U. and Muhlen, A. V. Z.: Hypogonadismas due to luteotropin-releasing hormone (LHRH) deficiency in a child with Prader-Labhart-Willi Syndrome. Deut. Med. Wschr., 99:1196–1198, 1974.

Mossberg, H. O.: Obesity in children: A clinical-prognostical investigation. Acta Ped., 35: Suppl. 2, 1–122, 1948.

Mullins, A. G.: The prognosis in juvenile obesity. Arch. Dis. Child., 33:307–314, 1958.

Nelson, R. A., Anderson, L. F., Gastineau, C. F., Hayles, A. B., and Stamnes, C. L.: Physiology and natural history of obesity. J.A.M.A., 223:627–630, 1973.

Newman, H. H., Freeman, F. N., Holzinger, K. J.: Twins: A study of heredity and environment. Chicago, University of Chicago Press, 1937.

Noorden, K. Von: Die Fettsucht. Nothnagel. Spec. Pathol. Ther., 7:1–156, 1900.

Oscai, L. B., Babirak, S. P., McGarr, J. A. and Spirakis, C. N.: Effect of exercise on adipose tissue cellularity. Fed. Proc., 33:1956–1958, 1974.

Parkin, J. M.: Syndrome of growth resistance, obesity and intellectual impairmeent with precocious puberty. Arch. Dis. Child, 48:86–87, 1973.

Parra, A., Cervantes, C. and Schultz, R. B.: Immunoreactive insulin and growth hormone responses in patients with Prader-Willi syndrome. J. Pediatr., 83:587–593, 1973.

Parra-Covarrubias, A., Rivera-Rodrigues, I. and Almaraz-Ugalde, A.: Cephalic phase of insulin secretion in obese adolescents. Diabetes, 20:800–802, 1971.

Pitts, G. C. and Bullard, T. R.: Some interspecific aspects of body composition in mammals. In: Body composition in animals and Man. Proc of a Symposium May 4–6, 1967 at Univ. of Missouri. Washington, D.C., Publ #1598, Natl. Acad. Sci., pp. 45–70, 1968.

Powley, T. L. and Opsahl, C.: Failure of vagotomy to reverse obesity in the genetically obese Zucker rat. Am. J. Physiol., 226:34–38, 1974a.

Powley, T. L. and Opsahl, C. A.: Ventromedical hypothalamic obesity abolished by subdiaphragmatic vagotomy. Am. J. Physiol., 226:25–33, 1974b.

Prader, A., Labhart, A. and Willi, H.: Ein Syndrom von Adipositas, Kleinwuchs, Kryptorchismus und Oligophrenie nach myotonie-artigem Zustand im Neugeborenenalter. Schweiz. Med. Wschr., 86:1260–1261, 1956. (abs)

Prader, A. and Willi, H.: Das Syndrom von Imbezillitat, Adipositas, Muskelhypotonie, Hypogenitalismus, Hypogonadismus und Diabetes mellitus mit "myatonie"– Anamnese. Second International Congress on Mental Retardation. S. Karger Basel, Part I., p. 353, 1963.

Pyke, D. A. and Please, N. W.: Obesity parity and diabetes. J. Endocrinol. 15:26–33, 1957.

Quaade, F.: Obese children: Anthropology and Environment. Copenhagen, Danish Science Press, Ltd., 1955.

Raiti, S., Trias, E., Levitsky, L. and Grossman, M. S.: Oxandrolone and human growth hormone. Comparison of growth-stimulating effects in short children. Am. J. Dis. Child, 126:597–600, 1973.

Renold, A. E., Kikuchi, M., Gutzeit, A. H., Amherdt, M. and Orci, L.: Relationship between obesity and spontaneous inappropriate hyperglycemia (Diabetes) in animals. In: Obesity in Perspective. Fogarty International Center Series on Preventive Medicine, Vol II, Part II (Bray, G. A., ed.) Washington, D.C., U.S. Government Printing Office, 1976.

Ridley, P. T. and Brooks, F. P.: Alterations in gastric secretion following hypothalamic lesions producing hyperphagia. Am. J. Physiol., 209:319–323, 1965.

Rony, H. R.: Obesity and leanness. Philadelphia, Lea and Febiger, 1940.

Rüedi, B.: Identical twins with marked weight dissimilarity. Helv. Med. Acta, 35:512–520, 1971.

Schemmel, R., Mickelsen, O. and Gill, J. L.: Dietary obesity in rats: Body weight and fat accretion in seven strains of rats. J. Nutr., *100*:1041–1048, 1970.

Schultz, R. B. and Parra, A.: Relationship between body composition and insulin and growth hormone responses in obese adolescents. Diabetes, *19*:492–501, 1970.

Sharp, J. V., Lynch, M. J. and Doohen, D. J.: Liposarcoma. Am. Surg., *35*:121–124, 1969.

Sheldon, J. H.: Maternal obesity. Lancet, *2*:869–873, 1949.

Shields, J.: Monozygotic twins brought up apart and brought up together. London, Oxford University Press, 1962.

Shukla, A., Forsyth, H. A., Anderson, C. M. and Marnah, S. M.: Infantile overnutrition in the first year of life: A field study in Dudley, Worcestershire. Br. Med. J., *4*:507–515, 1972.

Silverstone, J. T. and Stunkard, A. J.: The anorectic effect of dexamphetamine sulphate. Br. J. Pharmacol., *33*:513–522, 1968.

Sjostrom, L., Bjorntorp, P. and Vrana, J.: Microscopic fat cell size measurements on frozen-out adipose tissue in comparison with automatic determinations of osmium-fixed fat cells. J. Lipid Res., *12*:521–530, 1971.

Slaunwhite, W. R., III, Goldman, J. K. and Bernardis, L. L.: Sequential changes in glucose metabolism by adipose tissue and liver of rats after destruction of the ventromedial hypothalamic nuclei: Effect of three dietary regimens. Metabolism, *21*:619–631, 1972.

Soffer, L. J., Iannaccone, A. and Gabrilove, J. L.: Cushing's syndrome. Am. J. Med., *30*:128–146, 1961.

Stefanik, P. A., Heald, F. P., Jr. and Mayer, J.: Caloric intake in relation to energy output of obese and non-obese adolescent boys. Am. J. Clin. Nutr., 7:55–62, 1959.

Stevenson, J. A. F.: Neural control of food and water intake. *In*: The Hypothalamus, (Haymaker, W., Anderson, E., and Nauta, W. J. H., eds.). Springfield, Charles C Thomas, 1969, pp. 524–621.

Stuart, H. C. and Sobel, E. H.: Thickness of the skin and subcutaneous tissue by age and sex in childhood. J. Pediatr., *28*:637–647, 1946.

Stunkard, A. J.: Eating patterns and obesity. Psychiatr. Q., *33*:284–295, 1959.

Stunkard, J., D'Aquili, E., Fox, S. and Filion, R. D. L.: Influence of social class on obesity and thinness in children. J.A.M.A., *221*:579–584, 1972.

Stunkard, A. J. and Burt, V.: Obesity and the body image. II. Age at onset of disturbances in the body image. Am. J. Psychiat., *123*:1443–1447, 1967.

Stunkard, A. J. and Pestka, J.: The physical activity of obese girls. J. Dis. Child., *103*:812–817, 1962.

Stunkard, A. J. and Mendelson, M.: Obesity and the body image. I. Characteristics of disturbances in the body image of some obese persons. Am. J. Psychiatr., *123*:1296–1300, 1967.

Summers, W. E., Watson, R. L., Woolridge, W. H. and Langford, H. G.: Hypertension, obesity and fibromyomata uteri, as a syndrome. Arch. Intern. Med., *128*:750–754, 1971.

Suczek, R. F.: The group approach to weight reduction. 2. Psychologic aspects of obesity and group weight reduction. J. Am. Diet. Assoc., *30*:442–446, 1954.

Svolos, D. G.: Craniopharyngiomas. Acta Chir. Scand. (Suppl) *403*, 1969.

Swanson, D. W. and Dinello, F. A.: Follow-up of patients starved for obesity. Psychom. Med., *32*:209–214, 1970.

Taitz, L. S.: Infantile overnutrition among artificially fed infants in the Sheffield Region. Br. Med. J., *1*:315–316, 1971.

Tanner, J. M. and Whitehouse, R. H.: Standards for subcutaneous fat in British children: Percentiles for thickness of skinfolds over triceps and below scapula. Br. Med. J., *1*:446–450, 1962.

Tanner, J. M., Whitehouse, R. H. and Takaishi, M.: Standards from birth to maturity for height, weight, height velocity and weight velocity. Arch. Dis. Child, *41*:613–635, 1966.

Ten State Nutrition Survey. Washington, D.C. Department of Health, Education and Welfare Publication No. (HSM) 72–8131, 1972.

Tepperman, J. and Tepperman, H. M.: Gluconeogenesis, lipogenesis and the Sherringtoman metaphor. Fed. Proc., *29*:1284–1293, 1970.

Tolis, G., Lewis, W., Verdy, M., Friesen, H. G., Solomon, S., Pagalis, G., Pavlatos, F., Fessas, P. H. and Rochefort, J. G.: Anterior pituitary function in the Prader-Labhart-

Willi (PLW) syndrome. J. Clin. Endocrinol. Metab., 39:1061–1066, 1974.

Trygstad, O.: Childhood obesity with particular reference to etiological factors. World Med. J., 3:49–51, 1972.

Vague, J.: The degree of masculine differentiation of obesities: A factor in determining predisposition to diabetes atherosclerosis, gout and uric calculus disease. Am. J. Clin. Nutr., 4:20, 1956.

Vague, J. and Boyer, J.: The regulation of the adipose tissue mass. Excerpta Medica, (Amsterdam) 1974.

Von Verschuer, O.: Die vererbungsbiologische Zwillingsforschung. Ergeb. Inn. Med. Kinderheilk, 31:35–120, 1927.

Wade, G. N.: Gonadal hormones and behavioral regulation of body weight. Physiol. Behav., 8:523–534, 1972.

Waltzkin, L.: Weight gain among hospitalized mentally ill men. Behav. Neuropsychiat., 1:15–18, 1969.

Weinberg, N., Mendelson, M. and Stunkard, A.: A failure to find distinctive personality features in a group of obese men. Am. J. Psychiat., 117:1035–1037, 1961.

Weitze, M.: Hereditary adiposity in mice and the cause of this anomaly. Copenhagen, University of Copenhagen Press 1960, p. 96.

Werkman, S. L. and Greenberg, E. S.: Personality and interest patterns of obese adolescent girls. Psychosom. Med., 29:72–80, 1967.

West, K. M. and Kalbfleisch, J. M.: Influence of nutritional factors on prevalence of diabetes. Diabetes, 20:99–108, 1971.

Wick., G., Sundick, R. S. and Albini, B.: The obese strain (OS) of chickens: An animal model with spontaneous autoimmune thyroiditis. Clin. Immun., 3:272–300, 1974.

Widdowson, E. M. and McCance, R. A.: Some effects of accelerating growth I. General somatic development. Proc. Roy. Soc. Biol., 152:188–206, 1960.

Withers, R. F. J.: Problems in the genetics of human obesity. Eugen. Rev., 56:81–90, 1964.

Wolff, O. H.: Obesity in childhood. A study of the birth weight, the height and the onset of puberty. Q. J. Med., 24:109–123, 1955.

York, D. A. and Bray, G. A.: Dependence of hypothalamic obesity on insulin, the pituitary and the adrenal gland. Endocrinology, 90:885–894, 1972.

Young, C. M., Hutter, L. F. and Scanlan, S. S.: Metabolic effects of meal frequency in normal young men. J. Am. Diet. Assoc., 61:391–398, 1972.

Zárate, A., Soria, J. and Canales, E. S. et al.: Pituitary response to synthetic luteinizing hormone in Prader-Willi syndrome, prepubertal and pubertal children. Neuroendocrinol., 13:321–326, 1973/74.

Zondek, B.: Die Krankheiten der endokrinen Drüsen. Berlin, 1926.

Zucker, L. M. and Zucker, T. F.: Fatty, a new mutation in the rat. J. Hered., 52:275–278, 1961.

CHAPTER 6

THE RISKS AND DISADVANTAGES OF OBESITY

The disadvantages of increased body fat can be expressed in many ways. Overweight may decrease longevity, it may aggravate the onset and clinical progression of other diseases, and it may modify the quality of life associated with one's social or economic status. We shall review some of the data relating overweight and where possible, obesity, to one's life style in an effort to put the risks of obesity into proper perspective.

It must be kept clearly in mind that almost all of the data we shall review was collected and analyzed in terms of overweight. As noted in Chapter 1, overweight refers to deviations in body weight from some "standard weight" related to height. Being overweight does not necessarily imply being obese. This distinction is most critical in athletes, but also applies to other groups. The correlation between measures of body weight such as relative weight, percent overweight, ponderal index (ht/ $\sqrt[3]{wt}$) or body mass index (wt/ht^2 and skinfolds or body density is 0.8 or less. Until better methods of measuring obesity are available we must interpret with care the results of epidemiologic studies using only body weight.

BODY WEIGHT AND LIFE EXPECTANCY

Two kinds of studies have evaluated the effects of overweight on longevity. The most widely quoted and most extensive studies are the retrospective analyses of the effects of relative weight (i.e., weight in relation to height) on individuals having life insurance policies who were followed up in collaborative studies by the insurance industry Society of Actuaries (1913, 1929, 1959). The most recent study utiliz-

215

ing this data was published in 1959 by the Society of Actuaries with the title "Body Build and Blood Pressure." It is similar to the previous studies published by the insurance industry and provides a broad basis for analyzing the effect of overweight on longevity, (Baird, 1971; Donald, 1973; Downes, 1953; Goodman, 1955; Hutchinson, 1961; Sanders, 1959; Britten, 1933). The second kind of data involves prospective studies of carefully controlled populations. A number of such studies are available for analysis.

RETROSPECTIVE STUDIES ON OVERWEIGHT AND LONGEVITY

Life Insurance Industry

In most cases the applicant for life insurance must undergo a medical examination. Among the data which are routinely recorded are height, weight and blood pressure, although in many cases the height and weight are obtained from verbal reports by the patient and are not actually measured. The analysis of such data with all of its limitations (Seltzer, 1966, 1969) has provided us with the major retrospective studies on the effects of overweight on mortality and morbidity.

In evaluating these studies it is important to recognize that the population under study is selected. They are generally of above average economic circumstances, are Caucasian, are free of serious medical defects, and are usually engaged in "safe" occupations. Such a group represents a special segment of the population. Results from the analysis of this data may thus not be applicable to the entire population. That this is so is suggested by the fact that mortality among insured individuals is less than the mortality rate for the entire population at all ages between 15 and 70 years (Mann, 1971, 1974). However, this might have been expected since the insured subjects under study were in "safe" occupations and were free from major disease at the time the insurance policy was obtained.

Figure 6–1 summarizes the effect of deviations from normal body weight on death rate, (Bray, Davidson and Drenick, 1972). For this figure the death rate for each age group was taken as 100 percent, and the groups were subdivided into various percentage deviations from the mean for the entire age group. The death rate in each of these subgroups compared to the population as a whole is expressed as a percentage deviation from 100. The minimum death rate for these two age groups is slightly less than the average weight for the entire population. As body weight increases above the average for the group, there is a progressive increase in "excess mortality." There is, similarly, a small increase in excess mortality with very low body weight. This is more pronounced in the younger age group than in the older

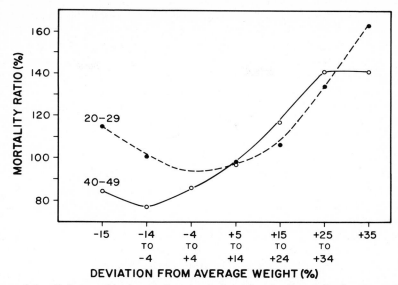

Figure 6–1. Relation of body weight to mortality. The death rate for deviations from the mean body weight has been plotted for persons aged 20 to 29 and 40 to 49. The 100 percent figure on the ordinate represents the number of deaths per 100,000 insured people of all weights in each age group. The deviations from this 100 percent figure represent greater or lesser numbers of deaths in the subgroups of the population whose deviations in body weight are plotted on the abscissa. (Reprinted from Bray, Davidson and Drenick, 1972, with permission from the Annals of Internal Medicine.)

one and may reflect the higher rate of tuberculosis which was a much more common disease at the time these insurance policies were issued.

The most recent study, performed by the Metroplitan Life Insurance Company, evaluated 26,000 policies on men and 25,000 policies on women issued between 1925 and 1934 on people who were overweight and between the ages of 20 and 64 at the time the policy was issued (Armstrong, 1951; Marks, 1960). These overweight policy holders were traced through 1950, and the results were expressed in relation to a much larger population who were not overweight and who obtained insurance policies at standard risks. The relation of actual deaths of these overweight men and women to the deaths expected for normal weight subjects is shown in Table 6–1. For the overweight men the death rate was one and a half times that for the normal weight men. It was nearly as high for women. Among the men the highest death rate was seen in the youngest age groups, but no similar effect of age was seen in the women. At all ages there was an increased death rate associated with overweight.

The factors involved in this excess mortality are summarized in Table 6–2. Diabetes mellitus, gallbladder disease, and cardiovascular-renal disease were the major causes of excess mortality.

TABLE 6–1.   *Effect of Overweight on Life Expectancy**

AGE AT INITIAL EXAMINATION	ACTUAL DEATHS AMONG OVERWEIGHT EXPECTED DEATHS OF NORMAL WEIGHT	
	Men	*Women*
20 to 29	180	134
30 to 39	169	152
40 to 49	152	150
50 to 64	131	138
All ages 20 to 64	150	147

*Adapted from Armstrong et al.: J.A.M.A., *147*:1007–1014, 1951.

Since cardiovascular diseases now account for more than half of the total deaths in the United States, the excess mortality associated with overweight could be a very important factor if confirmed by other studies. The degree of excess mortality associated with overweight rises with the degree of excess weight. It is greater among males than females, and is worse at younger than at older ages.

To make this more concrete, let me illustrate the effect of a 100 pound weight difference on life expectancy of a man aged 50. At 70 inches (179 cm) the suitable weight is 170 pounds (77 kg). Life expectancy for such a man is 25 years, and the death rate is 5 to 10/1000. If a man 70 inches tall weighed 270 pounds and were free of hypertension and diabetes mellitus his life expectancy would be only 18 years and the death rate increased 50 to 100 percent (i.e., 10 to 20/1000). If an overweight man has either diabetes mellitus or hypertension, life expectancy is shortened still further.

In a critical evaluation of the life insurance data, Seltzer (1966, 1969) pointed out that the effects on mortality only became significant when body weight was more than 30 percent above "desirable" levels. Converting the data from the Build and Blood Pressure Study into body mass index, we obtained the relationship shown in Figure 6–2. Note that only at a body mass index of more than 30 did excess

TABLE 6–2.   *Principal Causes of Death among the Overweight**

CAUSE	PERCENTAGE OF EXPECTED RATE	
	Men	*Women*
Diabetes mellitus	383	372
Gallbladder disease	206	284
Cardiovascular-renal	149	177
Accidents	111†	135
Cancer	97†	100†
Suicide	78†	73
Tuberculosis	21	35

*Adapted from Marks, H. H.: Bull. N.Y. Acad. Sci., *36*:296–312, 1960.
†Not statistically significant.

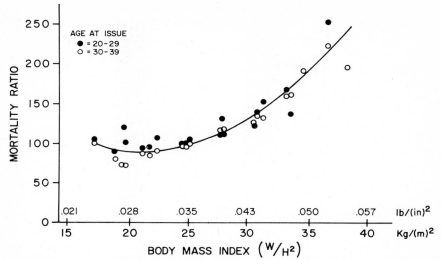

Figure 6–2. Relation of body mass index to mortality. (The data from the Build and Blood Pressure study have been replotted from the calculations of Seltzer: New Eng. J. Med., 274:254–259, 1966.)

mortality become prominent, although a body mass index of 27 is considered overweight (Chapter 1).

One other illustration may also help to dramatize the hazards to life of gross obesity. Drenick (1975) re-examined 127 grossly obese men who had originally been treated by fasting. Eighteen had died in the interval after leaving the hospital. The average age of this group was 41 years. For men of comparable age and standard weight, life insurance figures indicate that only three would be expected to die in the same length of time. The death rate was thus increased sixfold in this group of obese men.

If significant degrees of "overweight" are "hazardous to your health," does weight reduction improve longevity? Few data are available to help answer this question, except one study from the life insurance industry (Dublin, 1953; Dublin and Marks, 1951; Marks, 1960). These individuals came from a group of people who had initially received sub-standard insurance because they were overweight but who subsequently were issued other policies at the lower weight. Among policy holders who lost weight and maintained the loss, life expectancy improved to that of insured people with "standard" risk (Fig. 6–3).

Postmortem Correlation of Body Weight with Atherosclerosis

Several retrospective studies have examined the effects of overweight on atherosclerotic changes in the cardiovascular system.

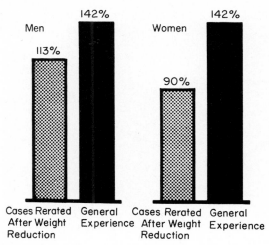

Figure 6–3. Effect of weight loss on mortality. The mortality ratio is calculated for overweight policy holders, relative to normal weight individuals and those who were reinsured after losing weight. Both men and women who lost weight and were reinsured had an improved life expectancy. (Reprinted from Marks, H. H.: Bull., N.Y. Acad. Sci., 36:296–312, 1960, with permission.)

Wilens (1947) reported on the incidence of atherosclerosis in 1000 consecutive autopsies to which were added 250 autopsies on "obese subjects." Of this total 395 were defined as obese on the basis of an autopsy protocol in which the abdominal panniculus was thicker than 3 centimeters. In the obese males the incidence of "severe" atherosclerosis was increased 2.5 times as compared to individuals with poor nutrition (i.e., an abdominal panniculus of less than 1 centimeter). The relationship between nutritional status and the incidence of atherosclerotic lesions was similar in each decade, and exclusion of the hypertensive patients did not change it.

In contrast to the data of Wilens are the data from Faber and Land (1949), Wilkens et al., (1959), Spain et al. (1953), and Kannel and Gordon (1974) (Table 6–3). Wilkins and his collaborators studied 500 consecutive autopsies, 153 of whom died with evidence of atherosclerotic disease. In this group obesity was expressed as the ratio of weight over height. By this criterion 47 males and 30 females were classified as overweight. In these patients obesity had a minor effect on atherosclerosis, except in the coronary artery and then only in men. The authors concluded ". . . obesity . . ., in general, exerts only a minor influence on the degree of atherosclerosis." Faber and Land found no effect of obesity on the atherosclerotic lesions in the aorta or on its cholesterol content. Spain et al. were also unable to detect a relationship between obesity and the presence of atherosclerotic lesions in the coronary arteries (Table 6–4) (see also Cramer et al., 1966).

TABLE 6–3. *Reported Associations of Overweight and Atherosclerosis Determined at Post Mortem Examination*

AUTHOR	YEAR	NO. SUBJECTS	CRITERION FOR OVERWEIGHT	ASSOCIATIONS WITH OVERWEIGHT
Wilens	1947	1250	panniculus >3 cm	↑Incidence of severe atherosclerotic lesions
Faber	1949	408	relative weight	No effect on weight of aorta or its content of cholesterol or calcium
Spain	1953	111	somatotype	No effect of obesity on coronary atherosclerosis
Wilkins	1959	500	wt/ht	Minor influence on atherosclerosis except in coronaries of males where it had significant effect
Kannel	1974	66	relative weight	↑Heart weight ↑Thickness of left ventricle No effect on atherosclerosis

Most recently Kannel and Gordon (1974) have examined the relationship of body weight to the findings on autopsy in patients participating in the Framingham study. Body weight was related to the weight of the left ventricle, as well as its thickness. Heavier patients had larger and heavier hearts (Amad et al., 1965). These effects of overweight on the heart were more prominent in the women than in men. These correlations of body weight, heart weight and thickness of the left ventricle were statistically significant and were independent of an association with blood pressure, hyperglycemia or hypercholesterolemia. However, there was little relation of body weight to the frequency of atherosclerotic lesions in the coronary arteries. It would thus appear that obesity had a weak atherogenic effect but a significant hemodynamic effect on the function of the myocardium as measured in patients dying in Framingham, Massachusetts.

PROSPECTIVE STUDIES OF OVERWEIGHT AND LONGEVITY

Several prospective studies have also examined the importance of overweight and obesity in the development of cardiovascular disease. Table 6–4 summarizes these associations from a number of studies. We will examine several of them in detail, including the Framingham study (Gordon and Kannel, 1973; Kannel and Gordon, 1974), The International Cooperative Study of Cardiovascular Epidemiology (Car-

TABLE 6–4. *Associations Between Body Weight, Morbidity and Mortality*

Author	Year	No. of Subjects	Sex	Type of Study	Criteria for Overweight or Obesity	Associations
Robinson and Brucer	1940	3436 2184	M F	Cross sectional	a. wt/ht $\frac{wt \times 100}{ht \times chest\ circumference}$ b.	Hypertension correlated with body build (criteria b) but uncertain correlation with obesity if build held constant.
Levy et al.	1946	22,741	M	Retrospective	wt/ht	Overweight associated with hypertension. Overweight *alone* did not increase mortality.
Garn et al.	1951	97	M	Retrospective	Body weight	Body weight similar in matched men with and without myocardial infarction.
Armstrong et al. Marks	1951 1960	25,998 24,901	M F	Retrospective	Relative weight	Overweight ↑ overall mortality by 1.5 times.
Stamler	1966	756	M	Prospective	Relative weight	Overweight doubled risk of developing coronary disease.
Spain et al.	1963	5000	M	Prospective (5 year report)	a. Relative weight b. Somatotype	Overweight individuals with hypertension or diabetes mellitus have higher prevalence of coronary disease. Uncomplicated overweight has no increased prevalence.
Dunn et al.	1970	13,148	M	Prospective (14 years)	Relative weight	Overweight (>25%) associated with hypertension or diabetes mellitus, not with coronary heart disease.

Author	Year	N	Sex	Type	Measure	Findings
Rosenman et al.	1970	3182	M	Prospective (4½ years)	Ponderal index $(ht^{/3}\sqrt{wt})$	Ponderal index alone is not a useful prediction of coronary heart disease.
Chapman et al.	1971	1859	M	Prospective (15 years)	Ponderal index $(ht^{/3}\sqrt{wt})$	Overweight associated with myocardial infarction in men under 40 but not those over 40. Angina pectoris increased in overweight men over 40.
Heyden, Cassel et al.	1971	3102	M	Prospective	$wt/(ht)^2$	Overweight associated with cerebro-vascular incidents. Among smokers overweight associated with coronary heart disease.
Cotton et al.	1972	91	M	Retrospective (98 matched men)	$wt/(ht)^2$	Overweight not associated with coronary heart disease.
Carlson et al.	1972	3168	M	Prospective	wt/ht	Wt/Ht had no prognostic significance for coronary heart disease.
Keys et al.	1972	2442 (U.S.) 2439 (N. Europe) 6519 (S. Europe)	M M M	Prospective	Relative weight Skinfolds $wt/(ht)^2$	Overweight and obesity associated with coronary heart disease in U.S. and S. European men. Effect mainly through association of overweight and hypertension.
Rimm et al.	1972	73,532	F	Retrospective	wt/ht	Overweight associated with hypertension, diabetes mellitus and gallbladder disease.
Kannel and Gordon	1974	5209	M+F	Prospective (18 years)	Relative weight	Overweight associated with sudden death and angina pectoris. Overweight is not a major independent prediction.

diovascular Disease in Seven Countries) (Keys, 1970, 1975, and the study of Evans County, Georgia by Cassel (1971a, b) (Heyden et al., 1971a, b).

The Framingham Study

One of the most widely quoted studies on the risk factors related to coronary artery disease was conducted on 5209 men and women living in Framingham, Massachusetts whose initial examinations were conducted between 1948 and 1950 (Dawber et al., 1957; Kannel et al., 1967; Kannel and Gordon, 1974). In this study participants were examined at two year intervals and the incidence of various forms of heart disease including angina pectoris, sudden death, myocardial infarction and cerebral vascular disease was related to relative body weight.

Two criteria have been used to define relative body weight. The first, called "Framingham relative weight," is based on the median weights for heights obtained from the initial examination carried out between 1948 and 1950. The median body weights on subjects in Framingham were almost identical with the upper limits for individuals with heavy frame in the tables provided by the Metropolitan Life Insurance Company (Chapter 1). In order to make the Framingham data more comparable with other data in the literature, Kannel et al. (1967) have also compared body weights to the median weight of the Metropolian Life Insurance table.

Using these "desirable weights" approximately 15 percent of the men and 20 percent of the women were at least 35 percent overweight, and 3 percent of men and 9 percent of the women were more than 50 percent overweight. The investigators in Framingham have also measured skinfold thickness and arm circumferences during the 18 years in which this study has been in progress. The correlations between relative body weight and skinfold thickness or arm circumference are greater than r=0.8 suggesting that the associations noted below between cardiovascular disease and "overweight" are reflections of the association with obesity.

In this study weight gain was associated with a rise in serum lipids, an increase in blood pressure, an impairment in glucose tolerance and a slight rise in uric acid (Kannel and Gordon, 1974). The overall mortality in the overweight participants of both sexes was lower than for those of normal body weight, but mortality from coronary artery disease, and especially sudden death, was substantially higher in the overweight. There was a higher incidence of coronary attacks, coronary insufficiency, cerebral vascular infarction and congestive heart failure in the overweight. There was, however, no effect of excess weight on the frequency of intermittent claudication.

By using multivariate analysis the investigators could assign a relative risk to each factor associated with cardiovascular disease. With this analysis it was clear that, in women, the net effect of overweight or obesity was small for all cardiovascular events except congestive heart failure. For males there was a significant relationship between overweight and cardiovascular mortality, even when such atherogenic factors as hypertension, smoking and family history were taken into account. Both angina pectoris and coronary attacks were significantly related to overweight in the men. The attack rate of myocardial infarction, however, had a less striking relation to overweight. This relatively small effect of excess body weight on the likelihood of developing a myocardial infarction has been observed in most of the prospective studies which have been conducted (Table 6–5). This difference in effects of overweight on the various manifestations of cardiovascular disease merits additional consideration and will be reviewed later.

In summary, "Although there is some unique effect, obesity (overweight) is clearly not a major independent predictor of cardiovascular incidence (disease) given knowledge of the major risk factors. This is not to say that overweight is an unimportant consideration in prophylaxis against cardiovascular disease, but rather that it is not particularly helpful in estimating risks." In general other risk factors such as sex, age, hypertension, elevated cholesterol, and smoking were better discriminators for coronary artery disease than is obesity.

The International Cooperative Study of Cardiovascular Epidemiology

This prospective study involved an international collaborative examination of coronary heart disease in fourteen cohorts of men in Holland and Finland (2439 men called the Northern European group), in Italy, Greece and Yugoslavia (6519 men called the Southern European group), and in railway workers in the United States (2442 men) (Keys, 1970, 1975; Keys et al., 1972). Men at entry into the study were between 40 and 59 years old. The assessment of body weight and fatness was based on the ratio of weight/(height) ^{2} (body mass index),

TABLE 6–5. *Effects of Weight Loss of "Atherogenic Traits"** *

Atherogenic Trait	Mean Decrease with 10 Percent Reduction in Body Weight in Males
Cholesterol	11 mg/dl
Blood pressure-systolic	5 mm/Hg
Blood glucose	2 mg/dl
Uric acid	0.4 mg/dl

*From Kannel and Gordon (1974), with permission.

and the obese were those individuals where the body mass index was greater than 27. Measurements of the triceps and subscapular skinfolds were also used, and obesity was defined as the sum of the skinfolds greater than 37 mm.

Using these criteria, over half (52.3 percent) of the United States railway men would be considered obese. This is substantially higher than the fraction of obese men in the Northern European group, but comparable to that in the Southern European group. Coronary events were divided into two subgroups: the "hard" events (by which was meant death from coronary heart disease or definite myocardial infarction); and the "soft" events (including classical angina pectoris, clinical judgment of definite heart disease or clinical judgment of possible heart disease). An examination of the data reveals the similarity between the body mass index for U.S. railmen and for the population in Southern Europe, and a sharp difference from that observed in the men from Northern European countries.

Among the men from the United States and Southern Europe, there were few, if any, significant relationships of body weight when "hard" events were the measure of coronary heart disease. However, there were statistically significant correlations between overweight and the "soft" criteria for coronary artery disease. Among the men from Northern Europe, the relationship was nearly reversed. There were statistically significant correlations between all measures of body weight and "hard" criteria for coronary artery disease among the males from Northern Europe, but no significant association with body weight and "soft" diagnostic criteria for coronary artery disease. This geographic difference is presently unexplained.

To explore this data further, a multivariate analysis was performed in which relative risk could be assigned to each factor investigated. A high correlation was observed between relative weight and blood pressure. This finding has been observed in almost all studies in which body weight and blood pressure have been measured. From this multiple variate analysis, Keys et al. (1972) concluded that in none of the relationships did the measures of relative weight or fatness have any independent value in predicting the risk of developing coronary heart disease. Thus as an independent predictor for coronary heart disease, body weight has little value.

However, excess weight is important because of its association with high blood pressure. It should be noted that the data of Keys et al. (1972) were obtained from a study of men aged 40 to 59 at the time of entry into the study. The data in Table 6–2 show that the effects of overweight diminished as the age at which life insurance was issued increased. This suggests that overweight may have its major influences on mortality in men under age 40 and thus may not have been detected by Keys et al. (1972).

Los Angeles Heart Study

A group of 1859 male civil servants (1552 white, 302 black and 5 oriental) have been re-examined for up to 15 years. During this time there were 242 new cases of heart disease among the 1503 men at risk, giving an annual rate of 10.7/1000 men. In this study the body weight and height were related using the ponderal index (ht/ $\sqrt[3]{wt}$). Men with a ponderal index of less than 12.0 were called obese. Although there was a trend for myocardial infarction to occur more frequently in the overweight men, this change was not consistent nor statistically significant.

Using sophisticated statistical analyses, Chapman et al. (1971) showed that body weight was associated with the development of coronary artery disease in men who were between 30 and 39 years of age at the beginning of the study. In men over 40 at entry, there was a significant relationship of body weight to the development of angina pectoris but not to myocardial infarction, and in men over age 50 body weight added no predictive value for discriminating the likelihood of developing coronary artery disease. In this study the principal effect of body weight on heart disease was in younger men aged 30 to 39 where it was predictive for developing myocardial infarction, and in men aged 40 to 49 for predicting angina pectoris. The lack of association in older men of overweight and heart disease is similar to the conclusion of the other two prospective studies, (Table 6–4).

Other Studies

Several other studies are listed in Table 6–4 but will be commented on only briefly, (Cotton 1972; Epstein, 1971; Stamler et al. 1966; Spain et al. 1963). Carlson and Bottiger (1972) studied 3168 men over a nine year period. In this group the ratio of weight over height (wt/ht) had no prognostic significance for the development of coronary artery disease in men in any age group. In a study of 3102 men living in Evans County, Georgia, body mass index (wt/(ht)^2) was used to assess overweight. Among this group of men several factors, including ethnic origin, social class, blood pressure, smoking and physical activity were all associated with the development of cardiovascular disease (Cassel, 1971a, b; Heyden et al., 1971a, b, c).

Among smokers there was a significant effect of excess body weight on the development of coronary heart disease. Among the overweight smokers the rate was twice that of the lean nonsmokers (150 vs 80/1000). There was no enhanced risk, however, among the overweight nonsmokers.

Overweight was also related to incidence of cerebral vascular disease, particularly among those who gained weight after age 20.

Among those who weighed less than 150 pounds (68 kg) at age 20 and who gained less than 30 pounds (14 kg) after that, the risk of developing a stroke (CVA) was only 40 percent that of the people weighing over 150 pounds (68 kg) at age 20 and who gained over 30 pounds (14 kg) after that (38/1000 vs 90/1000). In contrast, there was no relationship between weight at age 20 or weight gain following age 20 and the incidence of coronary heart disease among survivors in the same population.

Cotton et al. (1972) compared 91 men who were under age 65 and who had overt coronary heart disease with 98 healthy age-matched males. Body mass index (wt/(ht)^2) was not significantly different between these two groups. Among the variables examined, however, several were significantly different. They included the diastolic blood pressure, arcus senilis, baldness, cholesterol, a family history of diabetes, hypertension and xanthelasma, which were all predictive of a risk for developing coronary heart disease.

Garn et al. (1951), in a similar study, found body weight to be similar in a group of men with myocardial infarction and in a group of matched controls without coronary heart disease. Dunn and his collaborators (1970) provided a four and one half year follow up on 13,148 males who had 401 new coronary events during the course of the study. Among these men, relative weight was significantly associated with hypertension and with diabetes, but not with the development of coronary artery disease. Finally, Rosenman et al. (1970) reported data on 3182 subjects who participated in the Western Collaborative Group Study. Body weight had no effect on the risk of developing a heart attack, while such factors as family history, increased systolic and diastolic blood pressure, smoking and an increase in cholesterol were all shown to add significant risk.

The extensive literature on the relationship between overweight or obesity and the likelihood of developing atherosclerosis or other medical complications can be depicted in two ways (Rimm et al., 1972) (Fig. 6–4). There might be a relationship in which obesity is directly related to the onset of these other conditions as a cause and effect phenomenon (panel A in Fig. 6–4). This is the conclusion that might be reached from the various retrospective studies. The several prospective studies make any simple relationship unlikely (Chlouverakis, 1973). For this reason the diagram depicted in panel B of Figure 6–4 seems more likely. With this model, obesity and the various medical conditions with which it is frequently associated are independently related to one another. Under these circumstances, obesity could serve as a useful marker for the possible presence of these medical conditions, but obesity could also occur in their absence.

The data from the Framingham Study also suggests a significant and important relationship between overweight and sudden death. In

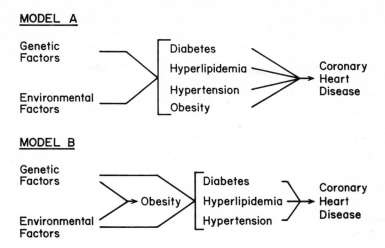

Figure 6–4. Relation of obesity to other disease. Model A shows obesity as a causative effect and Model B shows obesity as a phenomenon which is not directly related to the major risks of coronary artery disease. (Reprinted from Rimm et al.: Obesity and Bariatric Med., *1*:77–84, 1972, with permission.)

contrast, most other studies have not shown an association between overweight and the development of myocardial infarction. The principal exception to this statement is the study by Chapman et al. (1971) in which the ponderal index was a significant predictor for the development of myocardial infarction in men under age 40 but not in men over age 40. Overweight is also associated with the development of cerebral vascular accidents.

The findings in the Evans County Study that overweight and coronary artery disease had a significant relationship in smokers but not in nonsmokers, and the varying effects of overweight on sudden death, angina pectoris, coronary artery disease and cerebral vascular disease indicate the importance of defining the subgroups to be examined, and of examining the effects of overweight in various age groups. It may well be that the effects of excess weight are of more importance in younger men than when overweight develops in older men. Alternatively, in the men who are overweight early in life, the extra mortality may have been dissipated by the time they reach the age of 40.

The effects of body weight on vascular disease may be related to changes in body weight. Albrink and Meigs (1964) suggested that natural, lifelong obesity may be different from obesity acquired after-puberty. Bjurlf (1959) reached a similar conclusion from his study of atherosclerosis and the size and number of subcutaneous fat cells. He suggested that increased numbers of fat cells were genetically controlled and that large fat cells were acquired. The Los Angeles Heart Study also supports this conclusion. In men under 40 years of age,

those whose weight increased by 10 percent or more had a significantly greater risk of hypertension than men who gained less
weight.

The most convincing evidence for this proposition, however, are
the studies of Heyden et al. (1971b), reviewed above, and the data of
Abraham et al. (1971). Figure 6–5 shows the data of Abraham et al.
(1971) on the relation of childhood and adult weight to the incidence
of hypertensive and cardiovascular renal disease among 715 males
whose average age was 48. Childhood weight status was determined
from school records obtained between ages 9 and 13. The highest
prevalence for both conditions occurred in the men with the lowest
childhood weight who became overweight as adults (Fig. 6–5). It may
well be that changing weight categories during adolescence and early
adult years has more importance on the development of subsequent
diseases than maintaining a higher weight category throughout life.
Such an hypothesis awaits further research.

OVERWEIGHT AND MORBIDITY

Overweight and Blood Pressure

Hypertension can be defined as a blood pressure with the systolic
reading above 160 mmHg and a diastolic reading above 95mmHg. The
range of diastolic pressures between 90 to 95 is considered borderline
and only those below 90 mmHg are considered normal. For systolic

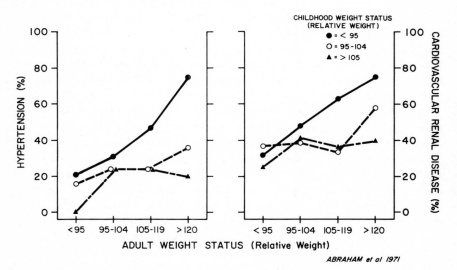

Figure 6–5. Relation of weight gain to hypertension and cardiovascular renal disease.
The individuals who gained weight in adult life and who had a normal (95 to 104) or low
(<95) weight status as children showed the highest incidence of both diseases as adults.
(Reprinted from Abraham et al.: HSMHA Health Reports, 86:273–284, 1971.)

pressure 140 to 160 mmHg is borderline and less than 140 mmHg normal. Technical problems in the measurement of blood pressure in obese subjects have proved troublesome and must be considered in evaluating the importance of any epidemiologic studies on this problem.

It is widely taught that readings of the indirect auscultatory method of obtaining blood pressure with an inflatable cuff tend to be higher in obese individuals than those obtained by direct intra-arterial measurement (Ragan and Bordley, 1941). This widely held belief has come in for critical re-evaluation as a result of two studies which failed to find a consistent difference between indirect and direct measurements of blood pressure. Both Rafferty and Ward (1968) and Holland and Hummerfelt (1964) failed to show that differences between intra-arterial measurements of blood pressure and those taken with a cuff were related to the circumference of the arm or to skinfold thickness. However, there was a significant correlation between the circumference of the arm and the measurements of direct intra-arterial pressure. (Pickering et al., 1954).

Berliner et al. (1961) showed that a large arm girth did not regularly distort the blood pressure reading in one direction or the other. A careful study of the various factors involved in the measurement of arterial blood pressure by King (1967) found that the length of the cuff bladder for the manometer was of prime importance. When the cuff was short, there were great differences between systolic and diastolic pressures measured by intra-arterial methods as compared with indirect measurements. When a long (42 cm) cuff was used, these differences became very small. In another study of the standard cuff type sphygmomanometer versus intra-arterial measurement Kvols et al. (1969) found that the cuff and the intra-arterial measurements were within 10 mmHg in one third of the patients. When a thigh cuff was used on the upper arm, the direct and indirect methods agreed in 50 percent of the patients. These authors concluded that the only reliable way to obtain an accurate reading of blood pressure in grossly obese individuals is by direct intra-arterial measurements.

Since the girth of the arm is correlated with intra-arterial blood pressure, it is likely that the studies using a long cuff will provide a reasonably accurate measurement of blood pressure for population studies. However, the more nearly the inflatable bladder of the pressure cuff surrounds the arm, the more reliable the indirect measurements will become.

Most population studies show a rise in blood pressure with an increase in body weight or other indices of body "fatness," (Levy et al., 1946; Master, 1953; Master and Lasser, 1958; Terry, 1923; Thomas and Cohen, 1955). A comprehensive review of the relation of overweight and hypertension has been published by Chiang, Perlman and Epstein (1969). It will suffice to emphasize only a few points. Robinson and Brucer (1940) examined the relationship between blood pressure and a modified ponderal index which included chest circumference (wt/ht × 100/chest circumference). Two points emerged: first, that overweight had a striking correlation with a lateral body build. Those individuals with a large chest circumference relative to their height and weight had a higher blood pressure than slender individuals. Hypertension was present in 37 percent of the broad chested men, but in only 3 percent of the slender men. Body build exerted an almost proportionate effect on systolic and diastolic blood pressure.

Second, when blood pressure was compared in groups with constant body build, there was no significant correlation between obesity and hypertension. The greatest correlation of blood pressure with obesity was observed in the men with a slender build. A much smaller correlation was found in the broad chested men. From these data it would appear that body build was more important than obesity per se in the positive correlation between blood pressure and body weight.

Retrospective data have also been obtained from life insurance companies in this country and abroad. Döring (1958) compared blood pressure and age for German men 170 to 174 cm tall. The lightest men had the lowest blood pressure at all ages and the highest blood pressure occurred in the heaviest men. Similar data from the United States showed that for men aged 40 to 44, diastolic blood pressure was 6 mm higher for men 25 percent or more overweight than for those 10 percent or more underweight.

Prospective studies have also shown the correlation between obesity and hypertension. In Tecumseh, Michigan and Framingham, Massachusetts there was a correlation of approximately $r = 0.3$ between blood pressure and relative weight (Chiang et al., 1969; Kannel et al., 1967). In a large Scandinavian study of over 67,000 adults, there was an increase in systolic pressure of 3 mmHg and a rise in diastolic pressure of 2 mmHg for every 10 kg (22 pounds) increase in body weight (Bjerkedal, 1957). Finally, the data of Keys et al. (1972) obtained from the men in the International Collaborative Study of Cardiovascular Epidemiology showed that the apparent effects of obesity on increased cardiac deaths could be accounted for by the relationship between obesity and blood pressures.

Even with the limitations in the techniques of measuring blood pressure by indirect auscultation, the available data almost uniformly indicate the important relationship between body weight and blood pressure. The increased blood pressure probably results from increased peripheral resistance, but as yet we have little insight into the mechanisms of the increased peripheral resistance (Bachman et al., 1973). The importance of the correlation between blood pressure and weight is emphasized by the reduction of blood pressure which frequently follows successful weight reduction. The epidemiologic data obtained during World War II revealed that during periods of caloric deprivation, hypertension was almost nonexistent (Brozek et al., 1948).

A number of clinical studies correlating changes in blood pressure with weight reduction have been summarized by Chiang et al. (1969). Fletcher (1954) studied the effect of weight reduction on blood pressure of 38 women who were more than 20 percent overweight. The mean weight loss in 6 months was 32 pounds (14.5 kg); the drop in systolic blood pressure averaged 32 mmHg, and the drop in diastolic blood pressure was 16.6 mmHg in the subgroup with initial diastolic pressures above 100 mmHg. Adlersberg et al. (1946) had similar results with 72 percent of the 54 patients showing a significant drop in blood pressure. Martin (1952), however, had a lower success rate.

More recently Heyden et al. (1971c) noted a drop in systolic and diastolic blood pressure in the patients they observed. The beneficial effects of weight loss on blood pressure, cholesterol, and uric acid are shown in Table 6–5 from the Framingham Study. It should be noted that weight reduction is more effective in lowering systolic blood pressure than diastolic pressure. Whether the therapeutic effect of weight reduction is related to the magnitude of the decline in body weight or to other environmental factors is unclear. However, weight reduction can produce significant reduction in blood pressure in approximately half or more of the hypertensive patients.

Overweight and Cardiovascular Function

The relationship between overweight and cardiovascular disease has been studied extensively (Prodger and Dennig, 1932; Alexander, 1963; Bachman et al., 1973). The obese individual shows an increase in intracellular and extracellular fluid volume. Blood volume also increases with excess weight (Alexander, 1963), but when expressed in terms of ideal weight it is normal (Bachman et al., 1973). Cardiac output is increased in relation to the high oxygen consumption associated with obesity (see Chapter 4) (Alexander, 1963). The increased cardiac output is in turn produced primarily by increasing the stroke volume of the heart, since resting heart rate usually remains in the normal range in the overweight patient. A major reason for the increased cardiac output is the increased blood flow to adipose tissue (Larsen et al., 1966).

When the blood volume and cardiac output are expressed per kilogram of body weight, they are only about 60 percent of the predicted value. As noted elsewhere, however, the use of gross weight does not allow correction for differences in the composition of the extra weight. Surface area probably provides a more appropriate basis for this comparison. Estimates of blood flow through various peripheral tissues (including renal blood flow and cerebral blood flow) of obese patients indicate that the rates are essentially normal. However, splenic blood flow tends to be high.

Studies of the heart itself have shown that the transverse diameter, as measured on routine chest x-ray, shows a positive correlation with body weight (Alexander et al., 1962). This radiographic data is supported by the fact that the weight of the heart increases with increasing body weight (Cermak, 1965; Cermak and Brozak, 1970; Schwalb and Schimert, 1970). This is mainly the result of myocardial hypertrophy (Kannel and Gordon, 1974). Because the circulation is overtaxed as body weight increases, congestive heart failure may occur in grossly obese individuals (Smith, 1928). Studies by Alexander et al. (1962) on 40 grossly obese patients showed that four of them had some evidence of congestive heart failure. Of those patients who underwent cardiac catheterization, three quarters had increased pulmonary hypertension at rest and during exercise.

Bachman et al. (1973) obtained different findings. They observed that pulmonary resistance was normal at rest, but that there was an impaired response to exercise. Essentially all of the abnormalities in vascular and cardiac function returned toward normal with weight loss (Alexander and Peterson, 1972). The heart rate, stroke volume, cardiac work and oxygen uptake are all reduced (Table 6–6). This table shows the cardiovascular findings before and after weight loss in 9 grossly obese patients. Note that every parameter improved. It thus appears that most of the cardiovascular changes observed in obese patients are a consequence of the obesity and, like hypertension, are ameliorated by weight reduction.

Overweight and Pulmonary Function

Measurement of pulmonary function in the obese individual shows a number of abnormalities (Barrera et al., 1967; Bedell et al., 1958; Cherniak, 1959; Sharp et al., 1964). At one extreme are the

TABLE 6–6.   *Effect of Weight Loss on Cardiovascular Function**

	BEFORE	AFTER
Weight (kg)	112 to 218	53kg loss
Heart rate (min^{-1})	73 ± 10	68 ± 8
Stroke volume (ml)	107 ± 15	92 ± 17
Left ventricular stroke work (g-m)	150 ± 29	110 ± 29
Left ventricular work (kg-m/min)	11.1 ± 3.9	7.4 ± 2.0
$^V O_2$ (ml/min)	360 ± 82	247 ± 43
Cardiac output (1/min)	7.9 ± 1.8	6.2 ± 1.2
Systemic arterial pressure (mmHg)	102 ± 16	87 ± 12
Blood volume (1)	7.8 ± 1.5	6.1 ± 1.4

*Adapted from Alexander and Peterson: Circulation, 45:310–318, 1972, by permission of the American Heart Association, Inc.

patients with the Pickwickian syndrome named by Burwell and his collaborators (1956) after Joe, the fat boy in Dickens' *Pickwick Papers* (Wallgren et al., 1965). At the other extreme are the impairments in work capacity due to the increased mass of fat (see Chapter 4). Table 6–7 shows data from normal, moderately obese and grossly obese males studied at the Harbor General Hospital. There is a fairly uniform decrease in expiratory reserve volume, i.e., that volume of air which can be blown out after the normal ventilation. There is also low maximum rate of voluntary ventilation, as well as a tendency toward a general reduction in lung volumes.

Studies on airway resistance, on the compliance of the lung, and on the oxygen cost of breathing have also revealed abnormalities. Lung compliance appears to be normal, but studies on the mechanics of breathing indicate that there is an increase in oxygen consumption associated with breathing because more work is required to move the mass of the obese chest. Finally,there appears to be some element of venous admixture; that is, segments of the lung which are not well perfused but are ventilated and other regions which are perfused but not adequately ventilated. This condition leads to the fairly consistent finding of modest degrees of decreased arterial oxygenation without corresponding increases in arterial carbon dioxide content. (Douglas and Chong, 1972).

Some obese patients show a diminished sensitivity of the respiratory center to the stimulatory effects of carbon dioxide. When breathing 5 percent CO_2, these patients do not show the usual and expected increase in the rate of respiration. This may play a role in the development of pulmonary abnormalities observed with the Pickwickian syndrome (Burwell et al., 1956). Lourenço (1969) prosposed one explanation for some of the pulmonary difficulties associated with obesity. He measured the activity of the diaphragm when the obese patient breathed increasing amounts of CO_2. The patients with hypoventilation showed less diaphragmatic activity, suggesting that inability of this muscle to function normally may play an important role in the pulmonary abnormality observed in obesity.

The Pickwickian syndrome is associated with a number of pulmonary abnormalities (Table 6–7). In almost all instances they have alveolar hypoventilation, thus providing less oxygen than normal to the blood. Maximal breathing capacity, vital capacity, functional residual capacity, respiratory work, thoracic compliance, lung compliance, diffusion of carbon monoxide, and pulmonary mixing are all significantly distorted in the obese individuals with severe hypoventilation and the Pickwickian syndrome.

The features of the Pickwickian syndrome as presented from a study of 22 patients at the Johns Hopkins Hospital are shown in Table 6–8. These patients are almost always sleepy, short of breath and cyanotic. There is a marked reduction in pO_2 and a substantial in-

TABLE 6–7.   *Pulmonary Function in Normal and Obese Males**

	Normal Weight	BODY WEIGHT Moderately Overweight	Grossly Obese
Age	27	27	25
Body weight (kg)	72	103	168
Vital capacity°	111.6	107.6	91.7
Expiratory reserve volume°	129.6	79.3	60.7
Inspiratory capacity°	102.8	118.6	107.7
Residual volume°	83.1	100.3	100.0
Total lung capacity°	105.7	101.8	93.2
Forced expiratory volume (percent in 1 second)	86.5	80.0	81.8
Maximal expiratory flow rate	463.9	562	466
Maximal breathing capacity	153.1	147	127
Diffusing capacity°	105.3	120.7	116.1
Functional residual capacity	108.8	87.6	—

*Adapted from Wasserman, Bray, Whipp and Koyal.
°Percent of normal.

crease in arterial pCO_2. Secondary polycythemia was frequent and right ventricular hypertrophy with signs of corpulmonale and right ventricular failure were often seen. The ventilatory response to increasing the CO content of the inspired air was tested in four of these patients and was clearly impaired in two (MacGregor et al., 1970).

Fatality among obese patients with the Pickwickian syndrome is common and occurred in nearly one third of these 22 patients. At autopsy no cause of death could be found in three patients; a myocardial infarction and pulmonary emboli accounted for the other two deaths. A number of serious complications occurred in 13 of these patients, including severe ventilatory insufficiency requiring tracheostomy, sudden unexpected death, pulmonary emboli and severe papilledema. Following the initiation of aggressive respiratory management, the number of deaths was strikingly reduced. Thus ag-

TABLE 6–8.   *Features of the Pickwickian Syndrome**

		NUMBER OF CASES
Number of Patients		22 (12 F; 10M)
Wt. (lbs)		209 to 588
Somnolence		21
Dyspnea		20
Cyanosis		15
Cardiomegaly		21
Arterial pCO_2	>50 mmHg	18
Hematocrit	>50 percent	14
pO_2	<mmHg	14

*Adapted from MacGregor, et al.: Bull. Johns Hopkins Hosp., *126*:279–298, 1970.

gressive therapy would appear to be appropriate in management of this form of respiratory insufficiency in grossly obese patients.

Overweight and Gallbladder Disease

Association of obesity or overweight with gallbladder disease has been suggested in several studies. One source is the insurance company statistics reviewed by Dublin et al. (1934). It has also been suggested in an autopsy study in which 612 gallbladder specimens were examined (Mentzer, 1926). Of these specimens 377 had gross disease with 44 of the diseased gallbladders coming from subjects weighing over 210 pounds.

In a detailed study of just over 73,000 respondents to a questionnaire issued by the TOPS* club, Rimm et al. (1972) found an increased incidence of gallbladder disease (Fig. 6–6). In this figure the patients have been divided into 10 groups with varying deviations in body weight. Level 1 is approximately 5.3 percent above ideal weight, whereas level 10 is 101 percent above ideal weight. Two facts emerge from this study: first, that a history of gallbladder disease increases with each decade from age 25 to more than 55 years of age; second, that within any age group, the frequency of gallbladder disease increases with the level of body weight. For women aged 25 to 34 years who are 100 percent or more overweight, 18 percent had gallbladder disease. Nearly 35 percent of the women aged 45 to 55 who were 100 percent or more overweight had gallbladder disease.

A third study demonstrating the relationship between weight and gallbladder disease was provided by the studies of Sturdevant, Pearce and Dayton (1973). The body weight of the subjects without gallstones was significantly less (p. <.01) than in the men with gallstones. The incidence of gallstones at autopsy in men who were more than 9.1 kg overweight was 43 percent (12/28); in the men who were less than 9.1 kg overweight, there was an incidence of only 16 percent (25/156). See Chapter 7 for a discussion of the mechanism.

Overweight and Diabetes

The relationship between diabetes mellitus and obesity is complex (Osserman 1951; Luft et al., 1968). (Details are reviewed in Chapters 5 and 7.) Rimm et al. (1972) have investigated this relationship among the more than 73,000 respondents to the TOPS Club questionnaire. Increasing body weight and age were both associated with a rising frequency of diabetes mellitus. Less than 1 percent of normal weight women aged 25 to 44 had diabetes mellitus, whereas 7 percent

---

*TOPS = Take Off Pounds Sensibly, Milwaukee, Wisconsin.

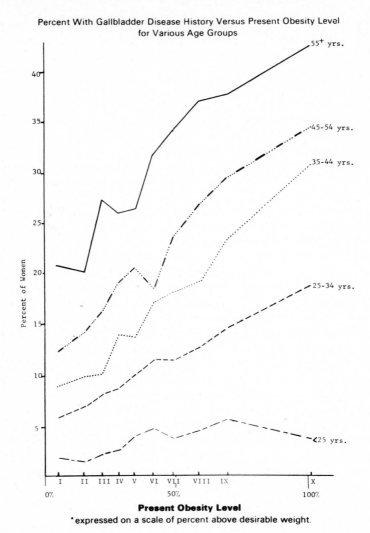

Percent With Gallbladder Disease History Versus Present Obesity Level
for Various Age Groups

Figure 6–6. Obesity and gallbladder disease. The percentage of women in various age groups who had a history of gallbladder disease rises with body weight. The weight categories divide the patients into 10 groups. Group X was 100 percent overweight. Group VII was 50 percent overweight. (Reprinted from Rimm et al.: Obesity and Bariatric Med., *1*:77–84, 1972, with permission.)

of those of the same age who were 100 percent overweight had this complication.

One explanation for the increased prevalence of diabetes mellitus in obese patients has been provided by studies in experimental animals. If the pancreas is slightly injured or partially removed, the induction of obesity in experimental animals is associated with the onset

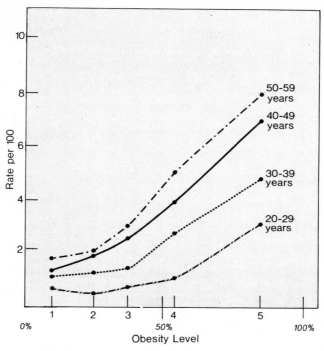

Percent With Adult Onset Diabetes Versus Present Obesity Level
for Various Age Groups

NOTE: Obesity level is expressed on a scale of percentage above ideal weight.

Figure 6-7.   Obesity and diabetes mellitus. The percentage of women in various age groups who had a history of diabetes mellitus rises with body weight. The weight categories divide the patients into groups according to percentage above ideal weight. Reprinted from Rimm, A. A., et al.: Relationship of obesity and disease in 73,532 weight-conscious women. Public Health Reports, *90*:44–51, 1975.

of diabetes. This can be understood in terms of the increased demands for insulin produced by obesity (see Chapter 7). Under these conditions the capacity to synthesize and release insulin by partially dam-

A similar conclusion can be drawn from two groups of clinical studies. The first is shown in Table 6–9. It shows the percentage increase in body weight for males and females between the ages of 25 and 60 in 4 different countries from data obtained in the late 1940's. The mortality from diabetes in these same populations is expressed on the right hand side of the same table. The mortality from diabetes mellitus was highest among females, who also had the greatest gain in aged pancreas is reduced, and the extra burden imposed by the extra body fat leads to pancreatic failure.

TABLE 6–9. *Relation of Mortality from Diabetes to Weight Gain after Age 25**

COUNTRY	PERCENT OF INCREASE IN WEIGHT BETWEEN AGES 25 AND 60		MORTALITY FROM DIABETES° (PERCENT)			
			OVER 45		ALL AGES	
	M	F	M	F	M	F
Japan	0.4	0.4	—	—	2.4	2.0
England	3.6	15.5	14.0	25.2	5.3	10.1
Canada	4.6	19.3	55.6	91.5	16.2	24.5
United States	8.1	15.0	67.7	111.6	20.7	34.0

*After Hundley: J. Am. Diet. Assoc., 32:417–422, 1956.
°Mortality rates per 100,000 population in 1948.

weight between ages 25 and 60. Moreover, Canada and the United States, whose populations had the greatest percentage increase in body weight between age 25 and 60, had the highest mortality from diabetes.

The "stress" to the pancreas imposed by obesity is also shown in data presented by Keen (1975). The siblings of diabetic patients were examined for the presence of diabetes and the results were related to the prevalence of obesity (Table 6–10). When the propositus with diabetes mellitus was overweight, the frequency of diabetes in the siblings was somewhat lower than when the propositus was not overweight. Morever, diabetes mellitus was present two to four times as often in the obese siblings of the diabetic family member who originally reported with diabetes as when the siblings were not obese. These data lend credence to the concept that, in the presence of obesity, diabetes develops more readily in individuals with pancreatic injury, (whether of genetic, chemical or viral origin) than in a similar individual who is not obese.

Changes in the Skin in Relation to Obesity

Two abnormalities in the skin have been associated with obesity. The first is a condition described as "fragilitas cutis inguinalis." Ganor and Even-Paz (1967) examined the resistance to stretching of the inguinal skin in 200 patients who were divided into three subgroups: lean, normal and fat. In 63 out of the 200 patients the inguinal skin ruptured in the linear fashion at right angles to the applied force. This phenomenon was restricted to the groin and was unrelated to the sex or age of the patient. It was clearly associated with obesity, however. Nearly 70 percent of the fat patients (as compared with 20 to 25 percent of the medium weight patients) showed this phenomenon. These authors also noted a positive relationship between the presence of

TABLE 6–10. *Frequency of Diabetes Mellitus*
Among the Siblings of Diabetics*

WEIGHT STATUS OF DIABETIC PROPOSITUS	FREQUENCY OF DIABETES AMONG SIBLINGS IN TWO WEIGHT GROUPS (PERCENT)	
	Obese	*Non-obese*
Obese	10.8	4.8
Non-obese	27.3	7.3

*Adapted from Keen: First International Congress on Obesity, 1975, p. 118.

stria and obesity, but not between the presence of stria and the tendency of the inguinal skin to rupture under stretching. The meaning of the relationship between the sensitivity of the inguinal skin in obese subjects to rupture during stretching is unclear.

Acanthosis nigricans is a second dermal abnormality having a significant association with obesity. Darkening of the skin in the creases of the neck and in the axillary region is important because it is sometimes associated with highly malignant cancers, usually an intra-abdominal adenocarcinoma occurring in middleaged and elderly patients. In the study of 100 patients by Brown and Winkleman (1968), 17 had the malignant form and 73 the benign form of acanthosis nigricans. In the patients with obesity and the benign acanthosis nigricans, most had stigmata of other endocrine diseases. These included hirsutism, acne, amenorrhea, abdominal straie and moon facies.

Hollingsworth and Amatruda (1969) re-examined the relationship of acanthosis and endocrine function in 28 massively obese patients, 14 of whom had associated acanthosis nigricans. In both groups the adrenal glands responded normally to injected ACTH. The suppression of adrenal secretion during treatment with low and high doses of dexamethasone showed no significant differences between obese patients with acanthosis nigricans and those without. However, the four female patients with acanthosis nigricans showed a loss of diurnal variation in plasma levels of 17-hydroxycorticosteroids, and more hirsutism and menstrual irregularities than those women without acanthosis nigricans.

Renal Function and Obesity

The recent description of the nephrotic syndrome in four patients with massive obesity has reawakened interest in the interrelation between obesity and renal function (Weisinger et al., 1974). The four patients in this report had proteinuria which ranged between 3.1 and 19.2 grams per day. However, hematuria was absent, and x-rays of the kidney in three of these patients showed a normal pattern in two and a horseshoe kidney in one. Renal biopsies obtained in two patients showed only minimal abnormalities and no definable pathologic cause for the nephrotic syndrome. Of particular importance was the relationship between the proteinuria and body weight. In all four patients, there was a significiant decline in protein excretion as the patients lost weight. These observations suggest that renal impairment similar to that observed in the experimental animal with hypothalamic lesions. (Brobeck, Tepperman and Long, 1943) may occur in obese patients with massive increases in body fat.

Obstetrics and the Overweight Patient

The relationship between body weight and reproductive function is discussed in Chapter 7. For the present discussion we will focus on the relationship between pre-pregnancy weight and the factors related to labor and the weight of the infant (Matthews and Der Brucke, 1938; Odell and Mengert, 1945). Peckham and Christianson (1971) performed a careful analysis on women in the Oakland clinic of the Kaiser-Permanente Medical Care Plan for whom pre-pregnancy weights were available. In this group there were 3939 white females who delivered babies between 1963 and 1965. At each height the lowest 10 percent, the middle 10 percent, and the highest 10 percent in body weight were selected for review. This technique provides the same distribution of heights in each of the three weight groups.

Among the "heavy" women body weight averaged 169 pounds. These individuals were older, averaging 29 years of age as compared to 25 years for the lightest women. Nearly 22 percent of the heavy women were over 35, but only 7.4 percent of the light women had attained this age. Moreover, 40 percent of the women in the "light" weight group were having their first pregnancies, but this percentage was much smaller in the heavy group. As noted earlier (Chapter 5), menarche occurred at a younger age in the heavy women and was somewhat delayed in the light weight women. By age 11, 27.5 percent of the heavy women had begun menstruating, but only 16.5 percent of the light ones had. In contrast, menstruation began after age 14 in 28 percent of the light weight women but in only 13.7 percent of the heavy women.

The frequency of toxinemia of pregnancy and hypertension were significantly increased among the heavy women. In addition, the duration of labor was longer. In over 7 percent of the heavy women labor lasted more than 24 hours. This occurred in only 0.8 percent of the light women. Cesarean section was performed in 5.5 percent of the heavy patients but in only 0.7 percent of the light ones. Thus more obstetrical complications were present in the heavy group than in the light one.

The weight of infants born to the heavy women was significantly heavier than the weights of babies born to the light women. A similar observation has been made by McKeown and Record (1957). The mean birth weight of the infants increased with maternal height and increasing maternal weight. However, McKeown and Record failed to observe any relationship between the duration of labor and the effect of body weight or body build.

The risk associated with operating on obese women with adenocarcinoma of the uterus has been examined by Prem, Mensheha and McKelvey (1965). The mortality rate following treatment of malignancy of the uterus was higher in obese women. Women weighing over 300 pounds had a 20 percent mortality, compared to 5 percent (1/18) for women weighing 250 and 299, and only 2 percent (1/65) for the women weighing between 200 and 249 pounds. This would thus bear out a long held clinical impression that marked obesity is associated with some enhanced risks of surgical mortality. Anesthesia also involves more risk in obese patients (Warner, 1968).

THE SOCIAL DISADVANTAGE OF OBESITY

Social Attitudes Toward the Obese

Obesity carries a social stigma in this country (Allon, 1975; Cahnman, 1968). This was most clearly shown by studies with children and adults who were asked to express a preference for various forms of disability, including obesity (Richardson, Hastorf, Goodman and Dornbusch, 1961; Goodman, Richardson, Dornbusch, and Hastorf, 1963). Children and adults were shown 6 pictures. These included: (1) a child with no disability; (2) a child with crutches and a brace on his left leg; (3) a child in a wheel chair with a blanket over his legs; (4) a child with a left hand missing; (5) a child who was disfigured around the left side of the mouth; and (6) an obese child. The sex of the drawings corresponded with that of the person who was shown the pictures.

In the first study, groups of boys and girls aged 10 to 11 from schools in New York City, Montana, and Northern California were asked to rate the pictures by selecting the child they would find most easy to like. This picture was removed and they were then asked to select the child they would find next most easy to like until all 6 pictures had been rated. The order of rating was the same for all groups of children regardless of their sex, socioeconomic status, racial background and whether they came from rural or urban communities. In all cases, the obese child was liked least. The number of children used in the original study by Richardson et al. (1961) was such as to leave little doubt about the social stigma attached to being an obese child.

In an extension of this study, Goodman et al. (1963) showed that a group of adults including physical therapists, occupational therapists, nurses, physicians and social workers rated the same six pictures exactly as did the children from rural and urban United States. Maddox, Back and Liederman (1968) provided confirmation of this data. They used the same group of pictures with patients from an outpatient clinic. The clinic population as a whole had almost the same rank order for the six pictures as the children and adults. Disabled adults and children did not like the obese child. These authors were surprised by the observation that black females who often value obesity rated the obese child as fourth from the top, not much improvement. When asked why the obese child was ranked at the bottom, many indicated that the other disabled children were the unfortunate victims of the environment. By implication the obese child was frequently thought to be "responsible" for his plight. In addition, many obese patients disliked the drawings of the obese child because it reminded them of themselves.

The potential disadvantages of obesity have been emphasized again in studies on social mobility and dating behavior. Elder (1969) indicated that physical appearance was the most important factor for women in attracting upwardly mobile men for marriage. Physical attractiveness was again the single most important factor in dating behavior among college age students (Walster, Aronson, Abrahams and Rottmann, 1966) Because of the importance of attitudes about physical attractiveness in our society and the relatively unattractive view of obesity by many children and adults, it is easy to understand the relative social positions and feelings of many obese individuals. This has been emphasized by Monello and Mayer (1963) in a study on the attitudes of obese adolescent girls. They observed that these individuals showed excessive concern with one's status, acceptance of dominant values in the culture, and passivity with a tendency towards withdrawal. These authors noted that all of these reactions are characteristics of minority groups, and they suggested that the obese adolescent girls may behave as a minority group in their responses toward the dominant culture.

Obesity as a social disability has been examined further by Maddox and his collaborators (Maddox, Anderson and Bogdanoff, 1966; Maddox and Liederman, 1969). In a study in the outpatient clinic at Duke University, the concordance between entries in the physician's chart concerning overweight and the actual degrees of overweight in the sample were compared. There was only about one chance in four that a patient who was more than 20 percent overweight would encounter a physician who would note in the medical record that his body weight was significantly increased and who would, in addition, propose a program for management of this problem.

The average weight of those who received no mention was 193 pounds and those whose weight was mentioned in the chart but for whom no proposal for management was made was 202 pounds. Those patients for whom a program of management was suggested weighed, on average, 212 pounds. An elevation in blood pressure or the presence of hypertension or coronary artery disease made it more likely that the weight problem would be noted and that a proposal for action would be initiated.

To explore the problem further; Maddox and Liederman (1969) submitted a questionnaire to 197 senior physicians, house officers and medical student clerks who were working in an outpatient clinic. Only 51 percent of the questionnaires were returned. Among the responding physicians, 93 percent said that their major source of knowledge was personal experience. Sixty-six percent indicated that personal research had contributed to their understanding of obesity; 50 percent had learned about obesity in medical conferences and a bare 22 percent stated that their sources of information included medical school lectures. More than half of the physicians admitted that they were usually unsuccessful in treating obesity. But 40 percent indicated that careful management was the preferred approach in spite of its relatively low success rate. In spite of this, less than half the number actually made proposals for treatment of patients who were more than 20 percent overweight, indicating that awareness on the part of the physician had not been activated by this degree of overweight.

A number of personal characteristics were assessed by severely obese persons and by the physicians. There were sharp differences in the overall assessment. In general, active, strong, successful and fast were descriptive adjectives applied by physicians to only 3 to 14 percent of the severely overweight persons. In contrast, self description by overweight persons used these adjectives between 31 to 45 percent of the time. Thus overweight individuals tended to assess themselves more positively than did the physicians caring for them. Moreover, there was a strong negative reaction to the obese patient on the part of many physicians. The intense negative judgment about obese patients was characterized by their weakness and unattractive features. They were frequently described as awkward and weak willed. These negative value judgments on the part of medical professionals working in an outpatient clinic are similar to those of the professionals working with disabled children who were assessing likeable characteristics of the disabled individuals.

Educational Disadvantages of Obesity

The low value with which the obese are viewed in the eyes of many might prejudice their educational opportunities. This has been suggested by Canning and Mayer (1966, 1967) who assessed obesity by measuring the thickness of the triceps of skinfold. Among high school students there were 81 obese males and 96 obese females. Obesity and intelligence were not correlated. The mean I.Q. for the group of obese and nonobese ranged between 112 and 114. Similarly the pre-college entrance Scholastic Aptitude Test (SAT) scores were similar for both groups. However, there were significantly fewer obese males in the top third of the high school class than there were lean males (21 percent versus 26 percent p <.01). Suggestive differences were also present for females, but this was not statistically significant (41 percent versus 32 percent for nonobese versus obese). Finally the mean high school range was lower for the obese than for the nonobese, but this was also not statistically significant.

In this study there were no differences in school attendance records nor in plans for jobs and education following graduation from high school. Yet when Canning and Mayer (1966) examined the frequency of obese and nonobese individuals in Ivy League colleges, they found a significantly lower number of obese females than of nonobese females. These data suggested that there might be a prejudicial admission policy toward the obese high school students. These authors noted that the obese and nonobese were equally interested in attending high ranking colleges and that evaluation of their capacities by objective data such as high school standing and intelligence quotient showed no significant differences. Louderback (1970) has explored this question more thoroughly in a book called *Fat Power*. In it he suggests the need for more tolerance towards the obese members of our society. (Allon, 1975).

Obesity and Employment

In a survey of public opinion in Southern California, television station KNXT found that nearly two thirds of the 500 respondents felt that employers were reluctant to hire fat people. Documentation of this, however, is difficult to obtain. One study suggests that fat bosses draw lower salaries than their lean counterparts. This study was conducted among 15,000 men who were known to an employment agency. Among the men who were greater than 10 percent overweight, only 9 percent were earning $25,000 to $40,000 per year. However, 40 percent of the men earning between $10,000 and

TABLE 6-11. *Frequency of Obese Men and Women in College**

EDUCATIONAL LEVEL	NUMBER OF STUDENTS		PERCENT OBESE		
	M	F	M	F	
High School	568	597	17.3	23.3	p < .001
College	1072	269	16.1	12.6	

*Adapted from Canning and Mayer: New Engl. J. Med., 275:1172–1174, 1966.

$20,000 per year were more than 10 percent overweight. This employment agency had had only one job request for an obese man, and that was to fill a job as an executive for a clothing company which made clothes for overweight men (Los Angeles Times, Jan. 2, 1974, Part I, p. 20). In the study on obesity and unemployment, it was observed that unemployment was associated with obesity mainly through the presence of such defects as arthritis, varicose veins, diabetes, hypertension and a history of gallbladder disease (Henschel, 1967).

Further observations on the economic difficulties associated with overweight have appeared in newspaper articles. A Federal judge recently ordered a major airline to pay back salary and interest to stewardesses who were dismissed because of overweight (Los Angeles Times, April 6, 1974, part 1, p. 2). This ended the dismissal of stewardesses because they did not meet weight limits. A candidate scoring near the top in her civil service examination was fired for being 50 pounds overweight (Los Angeles Times, November 11, 1974, part 1, p. 2). This patent discrimination in employment practices is being ended by action in the Federal courts. These instances serve to illustrate the significant economic and social hurdles which the obese must overcome in American society today.

REFERENCES

Abraham, S., Collins, G. and Nordsieck, M.: Relationship of childhood weight status to morbidity in adults. H.S.M.H.A. Health Reports, 86:273–284, 1971.

Adlersberg, D., Coler, H. R. and Laval, J.: Effect of weight reduction on course of arterial hypertension. J. Mt. Sinai Hosp. N.Y., 12:984–992, 1946.

Albrink, M. H. and Meigs, J. W.: Interrelationship of skin fold thickness, serum lipids and blood sugar in normal men. Am. J. Clin. Nutr., 15:255–261, 1964.

Alexander, J. K.: Obesity and the circulation. Mod. Concepts Cardiovasc. Dis., 32:799–803, 1963.

Alexander, J. K., Amad, K. H. and Cole, V. W.: Observations on some clinical features of extreme obesity with particular reference to the cardiorespiratory effects. Am. J. Med., 32:512–524, 1962.

Alexander, J. K. and Peterson, K. L.: Cardiovascular effects of weight reduction. Circulation, 45:310–318, 1972.

Allon, N.: The stigma of overweight in everyday life. In: Obesity in Perspective. Fogarty International Center Series on Preventive Medicine, Vol II, Part I and Part II. (Bray, G. A. ed.) Washington, D.C., U.S. Government Printing Office. In press 1976.

Amad, K. H., Brennan, J. C. and Alexander, J. K.: The cardiac pathology of chronic exogenous obesity. Circulation, 32:740–745, 1965.

Armstrong, D. B., Dublin, L. I., Wheatley, G. M. and Marks, H. H.: Obesity and its relation to health and disease. J.A.M.A., 147:1007–1014, 1951.

Backman, L., Freyschuss, U., Hallberg, D. and Melcher, A.: Cardiovascular function in extreme obesity. Acta Med. Scand., 193:437–446, 1973.

Baird, I. M.: Aetiological factors in coronary heart disease: Obesity and coronary heart disease. Postgrad. Med. J., 47:30–32, 1971.

Barrera, F., Reidenberg, M. M. and Winters, W. L.: Pulmonary function in the obese patient. Am. J. Med. Sci., 254:785–796, 1967.

Bedell, G. N., Wilson, W. R. and Seebohm, P. M.: Pulmonary function in obese persons. J. Clin. Invest., 37:1049–1060, 1958.

Berliner, K., Fujiy, H., Lee, D. H., Yildiz, M. and Garnier, G.: Blood pressure measurements in obese persons: Comparison of intra-arterial and auscultory measurements. Am. J. Cardiol., 8:10–17, 1961.

Bjerkedal, T.: Overweight and hypertension. Acta Med. Scand., 159:13–26, 1957.

Bjurlf, P.: Atherosclerosis and body build with special reference to size and number of subcutaneous fat cells. Acta Med. Scand. (Suppl. 349) 166:1–99, 1959.

Bray, G. A., Davidson, M. B. and Drenick, E. J.: Obesity: A serious symptom. Ann. Intern. Med., 77:779–795, 1972.

Britten, R. H.: Physical impairment and weight: Study of medical examination records of 3037 men markedly under or overweight for height and age. Publ. Hlth. Rep., 48:926–944, 1933.

Brobeck, J. R., Tepperman, J. and Long, C. N. H.: Experimental hypothalamic hyperphagia in albino rat. Yale J. Biol. Med., 15:893–904, 1943.

Brown, J. and Winkelmann, R. K.: Acanthosis nigricans: A study of 90 cases. Medicine, 47:33–51, 1968.

Brozek, J., Chapman, C. G. and Keys, A.: Drastic food restriction: Effect on cardiovascular dynamics in normotensive and hypertensive conditions. J.A.M.A., 137:1569–1574, 1948.

Burwell, C. S., Robin, E. D., Whaley, R. D. and Bickelmann, A. G.: Extreme obesity associated with alveolar hypoventilation—A Pickwickian Syndrome. Am. J. Med., 21:811–818, 1956.

Cahnman, W. J.: The stigma of obesity. Social. Quart., 9:283–299, 1968.

Canning, H. and Mayer, J.: Obesity—its possible effect on college acceptance. N. Engl. J. Med., 275:1172–1174, 1966.

Canning, H. and Mayer, J.: Obesity: An influence on high school performance. Am. J. Clin. Nutr., 20:352–354, 1967.

Carlson, L. A. and Bottiger, L. E.: Ischemic heart disease in relation to fasting values of plasma triglycerides and cholesterol. Lancet, 1:865–868, 1972.

Cassel, J. C.: Summary of major findings of the Evans County cardiovascular studies. Arch. Intern. Med., 128:887–889, 1971a.

Cassel, J. C.: Review of 1960 through 1962 cardiovascular disease prevalence study. Arch. Intern. Med., 128:890–895, 1971b.

Cermak, J.: Das Herzvolumen bei Fettleibigen. Arch. Kreislaufforsch., 47:234–245, 1965.

Cermak, J. and Brosak, V.: Das Herzvolumen bei Fettleibigen. Arch. Kreislaufforsch., 62:12–24, 1970.

Chapman, J. M., Coulson, A. H., Clark, V. A. and Borun, E. R.: The differential effect of serum cholesterol blood pressure and weight on the incidence of myocardial infarction and angina pectoris. J. Chronic Dis., 23:631–647, 1971.

Cherniack, R. M.: Respiratory effects of obesity. Can. Med. Assoc. J., 80:613–616, 1959.

Chiang, B. N., Perlman, L. V. and Epstein, F. H.: Overweight and hypertension: A review. Circulation, 39:403–421, 1969.

Chlouverakis, C. S.: Controversies in medicine—is obesity harmful? Obesity/Bariatric Med., 2:108–112, 1973.

Cotton, S. G., Nixon, J. M., Carpenter, R. G. and Evans, D. W.: Factors discriminating men with coronary heart disease from healthy controls. Brit. Heart J., 34:458–464, 1972.

Cramér, K., Paulin, S. and Werkö, L.: Coronary angiographic findings in correlation with age, body weight, blood pressure, serum lipids and smoking habits. Circulation, 33:888–900, 1966.

Dawber, T. R., Moore, F. E. and Mann, G. V.: Coronary heart disease in the Framingham Study. Am. J. Public Health, 47 (Suppl):4–24, 1957.

Donald, D. W. A.: Mortality rates among the overweight. In: Anorexia and Obesity (Robertson, R. F., ed.) Edinburgh, R.C.P., pp. 63–70, 1973.

Döring, H.: Die Blutdruckwerke in Abhangigkeit von Alter, Geschlecht und Korperbau. Lebensversicherungs-Medizin, 10:14–23, 1958.

Douglas, F. G. and Chong, P. Y.: Influence of obesity on peripheral airways patency. J. Appl. Physiol., 33:559–563, 1972.

Downes, J.: Association of the chronic disease in the same person and their association with overweight. Milbank Mem. Fd. Quart. Bull., 31:125–140, 1953.

Drenick, E. J.: Weight reduction by prolonged fasting. *In:* Obesity In Perspective. Fogarty International Center Series on Preventive Medicine, Vol. II, Part I and Part II. (Bray, G. A., ed.) Washington, D.C., U.S. Government Printing Office, In press 1976.

Dublin, L. I.: Relation of obesity to longevity. N. Engl. J. Med., *248*:971–974, 1953.

Dublin, L. I., Jimenis, A. O. and Marks, H. H.: Factors in the selection of risks with a history of gall bladder disease. Trans. Assoc. Life Insur. Med. Dir. Am., *21*:34–64, 1934.

Dublin, L. I. and Marks, H. H.: Mortality among insured overweights in recent years. Tr. Am. Life Insur. Med. Dir. Am., *35*:235–263, 1951.

Dunn, J. P., Ipsen, J., Elsom, K. O. and Ohtan, M.: Risk factors in coronary artery disease, hypertension and diabetes. Am. J. Med. Sci., *259*:309–322, 1970.

Elder, G. H., Jr.: Appearance and education in marriage mobility. Am. Sociol. Rev., *34*:519–533, 1969.

Epstein, F. H. and Ostrander, L. D., Jr.: Detection of individual susceptibility toward coronary disease. Prog. Cardiovasc. Dis., *13*:324–342, 1971.

Faber, M. and Land, F.: Human Aorta; influence of obesity on the development of arteriosclerosis in the human aorta. Arch. Path., *48*:351–361, 1949.

Fletcher, A. P.: Effect of weight reduction upon blood pressure of obese hypertensive women. Quart. J. Med., *23*:331–345, 1954.

Ganor, S. and Even-Paz, Z.: Fragilitas Cutis Inguinalis. A phenomen associated with obesity. Dermatologia, *134*:113–124, 1967.

Garn, S. M., Gertler, M. M., Levine, S. A. and White, P. D.: Body weight versus weight standards in coronary artery disease and a healthy group. Ann. Intern. Med., *34*:1416–1420, 1951.

Goodman, J. I.: Relationship of obesity to chronic disease. Geriatrics, *10*:78–82, 1955.

Goodman, N., Richardson, S. A., Dornbusch, S. M. and Hastorf, A. H.: Variant reactions to physical disabilities. Am. Sociol. Rev., *28*:429–435, 1963.

Gordon, T. and Kannel, W. B.: The effects of overweight on cardiovascular diseases. Geriatrics, *28*:80–88, 1973.

Henschel, A.: Obesity as an occupational hazard. Can. J. Public Health, *58*:491–493, 1967.

Heyden, S., Cassel, J. C., Bartel, A., Tyroler, H. A., Hames, C. G. and Cornoni, J. C.: Body weight and cigarette smoking as risk factors. Arch. Intern. Med., *128*:915–920, 1971a.

Heyden, S., Hames, C. G., Bartel, A., Cassel, J. C., Tyroler, H. A. and Cornoni, J. C.: Weight and weight history in relation to cerebrovascular and ischemic heart disease. Arch. Intern. Med., *128*:956–960, 1971b.

Heyden, S., Walker, L. and Hames, C. G.: Decrease of serum cholesterol level and blood pressure in the community. Seven to nine years of observation in the Evans County Study. Arch. Intern. Med., *128*:982–986, 1971c.

Holland, W. W. and Humerfelt, S.: Measurement of blood pressure: Comparison of intra-arterial and cuff values. Br. Med. J., *2*:1241–1243, 1964.

Hollingsworth, D. R. and Amatruda, T. T., Jr.: Acanthosis Nigricans and obesity. An endocrine abnormality? Arch. Intern. Med., *124*:481–487, 1969.

Hundley, J. M.: Diabetes; overweight: U.S. Problems. J. Am. Dietetic Assoc., *32*:417–422, 1956.

Hutchison, J. J.: Clinical implications of extensive actuarial study of build and blood pressure. Ann. Intern. Med., *54*:90–96, 1961.

Kannel, W. B. and Gordon, T.: Obesity and cardiovascular disease: The Framingham Study in "Obesity". (Burland, W., Samuel, P. D. and Yudkin, J. eds.) London, Churchill Livingstone, 1974.

Kannel, W. B., LeBauer, E. J., Dawber, T. R. and McNamara, P. M.: Relation of body weight to development of coronary heart disease. Circulation, *35*:734–744, 1967.

Keen, H.: The incomplete story of obesity and diabetes in "Recent Advances in Obesity Research": I. Proceedings of the first International Congress of Obesity. London, Newman Publishing Ltd., 1975, pp. 116–127.

Keys, A., et al.: Coronary heart disease: Overweight and obesity as risk factors. Ann. Intern. Med., *77*:15–27, 1972.

Keys, A. (ed.): Coronary heart disease in seven countries. Circulation, 41: (Suppl) 1–211, 1970.

Keys, A.: Overweight and the risk of heart attack and sudden death. In: Obesity in Perspective. Fogarty International Center Series on Preventive Medicine, Vol. II, Part II. (Bray, G. A. ed.) Washington, D.C., U.S. Government Printing Office. 1976.

King, G. E.: Errors in clinical measurement of blood pressure in obesity. Clin. Sci., 32:223–237, 1967.

Kvols, L. K., Rohlfing, B. M. and Alexander, J. K.: A comparison of intra-arterial and cuff blood pressure measurements in very obese subjects. Cardiovasc. Res. Cen. Bull., 7:118–123, 1969.

Larsen, O. A., Lassen, N. A. and Quaade, F.: Blood flow through human adipose tissue determined with radioactive xenon. Acta Physiol. Scand., 66:337–345, 1966.

Levy, R. L., White, P. D., Stroud, W. D. and Hillman, C. C.: Overweight: Its prognostic significance in relation to hypertension and cardiovascular renal diseases. J.A.M.A., 131:951–953, 1946.

Louderback, L.: Fat Power: Whatever You Weigh Is Right. New York, Hawthorn Books, Inc. 1970.

Lourenço, R. V.: Diaphragm activity in obesity. J. Clin. Invest., 48:1609–1614, 1969.

Luft, R., Cerasi, E. and Anderson, B.: Obesity as an additional factor in the pathogenesis of diabetes. Acta Endocrinologica, 59:344–352, 1968.

MacGregor, M. I., Block, A. J. and Ball, W. C., Jr.: Topics in clinical medicine. Serious complications and sudden death in the Pickwickian Syndrome. Bull. Johns Hopkins Hosp., 126:279–295, 1970.

Maddox, G. L., Back, K. W. and Liederman, V. R.: Overweight as social deviance and disability. J. Health Soc. Behav., 9:287–298, 1968.

Maddox, G. L., Anderson, C. F. and Bogdonoff, M. D.: Overweight as a problem of medical management in a public outpatient clinic. Am. J. Med. Sci., 252:394–402, 1966.

Maddox, G. L. and Liederman, V.: Overweight as a social disability with medical implications. J. Med. Educ., 44:214–220, 1969.

Mann, G. V.: Obesity, the nutritional spook. Am. J. Public Health, 61:1491–1498, 1971.

Mann, G. V.: The influence of obesity on health. (First of two parts). N. Engl. J. Med., 291:178, 1974.

Marks, H. H.: Influence of obesity in morbidity and mortality. Bull, N. Y. Acad. Sci., 36:296–312, 1960.

Martin, L.: Effect of weight reduction on normal and raised blood pressures in obesity. Lancet, 2:1051–1053, 1952.

Master, A. M., Jaffe, H. L. and Chesky, K.: Relationship of obesity to coronary disease and hypertension. J.A.M.A., 153:1499–1501, 1953.

Master, A. M. and Lasser, R. P.: Relationship of the blood pressure to weight, height and body build in apparently healthy subjects, 65–106 years of age. Am. J. Med. Sci., 235:278–289, 1958.

Matthews, H. B. and Der Brucke, M. G.: "Normal expectancy" in the extremely obese pregnant women. J.A.M.A., 110:554–559, 1938.

McKeown, T. and Record, R. G.: The influence of body weight on reproductive function in women. J. Endocrinol., 15:410–422, 1957.

Mentzer, S. H.: Clinical and pathological study of cholecystitis and cholelithiasis. Surg. Gynec. Obstet., 42:782–793, 1926.

Monello, L. F. and Mayer, J.: Obese adolescent girls: An unrecognized "minority" group. Am. J. Clin. Nutr., 13:35–39, 1963.

Odell, L. D. and Mengert, W. F.: The overweight obstetric patient. J.A.M.A., 128:87–89, 1945.

Osserman, K. E. and Dolger, H.: Obesity in diabetes: A study of therapy with anorexigenic drugs. Ann. Int. Med., 34:72–79, 1951.

Peckham, C. H. and Christianson, R. E.: The relationship between prepregnancy weight and certain obstetric factors. Am. J. Obstet. Gynecol., 111:1–7, 1971.

Pickering, G. W., Roberts, J. A. F. and Sowry, G. S. C.: Etiology of essential hypertension: effect of correcting for arm circumference on the growth rate of arterial pressure with age. Clin. Sci., 13:267–271, 1954.

Prem, K. A., Mensheha, N. M. and McKelvey, J. L.: Operative treatment of adenocarcinoma of the endometrium in obese women. Am. J. Obstet. Gynecol., 92:16–22, 1965.

Prodger, S. H. and Dennig, H.: Study of circulation in obesity. J. Clin. Invest., 11:789–806, 1932.

Rafferty, E. B. and Ward, A. P.: Indirect method of recording blood pressure. Cardiovasc. Res., 2:210–218, 1968.

Ragan, C. and Bordley, J., Jr.: Accuracy of clinical measurements of arterial blood pressure. Bull. Johns Hopkins Hosp., 69:504–528, 1941.

Richardson, S. A., Hastorf, A. H., Goodman, N. and Dornbusch, S. M.: Cultural uniformity in reaction to physical disabilities. Am. Sociol. Res., 26:241–247, 1961.

Rimm, A. A., Werner, L. H., Bernstein, R., and van Yserloo, B.: Disease and obesity in 73,532 women. Obesity Bariatric Med., 1:77–84, 1972.

Robinson, S. C. and Brucer, M.: Hypertension. Body build and obesity. Am. J. Med. Sci., 199:819–829, 1940.

Rosenman, R. H., Friedman, M., Straus, R., Jenkins, C. D., Zyzanski, S. J. and Wurm, M.: Coronary heart disease in the western collaborative group study: A follow-up experience of 4½ years. J. Chronic Dis., 23:173–190, 1970.

Sanders, K.: Coronary artery disease and obesity. Lancet, 2:432–435, 1959.

Schwalb, H. and Schimert, G.: Das Herz bei Fettsucht, Med. Klin., 65:1908–1913, 1970.

Seltzer, C. C.: Overweight and obesity. The associated cardiovascular risk. Minn. Med., 52:1265–1270, 1969.

Seltzer, C. C.: Some re-evaluations of the build and blood pressure study, 1959, as related to ponderal index, somatotype and mortality. N. Engl. J. Med., 274:254–259, 1966.

Sharp, J. T., Henry, J. P., Sweany, S. K., Meadows, W. R. and Pietras, R. J.: The total work of breathing in normal and obese men. J. Clin. Invest., 43:728–738, 1964.

Smith, H. L.: Relation of the weight of the heart to the weight of the body and of the weight of the heart to age. Am. Heart J., 4:79–93, 1928.

Society of Actuaries. Medico-Actuarial Investigation, 1913.

Society of Actuaries. Medical Impairment Study, 1929.

Society of Actuaries. Build and blood pressure study, 1959.

Spain, D. M., Bradeşs, V. A. and Huss, G.: Observations on atherosclerosis of the coronary arteries in males under the age of 46: A necropsy study with special references to somatotypes. Ann. Intern. Med., 38:254–277, 1953.

Spain, D. M., Nathan, D. J. and Gellis, M.: Weight, body types and the prevalence of coronary atherosclerotic heart disease in males. Am. J. Med. Sci., 245:63–69, 1963.

Stamler, J., Berkson, D. M. and Lindberg, H. A.: Coronary risk factors. Med. Clin. North Am., 50:229–254, 1966.

Sturdevant, R. A. L., Pearce, M. L. and Dayton, S.: Increased prevalence of cholelithiasis in men ingesting a serum-cholesterol-lowering diet. N. Engl. J. Med., 288:24–27, 1973.

Terry, A. J., Jr.: Obesity and hypertension. J.A.M.A., 81:1283–1284, 1923.

Thomas, C. B. and Cohen, B. H.: The familiar occurrence of hypertension and coronary artery disease, with observations concerning obesity and diabetes. Ann. Intern. Med. 42:90–127, 1955.

Wallgren, G., Bager, B. and Okmian, L.: Ventilatory insufficiency in an obese girl. Acta Paediat. Scand., 54:288–294, 1965.

Walster, E., Aronson, V., Abrahams, D. and Ratlmann, L.: Importance of physical attractiveness in dating behavior. J. Person. Soc. Psychol., 4:508–516, 1966.

Warner, W. A.: The obese patient and anesthesia. J.A.M.A., 205:102–103, 1968.

Weisinger, J. R., Kempson, R. L., Eldridge, F. L. and Swenson, R. S.: The nephrotic syndrome: A complication of massive obesity. Ann. Intern. Med., 81:440–447, 1974.

Wilens, S. L.: Bearing of general nutritional state on atherosclerosis. Arch. Intern. Med., 79:129–147, 1947.

Wilkens, R. H., Roberts, J. C., Jr. and Moses, C.: Autopsy studies in atherosclerosis III. Distribution and severity of artherosclerosis in the presence of obesity hypertension, nephrosclerosis, rheumatic heart disease. Circulation, 220:527–536, 1959.

CHAPTER 7

SOME METABOLIC EFFECTS OF OBESITY

The obese individual who is in a state of caloric equilibrium with his environment, that is, an individual who is neither gaining nor losing weight, demonstrates a number of endocrine and metabolic abnormalities. A list with some of these is shown in Table 7–1. Fasting blood sugar is often elevated, particularly in individuals who have been obese for many years. This is clearly demonstrated by the data of Ogilvie (1935) as replotted by Bierman et al. (1969) (Fig. 7–1). Glucose tolerance is also frequently impaired whether the challenge of glucose is given orally or intravenously (Embleton, 1938; John, 1934, Morse and Mahabir, 1964; Franckson et al., 1966). Obese individuals also usually demonstrate an elevation in serum insulin (Karam et al., 1963; Nikkilä and Taskinen, 1971; Deckert and Hagerup, 1967; Lambert et al., 1966). Several other metabolites may also be altered, and pyruvate, lactate and citrate are slightly elevated.

The effects of obesity on glucagon have not been entirely clarified and will be discussed in more detail below. Plasma free fatty acids are frequently elevated in obese individuals after an overnight fast, but the rise after 23 hours of fasting is greater in obese than in lean individuals. After exposure to the cold, many obese individuals show little or no rise in oxygen consumption in comparison with the rise in normal individuals. Adrenal corticosteroid excretion is often elevated, but plasma cortisol is generally normal. Cortisol production rates are also increased in most obese individuals. Growth hormone is usually reduced. We shall now consider in some detail the alterations in the pancreas, adrenal, pituitary and reproductive systems which are found in many obese patients.

TABLE 7–1. *Metabolic Changes in Obesity*

Parameter	Changes in Obese Patients Relative to Normal Weight Subjects
Carbohydrate Metabolism	
Fasting blood glucose	N or ↑
Glucose tolerance	
Intravenous	↓ or N
Oral	↓ or N
Glucose turnover	↑
Alcohol induced hypoglycemia	Smaller drop
Glycerol	↑
Lactate	↑
Pyruvate	↑
Citrate	↑
Amino Acids	
Arginine	↑
Leucine	↑
Tyrosine	↑
Phenylalanine	↑
Valine	↑
Others	N
Lipids	
Free fatty acids	↑
Turnover of free fatty acids	↑
Triglycerides	↑ or N
Cholesterol	N or ↑
Hormonal changes	
Insulin–basal	↑
Glucose	↑
Tolbutamide	↑
Glucagon	↑
Leucine	↑
Glucagon	N ?↑
Adrenal	
Cortisol concentration	N
Cortisol production	↑
Urinary 17-hydroxysteroids	↑
Thyroid	
Radioactive iodine uptake	N
Thyroxine (concentration)	N
Triiodothyronine (concentration)	N or ↑
Response to thyrotropin releasing hormone	N
Growth hormone	
Nocturnal rise	↓
Response to	
Glucose	↓
Insulin	↓
Arginine	↓
L-dopa	↓

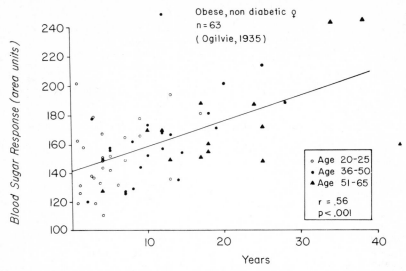

Figure 7–1. Glucose tolerance and the duration of obesity. The blood sugar response 2 hours after a 50g oral load. (Reprinted from Bierman et al.: Am. J. Clin. Nutr., *21*:1434–1437, 1968, with permission.)

THE PANCREATIC HORMONES: INSULIN AND GLUCAGON

INSULIN

Control of Secretion

The endocrine pancreas is located in the islets of Langerhans scattered throughout the acinar or digestive part of the pancreas. These islets of Langerhans are composed of several cell types which secrete different hormones. The alpha cells are currently thought to secrete glucagon, the beta cells to secrete insulin and the delta cells to secrete gastrin. Our understanding of the function of the pancreatic beta cells has been extended greatly by the application of modern techniques of radioimmunoassay and electronmicroscopy to obtain detailed information about the secretory dynamics of these cells (Bray et al., 1973). A schematic picture of the beta cell is shown in the accompanying figure (Fig. 7–2).

The sequence of events following exposure to a stimulus for insulin release has been carefully studied by Lacy (1970), Orci (1974) and Hellman (1970). The present concept involves the following sequence of steps. The first step is the secretion of the insulin which is stored in prepackaged granules by activation of the microtubular system in the membrane. As secretion begins, other granules migrate towards the cell wall and their contents are released into the extracellular fluid. As this process continues, the cell initiates the synthesis, storage and

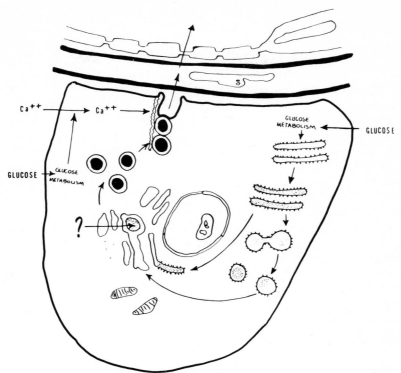

Figure 7–2. A diagram of the islet cell from the pancreas. Glucose stimulates the release of insulin (left side) and the synthesis of insulin (right side). The process of insulin synthesis involves the rough endoplasmic reticulum which becomes round in the process. The proinsulin which is formed is packaged into dense granules by the Golgi apparatus (near and to the left of the nucleus). Secretion involves calcium and the lining up of the insulin granules near the plasma membrane adjacent to the microtubular system. From Lacey, P. E. and Greider, M. H.: Handbook of Physiology, (Steiner and Frankel, ed.) 7, I, Washington, D. C., Am. Physiol. Soc., 1972, 77–89.

release of additional insulin molecules. The new insulin molecules are synthesized in the rough endoplasmic reticulum. They are synthesized as a single chain composed at one end of the alpha chain of insulin and at the other end of the beta chain with a connecting C-peptide joining the A and B chains. This single chain is termed proinsulin and is packaged by the Golgi apparatus into the insulin granules. These granules then migrate into the cytoplasm and toward the cell membrane. The action of a trypsin-like enzyme cleaves the C-peptide and leaves the active insulin molecules composed of the connected A and B chains. Since this cleavage appears to occur after packaging, one would expect that proinsulin would be secreted into the circulation along with insulin, a conclusion which has been demonstrated by Rubenstein et al. (1972). However, proinsulin accounts for only about 10 to 20 percent of the secreted insulin.

The secretory dynamics of the pancreatic beta cell have been examined in vitro and in vivo. This process can best be described as a "two-pool" system. That is, there is an initial rapid release of insulin after the beta cell is exposed to glucose, followed by a second phase of insulin release with continuous high rates of insulin secretion. The initial burst of insulin secretion is the result of release from storage granules while the slower phase represents release from granules plus an increasing fraction from newly synthesized insulin. With very low glucose concentrations (less than 5 mM), islets secrete very little insulin. As glucose concentration is increased, there is enhanced insulin output. The maximal effect of glucose occurs with a concentration of about 20 mM (approximately 360 mg/dl).

The role of glucose as a stimulator of insulin secretion has been intensively studied. Substances such as 2-deoxy-glucose which inhibit the metabolism of glucose also inhibit the secretion of insulin. Stimulation of insulin secretion by glucose is also inhibited by the 7-carbon sugar mannoheptulose, and by glucosamine, an amino derivative of glucose. These observations suggest that glucose must be phosphorylated as well as partially metabolized in order to stimulate the secretion of the insulin. Compounds such as manose and fructose which are metabolized more slowly than glucose, also stimulate insulin secretion but to a smaller degree. Lactose which is without effect on insulin secretion is not metabolized by the islet cells.

The other factors which influence insulin secretion can be divided into several groups. These include nutrients, hormonal factors, neural factors and drugs.

THE INFLUENCE OF NUTRIENTS.   Glucose is the major nutrient controlling the secretion of insulin. Second in importance are the amino acids. The studies of Fajans et al. (1967) have examined the effects of a protein meal and of individual amino acids on the secretion of insulin. A protein meal stimulates insulin secretion, and has a synergistic effect with glucose. The intravenous infusion of a mixture of 10 amino acids is a potent stimulator for insulin release (Table 7–2). Of these amino acids, arginine, lysine, leucine and phenylalanine are the most effective, with activities ranging between 86 and 32 percent of the activity of the total mixture (see Table 7–2). The remaining amino acids have a much smaller effect. Not only is the effect of a protein meal potentiated by glucose, but the infusion of glucose along with arginine also potentiates the release of insulin.

Fatty acids and ketone bodies may also stimulate insulin secretion. These substances, however, are much less potent than glucose or amino acids. Intravenous administration of acetoacetate or beta-hydroxybutyrate does not cause a rise in plasma insulin in man, but in experimental animals both free fatty acids and ketone bodies will cause insulin release. The magnitude of this effect, however, is small and the physiologic importance of these compounds is unclear.

THE HORMONAL FACTORS.   Table 7–3 divides the hormonal fac-

TABLE 7–2. *Effect of Amino Acids on Insulin Secretion**

AMINO ACIDS	RELATIVE POTENCY *(percent)*
Mixture of 10 amino acids	100
Arginine	86
Lysine	64
Leucine	34
Phenylalanine	32
Valine	12
Methionine	11
Threonine, isoleucine, tryptophan	10 to 30
Histidine	<1

*Adapted from Fajans et al.: Recent Prog. Horm. Res., 23:617–656, 1967.

tors which influence insulin secretion into two groups, the nutrients and hormones. The first group of hormones are those arising from other endocrine glands. The importance of gastrointestinal hormones was suggested as early as 1906, but has been brought into focus recently by studies comparing insulin secretion following oral and intravenous glucose (Perley and Kipnis, 1967). When glucose is administered orally, insulin concentrations rise promptly and then gradually return to baseline. When levels of glucose in plasma comparable to those produced by an oral load are achieved by infusing glucose intravenously, the secretion of insulin was only 30 to 40 percent of that seen after the oral load. Moreover, only 20 to 35 percent as

TABLE 7–3. *Factors which Modify the Secretion of Insulin and Glucagon*

FACTORS	DIRECTION OF CHANGE IN PLASMA	
	Insulin	*Glucagon*
Nutrients		
Glucose	↑	↓
Amino acids	↑	↑
Fatty acids	↑	↓
Hormones		
Intestinal		
Cholecystokinin-Pancreozymin	↑	↑
Gastrin	↑	–
Secretin	↑	↓
Glucagon	↑	–
Growth hormone	↑	–
Adrenal steroids	↑	–
Progestational agents	↑	–
Thyroid	↑	–
Epinephrine-norepinephrine	↑	–
Autonomic Nervous System		
Sympathetic	↓	?
Parasympathetic	↑	

much glucose is required by the intravenous route to duplicate the glucose concentrations achieved by an oral load of 100 g. These data suggest that some factor associated with the ingestion and absorption of glucose is important in stimulating insulin secretion in man.

Several hormones from the gastrointestinal tract have been implicated in this role, including secretion, cholecystokinin, pancreozymin and gastrin. Each of them can stimulate insulin when administered intravenously if given in large quantities. This raises doubts about their physiologic importance. Since these hormones have been purified, they produce smaller effects than the impure preparations, and this raises further doubts about whether any of these hormones plays an important role in modulating insulin secretion during absorption of glucose.

The other hormones involved in stimulating insulin secretion are also summarized in Table 7–3. Pharmacologic doses of glucagon given intravenously are followed by a rise of plasma immunoreactive insulin (Samols, Marri and Marks, 1965; Crockford et al., 1969; Karam et al., 1966; Grodsky et al., 1967; Sussman and Baugh, 1967). This effect of glucagon may well be mediated by the activation of adenylcyclase which may play a role in the secretion of insulin. Whether glucagon is involved in the physiologic control of insulin secretion is less clear.

Growth hormone also modifies insulin secretion. In individuals with congenital deficiency of growth hormone, insulin secretion in the basal state as well as following a glucose load tends to be subnormal (Merimee, Burgess and Rabinowitz, 1967). Treatment of these patients with growth hormone restores insulin levels to normal. This hormone also increases the basal levels of insulin in acromegalics (Cerasi and Luft, 1964; Ackerblom et al., 1969).

Adrenal steroids produce resistance to the peripheral actions of insulin after a glucose load. Glucose tolerance becomes impaired only when insulin reserves in the pancreas are impaired. These effects of adrenal steroids appear to be reversible since adrenalectomy usually returns pancreatic function to normal. In patients who produce excess quantities of aldosterone, glucose tolerance may also be impaired. Potassium replacement in these patients often restores glucose intolerance towards normal, and has led to the suggestion that the loss of potassium is the major cause for the glucose intolerance (Anderson et al., 1969).

Many oral contraceptives also increase basal insulin and the rise of insulin which follows glucose (Swerdloff et al., 1975). These pills usually contain both an estrogen and a progestational agent. The estrogens themselves are probably not responsible for the impaired glucose tolerance and the elevated levels of insulin since there was no deterioration of glucose tolerance in women treated for six months with estrogens alone. When various progestational agents are present, however, basal insulin was increased and glucose tolerance was impaired in a significant percentage of women (Swerdloff, 1975).

Thyroid hormone also influences secretion. In myxedema, glucose tolerance is improved and insulin secretion decreased. With excess thyroid hormone or in hyperthyroidism, the rise in insulin and the rise in glucose are frequently exaggerated (Bray and Jacobs, 1974).

THE NEURAL FACTORS.   The sympathetic and parasympathetic nervous system also modulate insulin secretion (Woods and Porte, 1974). The sympathetic nervous system appears to act primarily to reduce insulin secretion. During the infusion of epinephrine, Porte et al. (1966) found that plasma glucose concentrations rose, but that insulin release was inhibited. In subsequent studies, they demonstrated that the inhibition of insulin secretion by epinephrine could be prevented by simultaneous administration of phentolamine, an alpha-adrenergic blocking drug. This suggests that catecholamines interact with the beta cells of the islets of Langerhans to inhibit insulin release in the presence of glucose. Norepinephrine is also a potent inhibitor of insulin secretion in vivo, and with isolated islets in vitro. A physiologic role for the adrenergic (sympathetic) nervous system in controlling insulin secretion has been observed during "stress." After surgery or a heart attack, the release of insulin in response to the infusion of glucose is significantly reduced. Thus, glucose intolerance during stress would appear to reflect a decrease in the secretion of insulin due to increased circulating levels of catecholamines.

The parasympathetic nervous system supplies the pancreas through the vagus nerve. Stimulation of the vagus nerve increases insulin secretion (Kaneto et al., 1974; Frohman et al., 1967; Porte et al., 1973), and the magnitude of this rise is related to the level of blood glucose. If plasma glucose is elevated, vagal stimulation acts synergistically with the glucose to markedly increase insulin secretion. If glucose is not elevated, however, the rise in insulin after vagal stimulation is small (Bergman and Miller, 1973). Acetylcholine, the principal mediator of parasympathetic nervous system at the neuro-effector function, also enhances insulin secretion.

Insulin Secretion in Obesity

The islets of the pancreas are enlarged in obese patients. Ogilvie (1933) demonstrated that the islets of Langerhans obtained from 19 obese patients at autopsy were on average 65 percent larger than the normal islets. A similar hyperplasia of islet tissue has been demonstrated in experimental obesity produced by hypothalamic injury (Kennedy and Parker, 1963) as well as in genetically obese animals (York et al., 1972; Bray and York, 1971). Shortly after the development

of sensitive techniques for measuring plasma insulin by radioimmunoassay, Rabinowitz and Zierler (1962) found that obese patients
had increased levels of insulin. The elevation in insulin is correlated
with the degree of obesity (Bagdade et al., 1967) (Fig. 7–3). The authors of the study from which the data in Fig. 7–4 was obtained had
carefully controlled both the total caloric intake as well as the intake of
carbohydrates and the amount of exercise.

Stern et al. (1972) have obtained similar findings. In addition to
the increase in basal secretion of insulin, obese subjects almost uniformly show an increase in secretion of insulin after administration of
glucose (Ben-David et al., 1967; Bergstrand and Hellstrom, 1953;
Kreisberg et al., 1967; Martin and Martin, 1973; Sussman, 1966), the
injection of glucagon (Bendetti et al., 1967; Crockford et al., 1969), or
the infusion of L-leucine (Loridan et al., 1971; Johnson et al., 1973).
Patients with long-standing obesity show much more impairment than
those with recent onset of their obesity (Parra et al., 1971). Bagdade et
al. (1967) analyzed the rise in insulin of obese, normal and diabetic
subjects in response to glucose and demonstrated that the increment
in insulin following an oral glucose load was comparable if expressed
as a percentage increment above the fasting or basal level. These data
imply that the effects of obesity are manifested largely through the
increased basal levels of insulin. Studies by Karam et al. (1974) have
indicated that in obese subjects, the maximal rise in insulin is greater
than in normal subjects, but that the concentration of glucose required

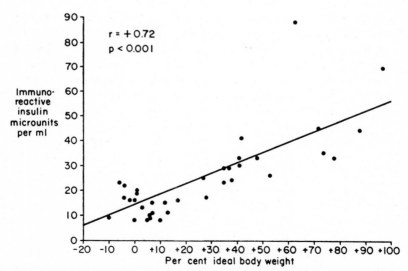

Figure 7–3.   Relation of insulin and ideal body weight. As the percentage of ideal body
weight increased, immunoreactive insulin also rose. (Reprinted from Bagdade et al.: J.
Clin. Invest., 46:1549–1557, 1967, with permission.)

to produce 50 percent of the maximal rise remains the same. This concentration is 140 mg/dl. From these studies, it would appear that there is an increase in the number of islets rather than an increase in the sensitivity of a few islets.

The data from obese patients showing increased levels of insulin in response to a challenge with glucose, glucagon and L-leucine raise two important questions: (1) by what mechanism does obesity produce hyperinsulinemia, and (2) by what mechanisms does the body prevent the drop in glucose in the presence of increased circulating levels of insulin? One explanation for the increased concentration of insulin in obesity would be provided if proinsulin represented a large fraction of the circulating radioimmunoassayable insulin.

As noted above, the conversion of proinsulin to insulin involves cleavage of a connecting peptide (C-peptide) which joins the alpha and beta chains during synthesis of insulin. Most antibodies to insulin cross-react with proinsulin as well as with insulin itself, yet the biological activity of proinsulin is only 1 to 2 percent that of native insulin. Secretion of proinsulin would be detected as an increase in circulating insulin by most immunoassays. The possibility that obese patients secrete increased amounts of proinsulin has been examined by Gordon and Roth (1969) and Melani et al. (1970). Normally, proinsulin accounts for no more than 10 percent of the total radioimmunoassayable insulin. A similar proportion is present in obesity. During stimulation of insulin secretion with glucose, both insulin and proinsulin rise, but the relative amounts do not differ from normal. Thus, the insulin which is secreted in obesity appears to contain approximately the same proportions of proinsulin as observed in normal subjects. This conclusion is supported by the data shown in Fig. 7–4. Glucose tolerance tests for normal individuals are shown in the three upper panels and from three obese patients in the lower panels. Although the rise in the total insulin is greater in several of the obese subjects, there was little or no difference in the fraction of proinsulin, as indicated by the heights of the solid bars.

A decrease in insulin turnover could also explain the higher levels of basal insulin. The available data on the turnover and metabolism of insulin in obesity, however, does not support this possibility. Insulin degradation has been examined in experimental animals and is not altered either in vivo or in vitro (Welsh et al., 1956). That is, the removal of insulin from the circulation is related to the circulating concentration of the hormone. As the concentration of insulin in the circulation increases, the quantity removed also rises because the turnover rate remains constant.

Genuth (1972) has recently re-examined this question in normal and obese subjects. Peripheral removal was estimated from specific activity of insulin after infusing radioactive insulin for three hours. The removal of insulin in the normal individual was correlated with

STARVATION GLUCOSE TOLERANCE TEST

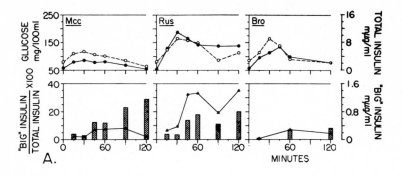

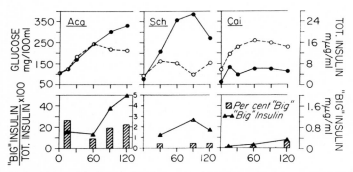

Figure 7-4. Big and little insulin during a glucose tolerance test in lean (top panels) and obese (lower panels) subjects. The glucose (solid lines) and insulin (broken lines) rose after the glucose load. The percentage rise in "big" insulin (proinsulin—lower half each pair of panels) was similar in lean and obese. (Reprinted from Gordon, P. and Roth, J.: J. Clin. Invest., *48*:2225–2234, 1969, with permission.)

surface area (r = .70). The obese subjects had a significantly higher clearance or removal of insulin than did the lean ones (278 ml/min vs. 223 ml/min). Short term fasting in the obese subjects lowered insulin concentrations from 25 to 15 μU/ml but did not alter the removal rate (Fig. 7–5). We must conclude, therefore, that the increased concentrations of insulin in obesity result from increased secretion of this hormone.

Since the increased basal levels of insulin reflect enhanced secretion, the question then becomes—by what mechanism is the secretion of insulin augmented? As we noted previously, the factors which modulate insulin secretion can be divided into three groups; nutrients, hormones and neural factors. Increased glucose concentration might be an important factor in enhancing the secretion of insulin in

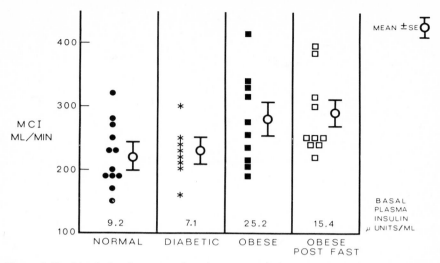

Figure 7–5. Metabolic clearance of insulin in normal, diabetic and obese patients. The obese subjects before and after a fast showed a higher clearance of insulin than lean subjects. (Reprinted from Genuth et al.: Diabetes, *21*:1003–1012, 1972.)

obesity. The fasting levels are higher in many obese individuals than in normal individuals (Sims et al., 1973). The small increases in glucose observed in obese individuals might be a reflection of their state of overnutrition and, in turn, might signal the pancreas to secrete more insulin.

INFLUENCE OF AMINO ACIDS. Increased concentrations of amino acids might also account in part for basal hyperinsulinemia of obesity. Felig et al. (1969) measured plasma amino acids in obese patients and found that arginine, leucine, tyrosine, phenylalanine and valine were increased. The remaining amino acids were not significantly different from normal. They suggested that this increase in amino acids might be responsible for the enhanced insulin output. Both arginine and leucine are potent stimulators of insulin secretion. Small increases in leucine might act synergistically with glucose to stimulate insulin secretion. Floyd et al. (1970) found that an infusion of amino acids potentiated the effects of glucose on the secretion of insulin. We have confirmed this finding (Fig. 7–6). An infusion of glucose 100 mg/min was given on one day, an infusion of a mixture of four insulin-stimulating amino acids was given on another day, and the combined infusion on a third day. It is clear that the insulin levels were much higher when the amino acids and glucose were given together.

Thus a small rise in glucose and a small rise in the concentration of leucine and arginine might be sufficient to account for the increased levels of insulin observed in the basal state in obese subjects. The

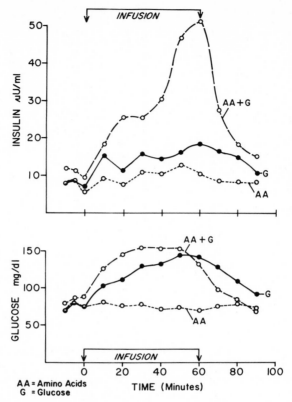

Figure 7–6. Effect of amino acids and glucose on plasma insulin. An infusion of a 27 g mixture of leucine, phenylalanine, valine, and isoleucine was given over a 60 minute interval, with and without a glucose infusion of 100 mg/minute. The combined infusion had a synergistic effect on insulin secretion. (Ogundipe and Bray, unpublished observations.)

sequence of events leading to hyperinsulinemia in obesity might be depicted as shown in Fig. 7–7. The consequences of increased caloric intake on the disposition of fatty acids, glucose and protein are presented.

NEURAL FACTORS.   The autonomic nervous system as a controller of basal insulin levels in obesity has been explored (Fiser and Bray, 1974). As noted earlier, the infusion of epinephrine into normal subjects increases glucose but blocks the rise in insulin. In obese patients an infusion of epinephrine increases the concentration of glucose and actually reduces the concentration of insulin below control levels. Blockade of the alpha receptors on the islet of Langerhans is associated with a rise in insulin in normal subjects (Robertson and Porte, 1973), implying that there is normally some sympathetic inhibition of insulin secretion.

In the obese patients, on the other hand, phentolamine did not

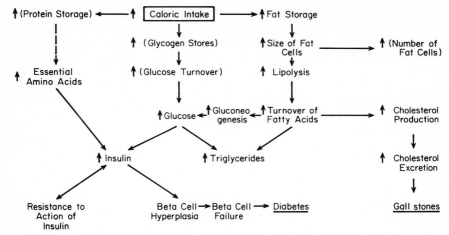

Figure 7–7. A schematic diagram for some of the metabolic consequences of ingesting excess calories. The brackets ( ) and broken lines indicate uncertainty about the proposed metabolic changes. This diagram allows a formulation of the pathogenesis of gallstones and diabetes, two of the major diseases associated with obesity.

significantly change the concentration of insulin, raising the possibility that tonic sympathetic activity was not suppressing insulin release in the obese patients. This would mean that a significant portion of the rise in basal insulin in obesity might represent withdrawal of tonic inhibition by the sympathetic nervous system. In addition, Parra and Schultz (1969) showed that an infusion of epinephrine did not change basal insulin but that an infusion of epinephrine and propranolol significantly reduced the basal level of insulin. The synergistic effect of a small increase in glucose and enhanced vagal release of acetylcholine might also enhance the basal level of insulin. These interrelations remain to be evaluated, however.

The second problem to be examined is the paradox of an elevated glucose along with high levels of insulin. Among the factors which might control the responsiveness to insulin are (1) the size of the adipocytes (Salans et al., 1974); (2) the total caloric intake (Sims et al., 1973); (3) the fraction of carbohydrate in the diet prior to testing the effects of insulin (Grey and Kipnis, 1971); (4) the presence of functional beta cells (Mahler and Szab, 1971); and (5) the degree of physical training (Bjorntorp et al., 1970; Fahlen et al., 1972; Bjorntorp, 1975).

Rabinowitz and Zierler (1962) approached this problem using a technique for perfusing the human forearm. With this method, blood samples are collected simultaneously from the brachial artery and from superficial and deep veins in the forearm. The deep venous channels drain primarily the muscles and the superficial veins drain mainly fat and skin. The obese subjects studied by Rabinowitz and

Zierler (1962; Rabinowitz, 1968, 1970) were approximately 20 percent overweight, but this degree of obesity is sufficient to double body fat. The uptake of glucose by muscles in the forearm before giving insulin was similar in the lean and obese subjects, even though the levels of insulin were significantly higher in the obese individuals. During the 26 minute intra-arterial infusion of insulin, however, the obese subjects showed a smaller uptake of glucose than did the lean subjects. These authors concluded that both muscle and adipose tissue of obese subjects were less responsive (i.e., "resistant") to the actions of insulin.

SIZE OF ADIPOCYTES.   Salans, Knittle and Hirsch (1968) used a second approach to examine the reduced effectiveness of insulin in obesity. They incubated an aspiration biopsy of adipose tissue in vitro before and after weight loss. The conversion of radioactivity from glucose-1-^{14}C to $^{14}CO_2$ in the presence and absence of insulin was used to measure the effects of this hormone. The difference between basal and insulin-stimulation rates of glucose oxidation was greater after weight loss than before. This difference was due largely to a decline in the basal oxidation of glucose when small fat cells were used. Maximal glucose oxidation in the presence of insulin showed little change with weight loss.

These authors interpreted their data to indicate that small adipocytes were more sensitive to insulin. An equally valid interpretation would be that basal glucose metabolism, i.e., in the absence of insulin, was reduced in the smaller adipocytes obtained after weight loss, but that the effects of insulin were not changed. Whichever interpretation one takes, the possibility that enlarged adipocytes were the mechanism for resistance to insulin has stimulated numerous studies to examine this hypothesis (see Chapter 3).

CALORIC INTAKE.   Total caloric intake in relation to energy needs also modifies the response to insulin. Adipose tissue from young growing animals has small fat cells which are more sensitive to the effects of insulin than adipose tissue from old adult animals with large fat cells. This difference might reflect differences in the size of fat cells but might also be due to the fact that growing animals are storing calories rapidly.

These possibilities were differentiated in experiments performed by DiGirolamo and Rudman (1968) and by Salans and Dougherty (1971), who showed that the large adipocytes from older animals can be made as sensitive as small adipocytes from young animals if the old animals are first fasted and then allowed to reaccumulate fat rapidly. Thus enlargement of adipocytes does not necessarily increase their resistance to insulin. A similar conclusion was reached in studies with adipose cells from obese humans (Bray, 1969a). The sensitivity of isolated human adipocytes to insulin could be enhanced by overfeeding obese patients with a high carbohydrate, high calorie diet containing 3500 calories or more for a period of two weeks. Conversely, brief periods of caloric restriction to 900 calories per day abolished the response to insulin, indicating the importance of controlling the total caloric intake of lean or obese subjects prior to obtaining fat to assess its response to insulin or other hormones (see Chapter 3 for details).

DIET COMPOSITION. The composition of the diet is another factor which influences the sensitivity to insulin. The magnitude of the response to insulin in small and large adipocytes is a function of the carbohydrate intake (Sims et al., 1973; Salans et al., 1974). Adipose tissue obtained from rats fed a high carbohydrate diet oxidizes more glucose in the presence of insulin in vitro than if adipose tissue is obtained from rats on a low carbohydrate diet. A similar effect occurs in humans.

When adipose tissue from lean subjects who have eaten a high carbohydrate diet is incubated with insulin, more glucose is oxidized to CO_2 than with fat from the same subjects fed a low carbohydrate diet. This is illustrated by the studies of Salans et al. (1974) who have recently re-examined the relation between the size of fat cells and the composition of the diet on glucose metabolism and the response to insulin. Fat cells were obtained by needle aspiration of subcutaneous tissue in volunteers who were fed diets of known carbohydrate content before and after weight gain and in obese patients who were also fed controlled diets before and after weight loss. Large fat cells from either group were less responsive to insulin than small fat cells. When the size of the fat cells remained constant, however, increasing carbohydrate in the diet increased both the basal and insulin-stimulation metabolism of glucose (see Chapter 3).

PRESENCE OF BETA CELLS. Intact pancreatic beta cells may be a fourth factor involved in regulating the resistance to insulin. Resistance to the hypoglycemic effects of exogenous insulin is a hallmark of the genetically obese mouse (ob/ob) (Bray and York, 1971). Destruction of the pancreatic beta cells in these animals by injecting alloxan restores the hypoglycemic effect of exogenous insulin. This occurs without a change in body weight and without a change in the size of the adipocytes. These observations by Mahler and Szabo (1971) suggest that something from the pancreas, either endogenous insulin or some other factor, is an essential element in the insulin resistance of these obese mice.

These studies have recently been repeated using streptozotocin to destroy the beta cells. After treatment with this drug, blood glucose rose in the lean animals but fell in the genetically obese mice. In contrast to the studies which used alloxan, the responsiveness of fat cells and muscle to insulin was unchanged and the progression of obesity was unaffected. This suggests that the hyperinsulinemia may not play an important role (Batchelor et al., 1975).

Although the size of the adipocyte is one factor in determining the resistance to insulin, it appears that total carbohydrate and calorie intake are at least as important. It seems unlikly that "resistance," i.e., reduced responsiveness of fat cells to the action of insulin, can provide the entire explanation for impaired effectiveness of this hormone in obese subjects. For one thing, the quantity of glucose metabolized by adipose tissue accounts for only a small fraction of total glucose metabolism (Rabinowitz, 1970). In addition, the studies of Rabinowitz and Zierler (1962) in obese subjects indicate that muscle is also resistant to the action of insulin. Finally, the utilization of glucose by the liver is also reduced in obese patients (Ahlborg et al., 1974), suggesting that resistance to the action of insulin occurs in all tissues (Olefsky et al., 1974).

The experiments of Sims and his colleagues at the University of Vermont (Sims et al., 1973) have provided a number of additional insights into the role of diet and weight gain on the development of insulin resistance in man. These investigators asked the following question: Can the endocrine profile of spontaneous obesity be reproduced when lean subjects gain weight by a period of self induced overeating? Groups of volunteers from the Vermont State Prison agreed to overeat until they gained between 15 and 25 percent of their initial body weight. All of these men were lean, none had been previously overweight, and they did not have a family history of diabetes. Initial measurements were obtained while the volunteers ate a diet calculated to maintain body weight. This was followed by several months of increased food intake. Body composition was calculated from measurements of density determined initially and again at the end of the studies (see Chapter 1). After the subjects had gained weight, they were placed on a second diet to maintain body weight and the tests that they had undergone at the beginning of the study were repeated.

The results of these studies are summarized in Table 7–4. Approximately 70 percent of the weight gained by these subjects was fat, and the remainder was water and protein (Sims et al., 1968). The fat was stored by increasing the size of preexisting adipocytes (Fig. 7–8). Plasma glucose was significantly increased. Of particular note is the fact that glucose was raised even when fat provided the entire caloric supplement used to produce weight gain (Sims et al., 1973). The basal levels of insulin were also increased after weight gain, regardless of the type of diet used to increase body weight. An increase in basal or fasting insulin is also observed when experimental animals become fat on a high fat diet if the carbohydrate content of the diet is controlled (Ogundipe and Bray, 1974). In addition, the insulin response of the normal volunteers to the administration of glucose was enhanced. Cortisol secretion was elevated (O'Connell et al., 1973) and the release of growth hormone in response to several stimuli was blunted (Sims et al., 1973). The concept that hyperinsulinemia and glucose intolerance are a consequence of excess caloric intake is consistent

TABLE 7–4.   *Endocrine and Metabolic Changes in Spontaneous and Experimental Obesity**

PARAMETERS	SPONTANEOUS OBESITY	EXPERIMENTAL OBESITY
Adipose tissue		
Cell size	↑	↑
Cell number	↑	U
Caloric balance		
Calories required to maintain obese state (kilocalories/sq m)	1300	2700
Return to starting weight	Rapid	Rapid
Spontaneous physical activity	↓	↓
Appetite late in the day	↑	↑
Fasting concentrations in blood		
Cholesterol	↑	↑
Triglycerides	↑	↑
Free fatty acids	↑	U or ↓
Amino acids	↑	↑
Glucose	N or ↑	↑
Insulin	↑	–
Glucagon	N	–
Growth hormone	N or ↓	U or ↓
Glucose tolerance		
Oral	↓	↓
Intravenous	↓	↓
Insulin release		
To oral glucose	↑	↑
To IV glucose	↑	↑
To IV arginine	↑	↑
Evidence of insulin resistance		
Insulin: glucose ratio	↑	↑
Adipose tissue metabolism		
Sensitivity to insulin in vitro	↓	↓
Sensitivity to insulin in vivo	↓	↓
Forearm muscle metabolism		
Insulin stimulated glucose uptake	↓	↓
Insulin inhibition of release of amino acid	–	↓
Hormones possibly affecting insulin resistance		
Glucocorticoids		
Plasma cortisol	N or ↓	U
Cortisol production rate	↑	↑
Urinary 17-hydroxycorticoids	↑	↑
Growth hormone		
Response to glucose	↓	↓
Response to arginine	↓	↓
Nocturnal rises	–	↓

*From Horton, E. S.: Epidemiologic aspects of obesity. *In*: Understanding and Successfully Managing Obesity. (L. D. Rubin, ed.). Proceedings of a symposium organized by World Health Information Services, supported by Merrell-National Laboratories, and published by Postgraduate Medicine Symposiums, 1974.

U = unchanged
N = normal

with the improvement in glucose tolerance (Newburgh and Conn, 1939) and the fall of insulin levels during weight loss (El-Khodary et al., 1972; Farrant et al., 1969; Drenick et al., 1972; Hellier, 1970; Bagdade et al., 1974).

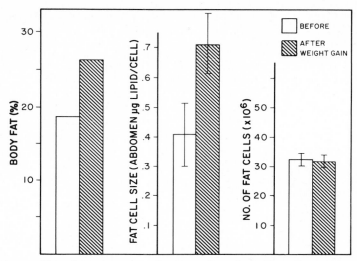

Figure 7–8.   Effect of weight gain on the size and number of fat cells. In normal weight men the storage of fat occurred entirely by increasing the size of fat cells. (Adapted from Salans et al.: J. Clin. Invest., 50:1005–1011, 1971.)

Resistance to the action of insulin was also demonstrated in studies perfusing the forearm and the liver of these volunteers before and after weight gain (Felig et al., 1973). At maximal weight, an intra-arterial infusion had a smaller response than before weight gain (Horton et al., 1974). This difference was similar to the insulin resistance of people with spontaneous obesity observed by Rabinowitz and Zierler (1962). Sims et al. (1973) have concluded that spontaneous obesity mimics the effects of dietary obesity observed in normal volunteers in the following aspects: (1) both have an increased level of basal insulin; (2) both show enhanced insulin secretion following glucose stimulation; (3) both have impaired glucose tolerance; (4) both show diminished response to insulin, as measured by glucose oxidation in adipocytes; (5) both demonstrate insulin resistance of forearm muscle to insulin; and (6) both have increased secretion of cortisol and diminished output of growth hormone.

GLUCAGON

Control of Secretion

The second pancreatic hormone is glucagon. It is a single chain peptide which contains 29 amino acids and is secreted by the alpha cell in the islet of Langerhans. The circulating concentration of this hormone can be changed by several means which have been summarized in Table 7–3. Amino acids increase the concentration of both insulin and glucagon. However, administration of glucose which increases insulin depresses the concentration of glucagon. All of the gastrointestinal hormones stimulate the output of insulin, but the response of glucagon is different. Cholecystokinin-pancreozymin stimulates the alpha-cell to release glucagon. Secretin, on the other hand, depresses glucagon output, and gastrin is without effect.

Glucagon appears to be a hormone which increases hepatic gluconeogenesis, and its level would be expected to relate to the needs for glucose formation by the liver. Thus, a glucose meal suppresses glucagon and a period of deprivation increases glucagon. Feeding a low carbohydrate diet also increases the concentration of glucagon, but a high carbohydrate diet lowers it (Unger, 1972).

Glucagon Secretion in Obesity

Studies on the effects of obesity on the basal and stimulated levels of glucagon have produced conflicting results. Wise et al. (1972, 1973) found that the basal level of glucagon was unchanged by obesity. After the infusion of alanine there was a smaller rise in glucagon in the obese subjects than in the lean ones, although plasma alanine levels were higher in the obese. Kalkhoff et al. (1973) used an infusion of arginine rather than alanine to stimulate a rise in the level of glucagon. With their procedure, the obese patients had a larger response than normal ones.

More recently, Schade et al. (1974) have used a method similar to that of Kalkhoff et al. (1973), but with contradictory results. In the obese patients infused by Schade et al. (1974), the rise in glucagon was smaller than in the normal subjects. One possible explanation for this difference is the prior diet. Since glucagon is a hormone of glucose need, the carbohydrate intake of the diet will change the basal levels as well as the stimulated level in obese and normal patients (Fiser and Bray, unpublished observations). Since the diets used by Kalkhoff et al. (1973) on the one hand, and Schade et al. (1974) on the other, cannot be readily compared, one might presume that differences in this variable accounted for differences in the basal and stimulated levels of glucagon in obese and lean subjects.

THE ADRENAL HORMONES IN OBESITY

Normal Pattern of Adrenal Response

The principal adrenal steroidal hormones can be divided into three groups: the glucocorticoids, represented in man primarily by cortisol (in some other species, corticosterone serves this function); the mineralocorticoids of which aldosterone is the most potent; and the androgenic precursors of which dehydroepiandrosterone (DHEA) and androstenedione are the major compounds. These steroidal hormones are synthesized from acetate or from cholesterol extracted from the blood perfusing the adrenal gland.

The secretion of adrenal steroids is almost entirely dependent on the presence of adrenocorticotropin (ACTH), a peptide containing 39 amino acids which is secreted by the pituitary gland. The release of ACTH is under hypothalamic control, although the chemical nature of the hypothalamic substance(s) which releases (or inhibits) ACTH secretion is unknown. Under normal conditions, the secretion of ACTH is highest in the early hours of the day and decreases to reach a minimum near midnight. This diurnal pattern of ACTH secretion is reflected in a diurnal pattern or rhythm for secretion of cortisol. The peak blood levels for cortisol are observed at approximately 6:00 a.m. and then decline during the day to reach a nadir at approximately midnight.

During the course of the day, the adrenal gland produces 15 to 20 mg of cortisol but the secretory pattern is periodic rather than continuous. That is, ACTH in the blood is continually oscillating about a mean figure, and consequently adrenal corticosteroid secretion shows similar oscillations. Over 90 percent of the cortisol secreted into the circulation is bound to an alpha globulin (transcortin), and only a small fraction is "free." Some of the circulating cortisol is removed during passage through the liver where two metabolic pathways are available for its disposition. It can be conjugated as a glucoronide or a sulfate to enhance its water solubility. The molecule can also be reduced by the addition of hydrogen at the 3-carbonyl and/or the 20-carbonyl group to produce tetrahydrocortisol or tetrahydrocortolone. These compounds have very little biologic activity but represent a significant fraction of the total corticosteroids excreted in the urine. Three to 10 mg of the conjugated tetrahydro-17-hydroxycorticosteroid along with a comparable amount of the tetrahydrocortolone are excreted in the urine each day.

Adrenal function can be assessed in a number of ways. Measurement of the concentration of cortisol and of its pattern of diurnal metabolism as well as the stimulation or suppression of the hormone concentration or excretion in response to various drugs may be helpful in this assessment. Stimulation can be accomplished by administering histamine or pyrogen and in many patients by the administration of lysine-vasopressin. Another drug, metyrapone, blocks the last step in the formation of cortisol and acts indirectly to increase the production of ACTH, which in turn stimulates the adrenal to secrete 11-deoxycortisol, the precursor of cortisol. Alternatively, the adrenal gland can be stimulated directly by the infusion or injection of ACTH itself.

TABLE 7-5. *Tests of Adrenal Function in Normal, Obese and Cushingoid Patients**

TEST		NORMAL	CUSHING'S SYNDROME	CUSHINGOID OBESITY	SIMPLE OBESITY
Cortisol Concentration 8 a.m. μg/dl		9.4 – 25.3	29.8 ± 2.5	17.6 ± 1.5	16.1 ± 1.7
4:30 p.m. μg/dl		4.5 – 13.8	26.3 ± 1.6	13.0 ± 1.1	12.2 ± 2.6
Cortisol Production Rate (THF) mg/m²/day		4.8 – 14.2	44.1 ± 5.2	14.5 ± 1.7	11.9 ± 1.8
Urinary 17-hydroxycorticoids mg/m²/day	M	7.3 – 13.0	21.1 ± 1.7	9.9 ± 0.8	7.6 ± 0.9
	F	4.8 – 11.3	—	—	—
Urinary 17-keto steroids mg/m²/day	M	7.0 – 11.8	11.7 ±	8.3 ± 0.7	5.9 ± 0.8
	F	3.8 – 9.9	—	—	—
Dexamethasone Suppression Overnight treatment	μg/dl	<5.1	19.7 ± 1.4	5.57 ± 1.01	3.33 ± 0.6
After 4 days of treatment	mg/24h.	<5.2	28.9 ± 3.1	6.9 ± 2.4	—
Metopirone Test percent increase in 17-OHCS		75 – 400 percent			
Transcortin Content		200–300			

*Data adapted from Vingerhoeds: Drukkerjielinknijk Utrecht, 1973, 148.

Adrenal Function in Obesity

The effects of "essential" obesity on the pattern of adrenal secretion have been compared in Table 7–5 with data on Cushing's syndrome, Cushingoid obesity and normal subjects (Prezio et al., 1964). Patients with Cushing's syndrome had all of the major features of the disease (Burke and Beardwell, 1973). Cushingoid obesity was diagnosed in patients with truncal obesity, i.e., centripetal obesity, with at least three of the following minor symptoms: round face (moon facies), reddish or purple striae, muscular atrophy, impotence, acne, easy bruisability, "buffalo" or dorsal hump, atrophy of the skin, psychiatric symptoms or menstrual abnormalities. All patients in this group were referred to the hospital with a diagnosis of "Cushing's syndrome," but at the time of classification there were insufficient criteria to make a definite clinical diagnosis (Vingerhoeds, 1973).

Essential obesity refers to patients who are overweight but have no other symptoms of Cushing's syndrome (Esanu et al., 1968). The concentration of cortisol (Dunkelman et al., 1964) in the circulation of obese patients is usually normal. In addition, the diurnal rhythm is preserved in patients (Schteingart et al., 1963; Martit et al., 1969) with simple obesity but the afternoon value was above normal in 7 of 19 patients with Cushingoid obesity.

Data from 10 obese patients hospitalized at our Clinical Research Center show higher afternoon values of plasma cortisol than normal. However, the morning values were suppressed with dexamethasone (Fig. 7–9). In the patients studied by Vingerhoeds, the suppression of cortisol after the administration of dexamethasone was normal in most of the ones with simple obesity (22/23) but was abnormal in 6 of 24 patients with Cushingoid obesity. Thus 1 mg of dexamethasone at midnight followed by measurement of cortisol the next morning is a good screening test (Schteingart et al., 1963). The obese patients who do not suppress are a small group for whom more complex procedures are needed to exclude the possibility of Cushing's syndrome. The response to most provocative stimuli is normal in the patients with simple or essential obesity. The rise in plasma cortisol in response to injected ACTH is normal (Schteingart et al., 1963) or slightly increased (Dunkelman et al., 1964). The response to metyrapone is also normal or slightly decreased (Laurian et al., 1966; Schteingart et al., 1963). Cortisol rises normally after the drop in blood sugar produced by injecting insulin (Bell et al., 1970; Goth and Gonezi, 1972).

Although plasma cortisol is usually normal, cortisol production rate (CPR) is frequently increased (Migeon et al., 1963; Garces et al., 1968). Since the secretory rate is correlated with the body weight of obese patients, expressing the data as mg/24 hours or mg/12 hours will usually distinguish between obese patients and the patients with Cushing's syndrome (Table 7–5) (Migeon et al., 1963; Copinschi et al.,

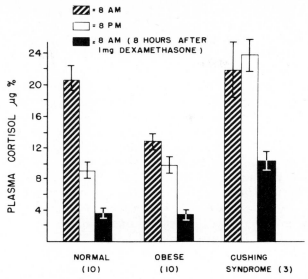

Figure 7–9. Plasma cortisol in obese patients and those with Cushing's syndrome. Diurnal rhythm (8 AM and 8 PM) was reduced in both groups of patients. Suppression with dexamethasone was normal in the obese patients but not in those with Cushing's syndrome.

1966; Konishi, 1970). The increased output of adrenal steroids is metabolized by the liver and the increased quantity of metabolites is excreted in the urine. Urinary free cortisol is, however, normal in obesity (Schteingart et al., 1963). The concentration of urinary 17-hydroxycorticosteroids and ketogenic steroids are thus often elevated in the urine of obese individuals (Dunkelman et al., 1964; Garces et al., 1968; Schteingart et al., 1963). When the quantity of urinary 17-hydroxycorticosteroids is related to surface area (Migeon et al., 1963) or to creatinine excretion (Konishi, 1970), the difference between obese and lean patients disappears.

Vingerhoeds (1973) has suggested that fasting may distinguish between patients who have Cushingoid obesity and those with Cushing's syndrome. During a fast of at least 10 days, eight patients with simple obesity were compared with six patients having Cushing's syndrome and ten with Cushing's obesity. Cortisol production and transcortin were unchanged by fasting (Schultz et al., 1964; Garces et al., 1968; Schachner et al., 1965). Some workers have also observed that, in obese patients, starvation restores the indices of adrenal function toward normal while the other workers have found no change (Sabeh et al., 1969). The decline in cortisol after oral dexamethasone returned to normal with fasting. The urinary 17-hydroxycorticosteroids declined in the patients with Cushingoid obesity but not in the patients with Cushing's syndrome. Thus it appears that a small group of patients with Cushingoid obesity may require a 5 to 7 day fast to distinguish their disease from Cushing's syndrome (Vingerhoeds, 1973; Garces et al., 1968).

The studies of O'Connell et al. (1973) on adrenal function of normal volunteers who gain weight (Sims et al., 1973) is in harmony with the changes in adrenal function observed in patients with spontaneous obesity. Cortisol production rate was increased in nine subjects and the excretion of 17-hydroxycorticosteroids was elevated in five of the normal subjects after gaining weight. Plasma cortisol, its diurnal rhythm and urinary metabolites were, however, unchanged. Excretion of urinary 17-ketogenic steroids declines with weight loss (Jacobsen et al., 1964) but may not return to normal (Dunkelman et al., 1964). The increased secretion of cortisol in obesity implies an increased secretion of ACTH, but the stimulus for the increased adrenal output, in the face of a normal concentration of plasma cortisol, is unknown. A thorough study of cortisol and ACTH in obese patients would provide important insights into this paradox.

Another feature of steroid physiology and obesity which deserves mention is that obese individuals excrete significantly less dehydroepiandrosterone (DHEA) than do control subjects. This steroid is a potent inhibitor of glucose 6-phosphate dehydrogenase and is also an hypocholesterolemic agent in rats (Lopez-S and Krehl, 1967; Ben-David et al., 1967). Glucose 6-phosphate dehydrogenase is the entry point into the pentose phosphate cycle which provides about two thirds of the NADPH needed for lipogenesis (Chapter 3). It is evident, therefore, that any drug or chemical which reduces the activity of the pentose phosphate cycle by inhibiting glucose 6-phosphate dehydrogenase might inhibit lipogenesis.

Conversely, deficiency of a substance which could block a process which normally inhibits lipid formation might accelerate fat deposition. Lopez-S and Krehl (1967) reported a urinary excretion of 1.13 mg for DHEA in the least obese and 0.75 mg in the most obese subjects. Corresponding concentrations of glucose 6- phosphate dehydrogenase in erythrocytes from these subjects were 384 and 450 units. Weight reduction in the obese patients restored both of these figures toward normal. The physiological and potential therapeutic significance of this finding are unknown and additional studies are needed to clarify it.

The discussion of aldosterone secretion in obesity will be considered when discussing the metabolism of water and electrolytes.

GROWTH HORMONE SECRETION IN OBESITY

Normal Physiology of Growth Hormone Secretion

Growth hormone plays a central role in growth and development of most mammalian species. This hormone is a large polypeptide with

191 amino acids (Kostyo, 1974). It represents approximately 1 percent of the dry weight of the pituitary gland and shows significant differences in its composition in various species. Thus, growth hormone from pigs or cattle is ineffective in stimulating growth in man, whereas growth hormone from human pituitaries will cause growth. On the other hand, growth hormone from human, monkey, pig and cattle pituitaries will stimulate growth in rats. Deficiency of growth hormone in the growing child retards growth and leads to an increased deposition of body fat (Tanner and Whitehouse, 1967). Administration of growth hormone to deficient children is followed by enhanced linear growth and a decrease in body fat.

A variety of factors control the secretion of growth hormone. Shortly after the development of a radioimmunoassay which was sensitive enough to detect circulating levels of this hormone, Roth et al. (1964) demonstrated that insulin-induced hypoglycemia was an effective way for increasing the level of growth hormone. This rise in hormonal level resulted from secretion and not from a decrease in the rate at which the hormone was removed or degraded since the metabolic clearance rate of growth hormone in plasma was unaltered. Many physiologic and pharmacologic agents are effective in stimulating growth hormone secretion.

Among the physiologic effects which increase growth hormone are exercise, sleep, a protein meal and a fall in the level of plasma free fatty acids. The increase in growth hormone with sleep occurs shortly after the induction of sleep and was originally thought to coincide with rapid eye movement sleep (REM) but is now known to be associated with the initial induction of deep sleep. An increase in growth hormone concentration is usually observed 4 to 5 hours following a glucose meal. Glucose initially suppresses growth hormone and the rebound which occurs approximately 4 hours later may be due to the early fall in free fatty acids (Fig. 7–10). This figure shows the effect of an oral glucose load on plasma glucose, insulin, free fatty acids and growth hormone of obese and lean children. Note that the early suppression of free fatty acids and growth hormone with a late rebound after insulin has returned to its initial level. Growth hormone is also stimulated by ingestion of a protein meal. A number of amino acids will also increase the output of growth hormone when infused intravenously, but arginine is the most potent.

Among the pharmacologic agents which can stimulate insulin secretion, L-dihydroxyphenylalanine (L-dopa) is of particular interest. This drug, now in wide use for treatment of a neurologic condition known as Parkinson's disease, will stimulate a rise in growth hormone. L-dopa can cross the blood-brain barrier and is a precursor of the two catecholamines, norepinephrine and dopamine. The stimulation of growth hormone by L-dopa suggests that one or another of these catecholamines is involved as a transmitter of information which stimulates the secretion of growth hormone.

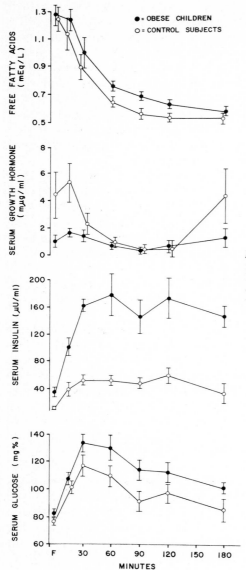

Figure 7–10. Effect of glucose on free fatty acids, growth hormone and insulin in normal weight and obese children. (Milunsky, Bray and Londono, unpublished observations.)

Elevation of free fatty acids during the administration of glucose prevents the later rise in growth hormone. Conversely, reduction of plasma free fatty acids with nicotinic acid is followed after a two hour lag by a rise in growth hormone (Irie et al., 1970; Quabbe et al., 1972). The secretion of growth hormone can also be inhibited by a peptide called somatostatin which has been isolated from the hypothalamus. It is a peptide with 14 amino acids and is a potent inhibitor of growth hormone secretion as well as insulin and glucagon. Its physiological role is still to be elucidated.

The biologic effects of growth hormone have been extensively investigated but are still incompletely understood (Kostyo, 1974). Evidence at hand suggests that its hormonal effects on growth are dependent upon an intermediary known as sulfation factor. Sulfation factor, also called somatomedin, may be produced by the liver in the presence of growth hormone (Van Wyk et al., 1974). This substance has insulin like activity as well as its effects on stimulating the accumulation of sulfate by cartilage. This substance presumably mediates the effects of growth hormone in most mammalian species.

Growth Hormone and Obesity

The effects of obesity on growth hormone have been studied extensively. The basal concentrations of growth hormone are normal or reduced in obese subjects. The induction of hypoglycemia with insulin usually does not stimulate a significant rise in growth hormone in obese patients (Fig. 7–11), and a reduced response to arginine has been demonstrated in a number of laboratories (Beck et al., 1964; Burday et al., 1968; Londono et al., 1969; Copinschi et al., 1967). The nocturnal rise in growth hormone associated with sleep is significantly reduced in obese children and is nearly absent in obese adults (Quabbe et al., 1971; Bray, unpublished observations). Exercise which also stimulates a rise of growth hormone in normal individuals fails to do so in the obese (Hansen, 1973; Schwarz et al., 1969).

Figure 7–11. Effect of hypoglycemia on plasma growth hormone. Insulin (0.1 U/kg) was given to 16 obese and 7 lean subjects. Both groups had a similar drop in blood glucose but the rise in growth hormone was much less in the obese. (Reprinted from Londono et al.: Metabolism, *18*:986–992, 1969.)

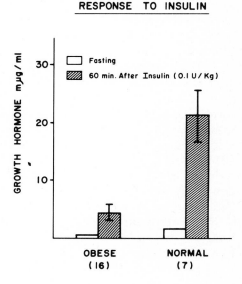

In normal subjects, an acute reduction in plasma free fatty acids is followed by a secondary rise in growth hormone two hours later. In obese subjects, a reduction in fatty acids has no significant effect on the level of growth hormone (Irie et al., 1970). The response to L-dopa, like the responses mentioned above, is also blunted in the obese (Mims et al., 1973; Fingerhut and Krieger, 1974). Thus as a general rule, obesity blunts the responsiveness to all factors which normally stimulate the release of growth hormone. These observations raise two critical questions: (1) is the reduction response of growth hormone a consequence of obesity, and (2) by what mechanism does this effect occur?

The studies of Sims and his collaborators (1973) demonstrate conclusively that growth hormone dynamics are altered by weight gain in normal volunteers. Three provocative tests were used: the late rise in growth hormone after a glucose tolerance test, the response to an infusion of arginine, and the rise during sleep. With all three stimuli, the rise of growth hormone was blunted after the lean volunteers had gained 15 to 25 percent above their initial body weight. Conversely, responsiveness of growth hormone was restored after weight loss in normal volunteers and in obese patients (Ball et al., 1972; El-Khodary et al., 1971; Londono et al., 1969). In addition, growth hormone concentration in very muscular but overweight men rose during an infusion of arginine, whereas obese patients showed very little response (Kalkhoff et al., 1971).

Growth hormone is lipolytic and enhances the utilization of fat as fuel for growth (see Chapter 3). The low levels of this hormone in obesity might tend to perpetuate the excess weight. This possibility has stimulated studies on the actions of growth hormone in obese individuals. Mautalen and Smith (1965) observed that the rise in free fatty acids produced by growth hormone was comparable in lean and obese patients when the doses of growth hormone were given in relation to body weight. At a dose of 0.1 mg/kg, the lean subjects showed a rise of 513 μEq/1 (range 563 to 1017). Thus obese patients respond normally to exogenous growth hormone.

During prolonged treatment with this hormone, obese subjects showed a significant increase in oxygen consumption (see Chapter 4). The calorigenic effect of this hormone enhances the rate at which fatty acids from adipose tissue are catabolized (Bray, 1969b; Bray et al., 1971). During prolonged treatment, growth hormone can significantly reduce nitrogen excretion and reverse the catabolic effects on nitrogen breakdown observed during treatment with tri-iodothyronine (Bray et al., 1971).

The most striking metabolic effects of exogenous growth hormone, however, have been observed when it is given during prolonged fasting in obese subjects. After fasting for more than 14 days, the administration of growth hormone produces nausea, vomiting and ketosis, which are associated with the development of acidosis (Drenick et al., 1970; Schwarz et al., 1972; Felig et al., 1971). This observation suggests that the relative resistance to ketosis in obese subjects may be the result of low levels of growth hormone. This concept has been tested by fasting obese subjects with and without pretreatment with growth hormone. The development of ketosis was not altered by the treatment with growth hormone (Schwarz et al., 1972; Bray, unpublished observations).

THE REPRODUCTIVE SYSTEM IN OBESITY

The control of reproductive function in the normal male and female is a complex process (Odell and Moyer, 1971). In the male the system consists of a gonad producing testosterone, which acts on the hypothalamus to regulate the secretion of the gonadotropins LH and FSH (LH = luteinizing hormone and FSH = follicle stimulating hormone). The production of testosterone in the male occurs almost entirely in the Leydig cells of the testis and is controlled primarily by LH. FSH, on the other hand, is principally concerned with the control of spermatogenesis.

In the female the system is considerably more complex due to the development of ova, their release at midcycle and the subsequent development of a corpus luteum. In the preovulatory phase, LH is low and FSH shows a small rise and then a fall. Estradiol, the major steroidal hormone from the ovary, rises slowly during the preovulatory phase and reaches a peak just before ovulation. The rise in estradiol levels, along with the rise in 17-alpha-hydroxyprogesterone, trigger the hypothalamus to release luteinizing releasing hormone (LRH), a peptide which stimulates the release of LH and FSH from the pituitary. In the luteal phase which follows ovulation, low levels of LH maintain the concentrations of progesterone produced by the corpus luteum.

In obesity, the onset of menstruation (menarche) and the regularity of menses may be deranged. The onset of menarche in obese girls frequently occurs at a younger age than in girls of normal weight (see Chapter 5). An explanation for this phenomenon has recently been provided by Frisch (1972) (Frisch and McArthur, 1974). She showed that menstruation is initiated when body weight reaches a critical mass. As the rate of growth accelerates in late childhood, the entrance into this critical weight range initiates the pubertal process. The growth spurt begins at a body weight of 31 kg. The maximum rate of weight gain occurs at 39 kg, and menstruation begins when body weight is 48 kg (22 percent body fat). Other data (Osler and Crawford, 1973) are basically in agreement with the formulation of Frisch. Since obese girls grow faster and enter this critical mass at a younger age than normal ones, menstruation starts at an earlier age.

The effect of body mass on sexual maturation has been studied in experimental animals by Kennedy and Mitra (1963a, b). They showed that in nutritionally deprived rats, the age of onset of the estrus cycle was delayed as compared with rats which were normally fed. The weight at which estrus cycles occurred, however, was the same in both groups, indicating that in this experimental animal the body weight played an important role in initiating estrus cycles. If the underfeeding is chronic, the estrus cycles become abnormal. Follicular cysts and persistent vaginal cornification may occur.

The obese patient often shows a decrease in the regularity of menstrual cycles and an increase in the frequency of menstrual abnormalities. In one study, 43 percent of the 100 women with menstrual disorders (which included amenorrhea, functional uterine bleeding, premature menopause and infertility) were overweight (i.e., 20 percent above standard weight) (Rogers and Mitchell, 1952). In contrast, only 13 percent of 201 women with no menstrual abnormalities were overweight. Of those women with amenorrhea, 48 percent were overweight. Of the 19 patients with functional uterine bleeding, 58 percent were obese.

In a follow-up study, 32 women with amenorrhea were evaluated for the effects of a therapeutic weight reduction program (Mitchell and Rogers, 1953). All women were initially at least 20 percent overweight and 20 were 50 percent or more above the standard weight. Of the 32 patients, 13 lost weight and, coincidentally, began to menstruate. The weight loss ranged from 13 to 69 pounds (5.9 to 31.5 kg), and in general the onset of menses occurred at intervals between 1 and 4 months after initiating the 1200 calorie diet. Thus it appears that alterations in body weight can influence both the onset of menstruation as well as the subsequent initiation of menstruation in women who have developed secondary amenorrhea.

An analysis of the menstrual cycle in 6 obese women has been published by Sherman and Korenman (1974). These obese women had two abnormalities. First, the rise in FSH in the first half of the cycle was lower than normal. Second, progesterone failed to rise normally in the second half of the menstrual cycle. The mechanism of these distortions in obese women is unknown, but they are reversible after weight loss.

In contrast with these studies in females there is almost no data dealing with the effects of obesity on function of the reproductive system in males.

THE METABOLISM OF SALT WATER AND ALDOSTERONE

The inability of many obese patients, particularly those with extreme weight problems, to excrete both salt and water is now generally recognized (Bansi and Olsen, 1959; Fineberg, 1964). The magnitude of the difficulty is illustrated in the accompanying figure on one of our patients hospitalized in the Clinical Research Center for many months (Fig. 7–12). During much of the time she was maintained on a 900 calorie liquid diet. The long plateau in her weight curve lasted in excess of 30 days. This was followed by a period of rapid weight loss. During the course of these studies, frequent measurements of her oxygen consumption demonstrated to us that her daily caloric requirements were nearly 2700 kCal. She had no family and, because of her age and obesity, was unable to ambulate effectively. Thus there was no possibility for her to obtain extra food. On an intake of 900 kCal/day the metabolism of 225 g of fat supplied the 1800 calorie difference between her intake and body need. Therefore, we expected her to lose 1 kg every 4 to 5 days. Over the long term, her body weight reached the expected level, but the long plateau provided a frustrating experience for both physician and patient.

The problem of water retention in obesity is aggravated by carbohydrate intake (Bloom 1962; 1967; Bortz et al., 1967). Elsbach and Schwartz (1961) have investigated this problem in detail and demonstrated that both fluid and electrolytes, particularly sodium chloride,

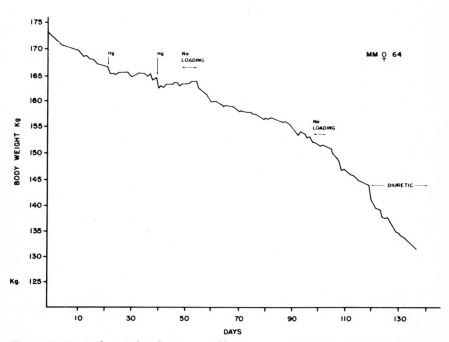

Figure 7–12. Body weight of a 64 year old woman maintained on a 900 calorie liquid formula diet. Note the plateau in weight between days 20 and 50, followed by a rapid weight loss. Hg = injection of mercurial diuretic.

are retained by obese subjects. This problem becomes more severe with refeeding at the end of a period of starvation. With the onset of fasting, there is an enhanced excretion of sodium, chloride and potassium which peaks at 2 to 4 days and then gradually subsides (Stinebaugh and Schloeder, 1966; Rappoport et al., 1965; Veverbrants and Arky, 1969; Boulter et al., 1973a). With refeeding carbohydrate (Bloom, 1967) or protein (Katz et al., 1968), sodium excretion falls to essentially zero and fluid retention occurs.

Several hypotheses have been advanced to explain the mechanism for salt loss during starvation and the retention of salt and water during refeeding with carbohydrate. Since sodium excretion is partly under the control of aldosterone, changes in the circulating level of this hormone or in its action on the kidney could explain the alterations in sodium excretion. With short term starvation, the secretion of aldosterone rises slowly and then gradually returns toward normal. With refeeding, aldosterone may rise. In one study, the sodium retention with refeeding was blocked by spironolactone, a drug which inhibits the action of aldosterone (Boulter et al., 1973b) but in an earlier study, there was no effect (Gersing and Bloom, 1962). The injection of aldosterone after 7 days of fasting reduced sodium excretion, indicating that the renal tubule can still respond to this hormone (Kolanowski et al., 1970).

The implication of aldosterone has also raised the possibility that renin may be involved. Renin, an enzyme which is secreted by the kidney, can increase aldosterone secretion by raising the concentration of angiotensin, a small peptide which directly stimulates aldosterone production. Measurement of plasma renin showed no consistent changes during fasting, but a small rise is observed after refeeding (Verdy and Marc-Aurele, 1973).

The acidosis which develops during starvation may play a role in the loss of sodium (Schloeder and Stinebaugh, 1966). If a metabolic acidosis was induced by giving ammonium chloride, the loss of sodium during subsequent starvation was markedly reduced.

Finally, Saudek et al. (1973) have proposed that glucagon may be important in the loss of sodium in starvation. During starvation both glucagon and sodium excretion rise in parallel. More important is the observation that infusing glucagon to achieve the levels reached during fasting enhances sodium excretion. From these data the following sequence may be constructed. The early loss of sodium with starvation occurs to provide cations for excretion of anions during the development of acidosis. If acidosis is produced before starvation begins, most of the initial salt loss is prevented. The retention of sodium with refeeding can be inhibited by spironolactone, a drug which blocks the effects of aldosterone on the renal tubule. This implies that aldosterone plays an important role in the retention of sodium after carbohydrate or protein (but not fat) are given. The special effect of carbohydrate in shutting off sodium loss suggests that it may provide a necessary source of energy to the aldosterone mediated transport of sodium in the renal tubule.

LIPID METABOLISM IN OBESITY

In Chapter 3 we examined the role of adipose tissue in the formation, storage and release of fatty acids. In the section below we will examine the transport and disposition of the two principal groups of lipids which circulate in the blood. Because long chain fatty acids, triglycerides and cholesterol are insoluble in water, these substances are transported in the blood as complexes with proteins. The free fatty acids are bound to albumin and the triglycerides and cholesterol are transported as lipoproteins.

Free Fatty Acids

The free fatty acids released from adipose tissue are a mixture of carbon chains which are 14, 16 or 18 carbons in length. During transport through the vascular compartment they are bound principally to serum albumin. Fatty acids are taken up by all tissues except possibly brain and erythrocytes. Three metabolic pathways are available for these circulating free fatty acids: (1) they can be oxidized; (2) they can be reaccumulated in adipose tissue (and in other tissues to a small degree); and (3) they can be taken up by the liver, metabolized to ketones or to triglyceride and secreted as lipoproteins or ketones into the circulation.

Several hours after the completion of a meal, oxidation of fatty acids provides more than 50 percent of the total fuel utilized for energy. The concentration of free fatty acids is usually between 300 and 600 μEq/1, and the turnover rate for oleic acid (^{c}18:1) is 231 mM/min, indicating that 29 percent of the concentration in the blood is removed and replaced each minute. The rate of removal or turnover is increased by exercise (Ahlborg et al., 1974) or starvation (Bolinger et al., 1966).

Fatty acids can also be reaccumulated by adipose tissue and stored as triglyceride (see Chapter 3). Fatty acids which enter the liver have several routes of metabolism. First, they can be oxidized to provide energy. Second, they can be esterified with glycerol and incorporated into lipoproteins which are secreted into the circulation. Third, the fatty acids can be converted to ketones which are secreted into the circulation. The ketones can enter other tissues and be metabolized or they can be excreted in the urine.

METABOLISM OF FREE FATTY ACIDS IN OBESITY

Free fatty acids are frequently elevated in obesity (Gordon, 1970; Bortz, 1969). Dole (1956) noted that 94 percent of the obese patients had fasting levels of free fatty acids which were above 600 μEq/1. In contrast, only 18 percent of the normal subjects had values above 600 μEq/1. This finding of increased free fatty acids in obese subjects has been confirmed many times. (Gordon, 1970; Opie and Walfish, 1963; Reitsma, 1967; Glennon et al., 1965). Hanley et al. (1967) observed that the fasting level of free fatty acids increased by 26 μEq/1 for each 10 percent increase in body weight.

After a fast of 24 hours or more the level of free fatty acids in obese subjects is often lower than in lean ones. (Beck et al., 1964; Pinter and Patee, 1968; Opie and Walfish, 1963). In addition, exposure to the cold (Glennon et al., 1965; 1967) or muscular exercise (Opie and Walfish, 1963) produce a smaller rise in free fatty acids in obese subjects than in lean ones. The initial interpretation of these blunted responses to fasting and cold was that obese subjects had a defective system for mobilizing fatty acids. Re-evaluation of this problem, however, has not confirmed this concept. Present data indicate that the elevated fasting levels of free fatty acids in obese subjects are probably the result of increased release of free fatty acids from adipose tissue, as well as increased peripheral rates of turnover (Issekutz et al., 1968) (Chapter 3).

Two groups of studies support this newer concept. The first are the careful studies on the rise in free fatty acids of obese subjects given catecholamines. Glennon et al., (1965) injected epinephrine into normal and obese subjects. The absolute rise in free fatty acids was slightly less in the obese patients, but the initial fasting levels were significantly higher. More detailed studies by Balasse (1968) showed that infusions of norepinephrine into obese subjects produced a greater rise in free fatty acids than in lean subjects, regardless of whether the norepinephrine was given on the basis of body weight or on the basis of estimated lean body weight. These recent data on the lipolytic response to epinephrine and norepinephrine thus failed to show any defect in the mobilization of fatty acids from adipose tissue depots.

The second line of evidence has come from the studies on the turnover of free fatty acid in lean and obese subjects. (Birkenhager and Tjabbes, 1969; Miller et al., 1968; Bjorntorp et al., 1969; Paul and Bortz, 1969; and Nestel and Whyte, 1968). These groups of investigators used infusions of radioactively labeled free fatty acid to achieve steady levels of radioactivity in the plasma. Under these conditions one can measure the ratio of radioactivity in free fatty acid to the total concentration of free fatty acid and thus estimate the rate at which free fatty acids are released from adipose tissue.

Birkenhager and Tjabbes (1969) showed a turnover rate of 837 μEq/min in the obese subjects, and a rate of 533 μEq/min in the lean subjects. This difference was even greater when the data were expressed in terms of lean body mass. Bjorntorp et al. (1969) made similar observations on the turnover of free fatty acid at rest, which was 505 μEq/min in the control subjects and 994 μEq/min in the obese subjects (Figure 7–13). This figure shows the body fat, plasma concentration of free fatty acids and the metabolic rate. In the study by Nestel and Whyte (1968) the turnover rate for fatty acids in nonobese men was 455 to 465 mM/min and in the obese men it was 656 mM/min. These authors observed a significant correlation between the concentration of plasma free fatty acids and plasma turnover rates of fatty acids. From these studies, we can conclude that the turnover rate of fatty acids is significantly related to the amount of body fat. The following sequence of events would appear to integrate these findings: large fat cells release more free fatty acids, which are in turn metabolized more rapidly (see Figure 7–8).

Lipoprotein

Lipoproteins are quantitatively the most important transport mechanism for triglyceride and cholesterol (Levy et al., 1972). Our understanding of the functional importance of these substances has

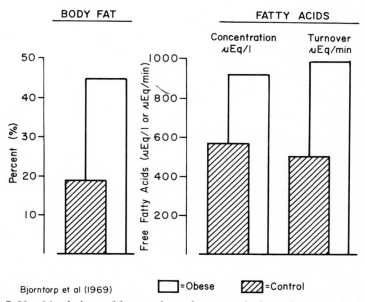

Figure 7–13. Metabolism of fatty acids in obesity. Body fat is shown on the left. The turnover and concentration of fatty acids were increased in obese subjects. (Adapted from Bjorntorp et al.: Acta Med. Scand., *185*:351, 1969, with permission.)

been greatly expanded by the technique of lipoprotein elec-
trophoresis and by the chemical techniques for peptide separation and
ultracentrifugation. Chylomicrons, one of the major classes of lipoproteins, are large particles containing predominantly triglyceride with
small amounts of cholesterol and phospholipid. The gastrointestinal
tract is the primary site for the formation of chylomicrons, which are
then transported through the lymphatic channels in the abdomen and
chest and emptied into the venous circulation through the lymphatic
duct. Removal of chylomicrons from the blood stream occurs at various tissue interfaces where an enzyme called lipoprotein lipase hy-
drolyzes the triglyceride into free fatty acids and glycerol. The free
fatty acids are then transported into tissues for metabolism or storage
as triglycerides.

The second group of lipoproteins are the so-called very low density (VLDL) or pre-beta lipoproteins. These are smaller particles than
the chylomicrons, but are large in comparison with most other circulating substances. The VLDL are formed in the liver from triglyceride, phospholipid, cholesterol and a protein coat. Release into
the circulation is followed by clearance at peripheral tissue stores by a
mechanism similar to that described for the chylomicrons. The very
low density lipoproteins serve as a mechanism for transporting triglycerides formed in the liver to the peripheral cells for storage or
metabolism.

The third goup of lipoproteins, the so-called low density (LDL) or
beta lipoproteins are smaller still and have a much higher concentration of cholesterol and phospholipid, and a smaller concentration of
triglyceride. The formation of the low density lipoproteins involves
the conversion of VLDL to LDL through the action of lipoprotein
lipase. In this process the larger VLDL of hepatic origin interact with
lipoprotein lipase. They then release free fatty acids and glycerol, and
transfer some components from the VLDL lipoprotein to the high
density lipoproteins (HDL). The remaining LDL particle contains the
beta protein, a large quantity of cholesterol, and smaller amounts of
triglyceride and phospholipid. Its removal from the circulation is dependent upon the liver where cholesterol is converted to bile acids.

The fourth class of lipoproteins is the high density lipoproteins
(HDL) whose function is less clearly defined. They are rich in phospholipids, cholesterol and protein, but have very little triglyceride.

An increase in the level of triglyceride is found in many obese
individuals, and the mechanism for this has been the subject of intensive study (Robertson et al., 1973; Olefsky et al., 1974). Albrink and
Meigs (1965) suggested that hypertriglyceridemia is associated with
the acquired rather than the constitutional forms of obesity. This
hypothesis was based on the observation that individuals who gain
weight after the ageof 25, or those with truncal obesity, showed a good
correlation of triglyceride levels with obesity. Forearm fatness, on the

other hand, which is thought to reflect constitutional obesity, is not well correlated with the levels of triglyceride. A similar observation has been made by Harlan et al. (1963) who found that triglyceride levels in VLDL were significantly correlated with weight gain after age 24.

Epidemiologic studies of small populations have also shown a relation between obesity and hypertriglyceridemia. For example, Ford et al. (1968) performed glucose tolerance tests in 20 subjects with a wide range of plasma triglyceride levels. They observed a significant correlation between measures of obesity and the levels of glucose and insulin observed in glucose tolerance tests. From a multivariate analysis of the data they concluded that relative body weight and insulin were interrelated variables acting together to influence plasma triglyceride. Glucose levels were not correlated with other variables, but did influence triglyceride levels. They concluded that triglyceride levels are determined by blood levels of insulin and glucose, and that the insulin levels are in turn dependent upon the degree of obesity. This concept is supported by the observations of Sims et al. (1968, 1973). In normal subjects who gained weight by overeating, fasting levels of insulin and triglyceride were increased. This series of alterations suggests that the rise in insulin and triglyceride may be a consequence of obesity.

The mechanism for the relationship between obesity and the elevation of the triglycerides of VLDL has been the subject of intensive study. Farquhar, Reaven and their collaborators (1975) have proposed that the principal defect is at the cellular level. Where there is a diminished response to insulin, this so-called impedance (or resistance) to insulin decreases the utilization of glucose and increases the output of insulin by the pancreas. The higher circulating levels of insulin act on the liver to stimulate triglyceride formation and release. These investigators have documented the increased impedance (Shen et al., 1970).

One prediction from their study is that insulin and triglyceride levels should change in the same direction. We have tested this concept by varying the dietary intake of obese patients (Fiser and Bray, 1974). The basal levels of insulin varied with both the carbohydrate and calorie content of the diet. Insulin was highest when the calories and carbohydrate were highest. With the lower carbohydrate diet, insulin was reduced even though calorie intake was the same. Reduction in calories but holding carbohydrate constant also reduced basal insulin. Thus insulin was influenced by both the carbohydrate and calorie content of the diet. Triglycerides, however, were related only to the carbohydrate content of the diet. When carbohydrate intake was high, triglycerides were high, but when carbohydrate intake was reduced, the triglyceride level fell. These observations point up the importance of carbohydrate intake in determining triglyceride levels.

They also suggest that the association of insulin and triglycerides in obesity may be mainly the result of carbohydrate.

Studies by Bagdade, Porte and Bierman (1969) have also shown a positive correlation between obesity and the concentration of triglyceride. Reaven et al. (1967) suggested that the hypertriglyceridemia was the result of increased hepatic triglyceride secretion, but they were unable to find a positive correlation between hypertriglyceridemia and obesity, although such correlation was observed by Bagdade, Porte, and Bierman (1967). One explanation for this difference may be the weight range of the subjects under study. The wide weight range used by Bagdade et al. would be more likely to detect a correlation. Shen et al. (1972) have used the term impedance (i.e., the reciprocal of resistance) to suggest that the diminished effectiveness of insulin on peripheral tissues leads to increased levels of insulin which in turn are responsible for stimulating the hepatic production of triglyceride in obese subjects. This hypothesis has made possible a number of experimental studies designed to examine the interrelationships of peripheral resistance to insulin and triglyceride production.

One approach is the use of an infusion containing propranolol and epinephrine, glucose and insulin, which is designed to block endogenous secretion of insulin as well as the endogenous release of glucose by the liver. The glucose and insulin then reach a constant level and the relationship between glucose and insulin provides an index of the rate at which glucose is being removed from the circulation. In obese subjects the glucose levels at equilibrium are considerably higher than in normal subjects, suggesting that tissue resistance to insulin is present. With weight loss the sensitivity to insulin returns and triglyceride and insulin return toward normal. Study of the desert rat (Psammomys obesus), an animal model of obesity which becomes fat when fed laboratory chow, has also shed light on the relation of triglyceride and obesity (Robertson et al., 1973). There was a positive correlation between triglyceride levels and obesity in these animals. The elevated triglyceride was the result of increased hepatic production.

In another study Hollister, Overall and Snow (1967) observed a significant association between body fatness and elevations of triglyceride, cholesterol and uric acid in 104 patients. It has been noted in epidemiologic studies that patients with hypertriglyceridemia (Type IV of Frederickson, see Levy et al., 1972) are frequently obese and often have abnormal glucose tolerance tests (Levy et al., 1972). The triglyceride concentrations in these subjects are frequently increased by feeding glucose. Weight loss will usually diminish the hypertriglyceridemia (Olefsky et al., 1974).

Cholesterol is transported by many lipoproteins but the low density lipoproteins (LDL) are quantitatively the most important.

This lipoprotein is important in human physiology because it correlates with the risk of developing arteriosclerotic heart disease. In epidemiologic studies a relationship between serum cholesterol and body fatness was found in the survey of the population in Tecumseh, Michigan. Among 6500 male and female subjects, there was a low but significant correlation between measures of body fatness (including skinfold thicknesses) and serum cholesterol for males aged 15 to 39 and females aged 30 to 39 (see Chapter 6).

Cholesterol synthesis is increased in obesity. Miettinen (1974) estimates that for each additional kg of body fat, cholesterol formation rises by 20 mg/day. The increased formation of cholesterol in obesity may be linked to the increased turnover of fatty acids. This is depicted in Figure 7–7. Obesity is also associated with an increased incidence of gallstones. An explanation for this association has been proposed recently by Grundy et al. (1974). The composition of bile from obese patients favors the precipitation of cholesterol with the formation of gall stones (Figure 7–14). The principal constituents of bile are bile salts, cholesterol and phospholipids. They are soluble only over a limited range of concentrations. If the concentration of any of these constituents exceeds this level, the bile will tend to separate and favor the formation of stones. The concentration of cholesterol in the bile from obese patients is high relative to the other constituents, thus favoring separation into two phases. In terms of excess cholesterol, the bile from obese patients is more lithogenic than bile from patients with gallstones. After weight loss the composition of the bile returns to normal.

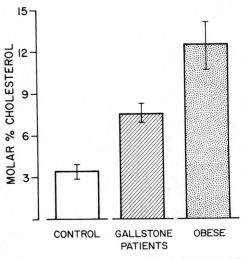

Figure 7–14. Relation of cholesterol in bile to the formation of gallstones. The percentage of cholesterol related to the sum of the phospholipids, bile acids and cholesterol in duodenal bile is shown for normal, stone forming and obese patients. (Adapted from Grundy et al.: Clin. Res., 22(3):49A, 1974, abs.)

GRUNDY et al 1974

REFERENCES

Ahlborg, G., Felig, P., Hagenfeldt, L., Hendler, R. and Wahren, J.: Substrate turnover during prolonged exercise in man. Splanchnic and leg metabolism of glucose, free fatty acids and amino acids. J. Clin. Invest., 53:1080–1090, 1974.

Akerblom, H. K., Newman, P. R., Meakin, J. W., Martin, J. M. and Simpson, W. J. K.: Insulin and growth hormone responses to glucose loading in treated acromegalics. Diabetologia, 5:183–187, 1969.

Albrink, M. J. and Meigs, J. W.: The relationship between serum triglycerides and skinfold thickness in obese subjects. Ann. N.Y. Acad. Sci., 131:673–683, 1965.

Anderson, J. W., Herman, R. H. and Newcomer, K. L.: Improvement in glucose tolerance of fasting obese patients given oral potassium. Am. J. Clin. Nutr., 22:1589–1596, 1969.

Bagdade, J. D., Porte, D., Jr. and Bierman, E. L.: The interaction of diabetes and obesity on the regulation of fat mobilization in man. Diabetes, 18:759–772, 1969.

Bagdade, J. D., Bierman, E. L. and Porte, D., Jr.: The significance of basal insulin levels in the evaluation of the insulin response to glucose in diabetic and non-diabetic subjects. J. Clin. Invest., 46:1549–1557, 1967.

Bagdade, J. D., Porte, D., Jr., Brunzell, J. D. and Bierman, E. L.: Basal and stimulated hyperinsulinism: reversible metabolic sequelae of obesity. J. Lab. Clin. Med., 83:563–569, 1974.

Balasse, E.: Influence of norepinephrine, growth hormone and fasting on FFA mobilization and glucose metabolism in lean and obese subjects. Diabetologia, 4:20–25, 1968.

Ball, M. F., El-Khodary, A. and Canary, J.: Growth hormone response in the thinned obese. J. Clin. Endocrinol. Metab., 34:498–511, 1972.

Bansi, H. W. and Olsen, J. M.: Water retention in obesity. Acta Endo., 32:113–122, 1959.

Batchelor, B. R., Stern, J. S., Johnson, P. R. and Mahler, R. J.: Effect of streptozotocin on glucose metabolism, insulin response and adiposity in ob/ob mice. Metabolism, 24:77–91, 1975.

Beck, P., Koumans, J H. T., Winterling, C. A., Stein, M. F., Daughaday, W. H. and Kipnis, D. M.: Studies of insulin and growth hormone secretion in human obesity. J. Lab. Clin. Med., 64:654–667, 1964.

Bell, J. P., Donald, R. A. and Espiner, E. A.: Pituitary response to insulin-induced hypoglycemia in obese subjects before and after feeding. J. Clin. Endocrinol. Metab., 31:546–551, 1970.

Ben-David, M., Dikstein, S., Bismuth, G. and Sulman, F. G.: Anti-hypercholesterolemic effect of dehydroepiandrosterone in rats. Proc. Soc. Exptl. Biol. Med., 125:1136–1140, 1967.

Benedetti, A., Simpson, R. G., Grodsky, G. M. and Forsham, P. H.: Exaggerated insulin response to glucagon in simple obesity. Diabetes, 16:666–669, 1967.

Bergman, R. N. and Miller, R. E.: Direct enhancement of insulin secretion by vagal stimulation of the isolated pancreas. Am. J. Physiol., 225:481–486, 1973.

Bergstrand, C. G. and Hellstrom, B. E.: The one-hour two-dose glucose tolerance test in normal and obese children. Acta Endocrinol., 14:335–340, 1953.

Bierman, E. L., Bagdade, J. D. and Porte, D., Jr.: Obesity and diabetes: the odd couple. Am. J. Clin. Nutr., 21:1434–1437, 1968.

Birkenhager, J. C. and Tjabbes, T.: Turnover rate of plasma FFA and rate of esterification of plasma FFA to plasma triglycerides in obese humans before and after weight reduction. Metabolism, 18:18–32, 1969.

Bjorntorp, P., Bergman, H. and Varnauskas, E.: Plasma free fatty acid turnover rate in obesity. Acta Med. Scand., 185:351–356, 1969.

Bjorntorp, P., DeJounge, K., Sjostrom, L. and Sullivan, L.: The effect of physical training on insulin production in obesity. Metabolism, 49:631–638, 1970.

Bjorntorp, P.: Effects of physical conditioning in obesity. In: Obesity in Perspective. Fogarty International Center Series on Preventive Medicine, Vol. II, Part II. (Bray, G. A. ed.) Washington, D.C., U.S. Government Printing Office. In press 1976.

Bloom, W. L.: Carbohydrates and water balance. Am. J. Clin. Nutr., 20:157–162, 1967.

Bloom, W. L.: Inhibition of salt excretion by carbohydrate. Arch. Int. Med., 109:26–32, 1962.

Bolinger, R. E., Schafer, M. E., and Kuske, T. T.: Effect of prolonged fasting on the expired $C^{14}O_2$ from palmitate and glucose in obese subjects. Metabolism, 15:394–400, 1966.

Bortz, W. M.: Metabolic consequences of obesity. Ann. Intern. Med., 71:833–843, 1969.

Bortz, W. M., Wroldson, A., Morris, P. and Issekutz, B., Jr.: Fat, carbohydrate, salt and weight loss. Am. J. Clin. Nutr., 20:1104–1112, 1967.

Boulter, P. R., Hoffman, R. S. and Arky, R. A.: Pattern of sodium excretion accompanying starvation, Metabolism, 22:675–683, 1973a.

Boulter, P. R., Spark, R. F. and Arky, R. A.: Effect of aldosterone blockade during fasting and refeeding. Am. J. Clin. Nutr., 26:397–402, 1973b.

Bray, G. A., Rimoin, D. L., Sperling, M. A., Fiser, R. H., Swerdloff, R. S., Fisher, D. A. and Odell, W. D.: The obese diabetic. A symposium on new developments. Calif. Med., 119:14–47, 1973.

Bray, G. A.: Effect of diet and triiodothyronine on the activity of sn-glycerol-3-phosphate dehydrogenase and on the metabolism of glucose and pyruvate by adipose tissue of obese patients. J. Clin. Invest., 48:1413–1422, 1969a.

Bray, G. A.: Calorigenic effect of human growth hormone in obesity. J. Clin. Endocrinol. Metab., 29:119–122, 1969b.

Bray, G. A. and York, D. A.: Genetically transmitted obesity in rodents. Physiol. Rev., 51:598–646, 1971.

Bray, G. A., Raben, M. S., Londono, J. and Gallagher, T. F., Jr.: Effects of triiodothyronine, growth hormone and anabolic steroids on nitrogen excretion and oxygen consumption of obese patients. J. Clin. Endocrinol., 33:293–300, 1971.

Bray, G. A. and Jacobs, H. S.: Thyroid activity and other endocrine glands. In: Handbook of Physiology, (Astwood, E. B. and Greep, R. O., eds.) American Physiological Society, Washington, D.C., 1974, pp. 413–433.

Burday, S. Z., Fine, P. H. and Schalch, D. S.: Growth hormone secretion in response to arginine infusion in normal and diabetic subjects: Relationship to blood glucose levels. J. Lab. Clin. Med., 71:398–911, 1968.

Burke, C. W. and Beardwell, C. G.: Cushing's syndrome. J. Med., 42:175–204, 1973.

Cerasi, E. and Luft, R.: Insulin response to glucose loading in acromegaly. Lancet, 2:769–772, 1964.

Copinschi, G., Cornil, A., Leclercq, R. and Franckson, J. R. M.: Cortisol secretion rate and urinary corticoid excretion in normal and obese subjects. Acta Endocrinol., 51:186–192, 1966.

Copinschi, G., Wegienka, L. C., Hane, S. and Forsham, P. H.: Effect of arginine on serum levels of insulin and growth hormone in obese subjects. Metabolism, 16:485–491, 1967.

Crockford, P. M., Hazzard, W R. and Williams, R. H.: Insulin response to glucagon: The opposing effects of diabetes and obesity. Diabetes, 18:216–224, 1969.

Deckert, T. and Hagerup, L.: Serum insulin in normal and obese persons. Acta Med. Scand., 182:225–232, 1967.

Di Girolamo, M. and Rudman, D.: Variations in glucose metabolism and sensitivity to insulin of the rats adipose tissue in relation to age and body weight. Endocrinology, 82:1133–1141, 1968.

Dole, V. P.: A relation between non-esterified fatty acids in plasma and the metabolism of glucose. J. Clin. Invest., 35:150–154, 1956.

Drenick, E. J., Brickman, A. S. and Gold, E. M.: Dissociation of the obesity-hyperinsulinism relationship following dietary restriction and hyperalimentation. Am. J. Clin. Nutr., 25:746–755, 1972.

Drenick, E. J., Gold, E. M. and Elrick, H.: Acute symptomatic ketoacidosis following growth hormone administration in prolonged fasting. Metabolism, 19:608–613, 1970.

Dunkelman, S. S., Fairhurst, B., Plager, J. and Waterhouse, C.: Cortisol metabolism in obesity. J. Clin. Endocrinol. Metab., 24:832–841, 1964.

El-Khodary, A. Z., Ball, M. F., Oweiss, I. M. and Canary, J. J.: Insulin secretion and body composition in obesity. Metabolism, 21:641–655, 1972.

El-Khodary, A. Z., Ball, M. F., Stein, B. and Canary, J. J.: Effect of weight loss on the growth hormone response to arginine infusion in obesity. J. Clin. Endocrinol. Metab., 32:42–51, 1971.

Elsbach, P. and Schwartz, I. L.: Salt and water metabolism during weight reduction. Metabolism, 10:595–609, 1961.

Embleton, D.: Glucose tolerance curves in 500 obese cases. Br. Med. J., 2:739–740, 1938.

Esanu, C., Oprescu, M., Mitrache, L., Cristoveanu, A., Tache, A. and Klepsch, I.: A clinical form of hypercortisolism differing from Cushing's Syndrome. Rev. Roum. Endocrinol., 5:267–286, 1968.

Fahlen, M., Stenberg, J. and Bjorntorp, P.: Insulin secretion in obesity after exercise. Diabetologia, 8:141–144, 1972.

Fajans, S. S., Floyd, J. C., Jr., Knopf, R. F. and Conn, J. W.: Effect of amino acids and proteins on insulin secretion in man. Recent. Prog. Horm. Res., 23:617–626, 1967.

Farquhar, J. W., Olefsky, J., Stern, M. and Reaven, G. M.: Obesity, insulin and triglycerides. In: Obesity in Perspective. Fogarty International Center Series on Preventive Medicine, Vol. II, Part II. (Bray, G. A. ed.) Washington, D.C., U.S. Printing Office. 1976.

Farrant, P. C., Neville, R. W. J. and Stewart, G. A.: Insulin release in response to oral glucose in obesity: The effect of reduction of body weight. Diabetologia, 5:198–200, 1969.

Felig, P., Marliss, E. B. and Cahill, G. F., Jr.: Metabolic response to human growth hormone during prolonged starvation. J. Clin. Invest., 50:411–421, 1971.

Felig, P., Marliss, E. and Cahill, G. F., Jr.: Plasma amino acid levels and insulin secretion in obesity. N. Engl. J. Med., 281:811–815, 1969.

Felig, P., Wahren, J., Hendler, R. and Brandin, T.: Obesity: evidence of hepatic resistance to insulin. Clin. Res., 21:623, 1973. (abs.)

Fineberg, S. K.: Massive obesity and water retention. G.P., 29:104–109, 1964.

Fingerhut, M. and Krieger, D. T.: Plasma growth hormone response to L-Dopa in obese subjects. Metabolism, 23:267–271, 1974.

Fiser, R. H., Jr. and Bray, G. A.: Effects of carbohydrate and calories on hormonal-metabolic parameters in obesity. Clin. Res., 22:467A, 1974.

Flatt, J. P.: Role of the increased adipose tissue mass in the apparent insulin insensitivity of obesity. Am. J. Clin. Nutr., 25:1189–1192, 1972.

Floyd, J. C., Jr., Fajans, S. S., Per, S., Triffault, C. A., Knopf, R. F. and Conn, J. W.: Synergistic effect of essential amino acids and glucose upon insulin secretion in man. Diabetes, 19:109–115, 1970.

Ford, S., Jr., Bozian, R. C. and Knowles, H. C.: Interactions of obesity and glucose and insulin levels in hypertriglyceridemia. Am. J. Clin. Nutr., 21:904–910, 1968.

Franckson, J. R. M., Malaise, W., Arnould, Y., Rasio, E., Ooms, H. A., Balasse, E., Conard, V. and Bastenie, P. A.: Glucose kinetics in human obesity. Diabetologia, 2:96–103, 1966.

Frisch, R. E.: Weight at menarche: Similarity for well-nourished and undernourished girls at different ages, and evidence for historical constancy. Pediatrics, 50:445–450, 1972.

Frisch, R. E. and McArthur, J. W.: Menstrual cycles: Fatness as a determinant of minimum weight necessary for their maintenance or onset. Science, 185:949–951, 1974.

Fröhman, L. A., Ezdinli, E. Z. and Javid, R.: Effect of vagotomy and vagal stimulation on insulin secretion. Diabetes, 16:443–448, 1967.

Garces, L .Y., Kenny, F. M., Drash, A. and Taylor, F. H.: Cortisol secretion rate during fasting of obese adolescent subjects. J. Clin. Endocrinol. Metab., 28:1843–1847, 1968.

Genuth, S. M.: Metabolic clearances of insulin in man. Diabetes, 21:1003–1012, 1972.

Gersing, A. and Bloom, W. L.: Glucose stimulation of salt retention in patients with aldosterone inhibition. Metabolism, 11:329–336, 1962.

Glennon, J. A., Brech, W. J. and Gordon, E. S.: Effect of a short period of cold exposure on plasma FFA level in lean and obese humans. Metabolism, 16:503–506, 1967.

Glennon, J. A., Brech, W. J. and Gordon, E. S.: Evaluation of an epinephrine test in obesity. Metabolism, 14:1240–1242, 1965.

Gorden, P. and Roth, J.: Plasma insulin; Fluctuations in the "Big" insulin component in man after glucose and other stimuli. J. Clin. Invest., 48:2225–2234, 1969.

Gordon, E. S.: Metabolic aspects of obesity. Adv. Metab. Disord., 4:229–296, 1970.

Goth, M. and Gonezi, J.: Effect of insulin-induced hypoglycemia on the plasma cortisol and growth hormone levels in obese and diabetic persons. Endokrinologie, 60:8–16, 1972.

Grey, N. and Kipnis, D. M.: Effect of diet composition on the hyperinsulinemia of obesity. N. Engl. J. Med., 285:827–831, 1971.

Grodsky, G. M., Bennett, L. L., Smith, D. F. and Schmid, F. G.: Effect of pulse administration of glucose or glucagon on insulin secretion in vitro. Metabolism, 16:222–233, 1967.

Grundy, S. M.: Effects of unsaturated fats in hypertriglyceridemia (Type IV). Clin. Res., 22(3):469A, 1974 (abs.)

Hanley, T., Lewis, J. G. and Knight, G. J.: The influence of fatness on the plasma NEFA response to glucose ingestion. Metabolism, 16:324–333, 1967.

Hansen, A. P.: Serum growth hormone response to exercise in non-obese and obese normal subjects. Scand. J. Clin. Lab. Invest., 31:175–178, 1973.

Harlan, W. R., Laszlo, J., Bogdonoff, M. D. and Estes, E. H., Jr.: Alterations in free fatty acid metabolism in endocrine disorders I: Effect of thyroid hormone. J. Clin. Endocrinol., 23:33–40, 1963.

Hellier, M. D.: The effects of prolonged starvation and refeeding on 24-hour urinary insulin levels in obese subjects. J. Endocrinol., 47:73–79, 1970.

Hellman, B.: Methodological approaches to studies on the pancreatic islets. Diabetologia, 6:110–120, 1970.

Hollister, L. E., Overall, J. E. and Snow, H. L.: Relationship of obesity to serum triglyceride, cholesterol and uric acid, and to plasma-glucose levels. Am. J. Clin. Nutr., 20:777–782, 1967.

Horton, E. S.: Epidemiologic aspects of obesity. In: Understanding and Successfully Managing Obesity. (Rubin, L. D., ed.) Postgrad. Med. Sympos., 1974, pp. 51–61.

Irie, M., Tsushima, T. and Sakuma, M.: Effect of nicotinic acid administration on plasma HGH, FFA and glucose in obese subjects and in hypopituitary patients. Metabolism, 19:972–979, 1970.

Issekutz, B., Jr., Paul, P., Miller, H. J. and Bortz, W. M.: Oxidation of plasma FFA in lean and obese humans. Metabolism, 17:62–73, 1968.

Jacobson, G., Seltzer, C. C., Bondy, P. K. and Mayer, J.: Importance of body characteristics in the excretion of 17-ketosteroids and 17-ketogenic steroids in obesity. N. Engl. J. Med., 271:651–656, 1964.

John, H. J.: Glucose tolerance studies in children and in adolescents. Endocrinol., 18:75–85, 1934.

Johnson, S., Karam, J. H., Levin, S. R., Grodsky, G. M. and Forsham, P. H.: Hyperinsulin response to oral Leucine in obesity and acromegaly. J. Clin. Endocrinol. Metab., 37:431–435, 1973.

Kalkhoff, R. and Ferrou, C.: Metabolic differences between obese overweight and muscular overweight men. N. Engl. J. Med., 284:1236–1239, 1971.

Kalkhoff, R. K., Gossain, V. V. and Matute, M. L.: Plasma glucagon in obesity. Response to arginine, glucose, and protein administration. N. Engl. J. Med., 289:465–467, 1973.

Kaneto, A., Miki, E. and Kosaka, K.: Effects of vagal stimulation on glucagon and insulin secretion. Endocrinology, 95:1005–1010, 1974.

Karam, J. H., Grodsky, G. M. and Forsham, P. H.: Excessive insulin response to glucose in obese subjects as measured by immunochemical assay. Diabetes, 12:197–204, 1963.

Karam, J. H., Grasso, S. G., Wegienka, L. C., Grodsky, G. M. and Forsham, P. H.: Effect of selected hexoses of epinephrine and of glucagon on insulin secretion in man. Diabetes, 15:571–578, 1966.

Karam, J. H., Grodsky, G. M. and Forsham, P. H.: Insulin secretion in obesity: Pseudodiabetes? Am. J. Clin. Nutr., 21:1445–1454, 1968.

Karam, J. H., Grodsky, G. M., Ching, K. N., Schmid, F., Burrill, K. and Forsham, P. H.: "Staircase" glucose stimulation of insulin secretion in obesity. Measure of beta-cell sensitivity and capacity. Diabetes, 23:763–770, 1974.

Katz, A. I., Hollingsworth, D. R. and Epstein, F.: Influence of carbohydrate and protein on sodium excretion during fasting and refeeding. J. Lab. Clin. Med., 72:93–104, 1968.

Kennedy, G. C. and Parker, R. A.: The islets of Langerhans in rats with hypothalamic obesity. Lancet, 2:981–982, 1963.

Kennedy, G. C. and Mitra, J.: Body weight and food intake as initiating factors for puberty in the rat. J Physiol., 166:408–419, 1963b.

Kennedy, G. C. and Mitra, J.: Hypothalamic control of energy balance and the reproductive cycle in the rat. J. Physiol., *166*:395–407, 1963a.

Kolanowski, J., Pizarro, M. A., deGasparo, M., Desmecht, P., Harvengt, C. and Crabbé,
J.: Influence of fasting on adrenocortical and pancreatic islet response to glucose
loads in the obese. Eur. J. Clin. Invest., *1*:25–31, 1970.

Konishi, F.: The relationship of urinary 17-hydroxycorticosteroids to creatinine in obesity. Metabolism, *13*:847–851, 1970.

Kostyo, J. L.: The search for the active core of pituitary growth hormone. Metabolism,
23:885–899, 1974.

Kreisberg, R. A., Boshell, B. R., DiPlacido, J. and Roddam, R. F.: Insulin secretion in
obesity. N. Engl. J. Med., *276*:314–319, 1967.

Lacy, P. E.: Beta cell secretion from the standpoint of a pathologist. Diabetes, *19*:895–
905, 1970.

Lambert, A. E., Hoet, J. J. and Ekka, E.: Plasma insulin levels during pregnancy, in
obesity and potential diabetes. Diabetologia, *2*:260–264, 1966.

Laurian, L., Herzberg, M. and Balas, L.: Metopirone test in overweight subjects. Acta
Endocrinol., *51*:264–267, 1966.

Levy, R. I., et al.: Dietary and drug treatment of primary hyperlipoproteinemia. Ann.
Intern. Med., *77*:267–294, 1972.

Londono, J. H., Gallagher, T. F. and Bray, G. A.: Effect of weight reduction,
triiodothyronine, and diethylstilbestrol on growth hormone in obesity. Metabolism,
18:986–992, 1969.

Lopez, A. and Krehl, W. A.: In vivo effect of dehydroepiandrosterone on red blood cells
glucose-6-phosphate dehydrogenase. Proc. Soc. Exptl. Biol. Med., *126*:776–778, 1967.

Loridan, L., Sadeghi-Nejad and Senior, B.: Hypersecretion of insulin after the administration of L-leucine to obese children. J. Pediatr., *78*:53–58, 1971.

Mahler, R. J. and Szabo, O.: Amelioration of insulin resistance in obese mice. Am. J.
Physiol., *221*:980–983, 1971.

Marti, H., Studer, H., Dettwiler, W. and Rohner, R.: Persistence of a physiological
circadian rhythm of plasma free 11-hydroxycorticosteroid levels in totally fasting
obese subjects. Experientia, *25*:320–321, 1969.

Martin, M. M. and Martin, A. L. A.: Obesity, hyperinsulinism, and diabetes mellitus in
childhood. J. Pediatr., *82*:192–201, 1973.

Mautalen, C. and Smith, R. W., Jr.: Lipolytic effects of human growth hormone in
resistant obesity. J. Clin. Metab., *25*:495–498, 1965.

Melani, F., Rubenstein, A. H. and Steiner, D. F.: Human serum proinsulin. J. Clin.
Invest., *49*:497–507, 1970.

Merimee, T. J., Burgess, J. A. and Rabinowitz, D.: Influence of growth hormone on
insulin secretion. Studies of growth hormone deficient subjects. Diabetes, *16*:478–
482, 1967.

Miettinen, T. A.: Current views on cholesterol metabolism. Horm. Metab. Res.(Suppl),
14:37–44, 1974.

Migeon, C. J., Green, O. C. and Eckert, J. P.: Study of adrenocortical function in obesity.
Metabolism, *12*:718–739, 1963.

Miller, H. I., Bortz, W. M. and Durham, B. C.: The rate of appearance of FFA in plasma
triglyceride of normal and obese subjects. Metabolism, *17*:515–21, 1968.

Mims, R. B., Stein, R. B. and Bethune, J. E.: The effect of a single dose of L-DOPA on
pituitary hormones in acromegaly, obesity and in normal subjects. J. Clin. Endocrinol. Metab., *37*:34–39, 1973.

Mitchell, G. W., Jr. and Rogers, J.: The influence of weight reduction on amenorrhea in
obese women. N. Engl. J. Med., *249*:835–837, 1953.

Morse, W. I. and Mahabir, R.: Changes in glucose tolerance and plasma free fatty acids
after fasting in obesity. Diabetes, *13*:286–290, 1964.

Nestel, P. J. and Whyte, H. M.: Plasma free fatty acid and triglyceride turnover in
obesity. Metabolism, *17*:1122–1128, 1968.

Newburgh, L. H. and Conn, J. W.: A new interpretation of hyperglycemia in obese
middle-aged persons. Am. Med. Assoc., *112*:7–11, 1939.

Nikkila, E. A. and Taskinen, M. R.: The insulin secretion rate in obesity. Postgrad. Med.
J. (June Suppl);412–417, 1971.

O'Connell, M., Danforth, E., Jr., Horton, E. S., Salans, L. and Sims, E. A. H.: Experimental obesity in man. III. Adrenocortical function. J. Clin. Endocrinol. Metab., 36:323–329, 1973.

Odell, W. D. and Moyer, D. L.: Hormone measurement. *In*: Physiology of Reproduction. St. Louis, The C. V. Mosby Co., 1971, pp. 1–13.

Ogilvie, R. F.: Sugar tolerance in obese subjects: A review of 65 cases. J. Med., 16:345–358, 1935.

Ogilvie, R. F.: The islands of Langerhans in 19 cases of obesity. J. Path., 37:473–481, 1933.

Ogundipe, O. O. and Bray, G. A.: The influence of diet and fat cell size on glucose metabolism, lipogenesis and lipolysis in the rat. Horm. Metab. Res., 6:351–356, 1974.

Olefsky, J., Reaven, G. M. and Farquhar, J. W.: Effects of weight reduction on obesity: Studies of lipid and carbohydrate metabolism in normal and hyperlipoproteinemic subjects. J. Clin. Invest., 53:64–76, 1974.

Opie, L. H. and Walfish, P. G.: Plasma free fatty acid concentrations in obesity. N. Engl. J. Med., 268:757–760, 1963.

Orci, L.: A portrait of the pancreatic β-cell. Diabetologia, 10:163–187, 1974.

Osler, D. C. and Crawford, J. D.: Examination of the hypothesis of a critical weight at menarche in ambulatory and bedridden mentally retarded girls. Pediatr., 51:675–679, 1973.

Parra, A. and Schultz, R. B.: Metabolic response to simultaneous infusion of epinephrine and propranolol in obese adolescents. Metabolism, 18:497–508, 1969.

Parra, A., Schultz, R. B., Graystone, J. E. and Cheek, D. B.: Correlative studies in obese children and adolescents concerning body composition and plasma insulin and growth hormone levels. Pediatr. Res., 5:605–613, 1971.

Paul, P. and Bortz, W. M.: Turnover and oxidation of plasma glucose in lean and obese humans. Metabolism, 18:570–584, 1969.

Paulsen, E., Richenderfer, L. and Ginsberg-Fellner, F.: Plasma glucose, free fatty acids and immunoreactive insulin in sixty-six obese children. Diabetes, 17:261–269, 1968.

Perley, M. J. and Kipnis, D. M.: Plasma insulin responses to oral and intravenous glucose: Studies in normal and diabetic subjects. J. Clin. Invest., 46:1954–1962, 1967.

Pinter, E. J. and Pattee, C. J.; Some data on the metabolic function of the adrenergic nervous system in the obese and during starvation. J. Clin. Endocrinol., 28:106–110, 1968.

Porte, D., Jr., Girardier, L., Seydoux, J., Kanazawa, Y. and Posternak, J.: Neural regulation of insulin secretion in the dog. J. Clin. Invest., 52:210–214, 1973.

Porte, D., Jr. Graber, A. L., Kuzuya, T. and Williams, R. H.: The effect of epinephrine on immunoreacting insulin levels in man. J. Clin. Invest., 45:228–236, 1966.

Prezio, J. A., Carreon, G., Clerkin, E., Meloni, C. R., Kyle, L. H. and Canary, J. J.: Influence of body composition on adrenal function in obesity. J. Clin. Endocrinol. Metab., 24:481–485, 1964.

Quabbe, H. J., Bratzke, H. J. and Siegers, U.: Studies on the relationship between plasma free fatty acids and growth hormone secretion in man. J. Clin. Invest., 51:2388–2398, 1972.

Quabbe, H. J., Helge, H. and Kubicki, S.: Nocturnal growth hormone secretion: Correlation with sleeping EEG in adults and pattern in children and adolescents with non-pituitary dwarfism, overgrowth and with obesity. Acta Endocrinol., 67:767–783, 1971.

Rabinowitz, D.: Hormonal profile and forearm metabolism in human obesity. Am. J. Clin. Nutr., 21:1438–1444, 1968.

Rabinowitz, D.: Some endocrine and metabolic aspects of obesity. Ann. Rev. Med., 21:241–258, 1970.

Rabinowitz, D. and Zierler, K. L.: Forearm metabolism in obesity and its response to intra-arterial insulin. Characterization of insulin resistance and evidence for adaptive hyperinsulinism. J. Clin. Invest., 41:2173–2181, 1962.

Rapoport, A., From, G. A. and Husdan, H.: Metabolic studies in prolonged fasting. I. Inorganic metabolism and kidney function. Metabolism, 14:31–58, 1965.

Reaven, G. M., Lerner, R. L., Stern, M. P. and Farquhar, J. W.: Role of insulin in endogenous hypertriglyceridemia. J. Clin. Invest., 46:1756–1767, 1967.

Reitsma, W. D.: The relationship between serum free fatty acids and blood sugar in non-obese and obese diabetics. Acta Med. Scand., 182:353–361, 1967.

Robertson, R. P., Gavareski, D. J., Henderson, J. D., Porte, D., Jr. and Bierman, E. L.: Accelerated triglyceride secretion: A metabolic consequence of obesity. J. Clin. Invest., 52:1620–1626, 1973.

Robertson, R. P. and Porte, D.: Adrenergic modulation of basal insulin secretion in man. Diabetes, 22:1–8, 1973.

Rogers, J. and Mitchell, G. W., Jr.: The relation of obesity to menstrual disturbances. N. Engl. J. Med., 247:53–55, 1952.

Roth, J., Glick, S. M., Yalow, R. S. and Berson, S. H.: The influence of blood glucose on the plasma concentration of growth hormone. Diabetes, 13:355–361, 1964.

Rubinstein, A. H., Melani, F. and Steiner, D. F.: Circulating proinsulin: Immunology measurement and biological activity In: Handbook of Physiology, (Steiner, D. F. and Freinkel, M., eds.) Vol. I. Am. Physiol. Soc., Washington, D.C., 1972, pp. 515–528.

Sabeh, G., Alley, R. A., Robbins, T. J., Narduzzi, J. V., Kenny, F. M. and Danowski, T. S.: Adrenocortical indices during fasting in obesity. J. Clin. Endocrinol., 29:373–376, 1969.

Salans, L. B., Bray, G. A., Cushman, S. W., Danforth, E., Jr., Glennon, J. A., Horton, E. S. and Sims, E. A. H.: Glucose metabolism and the response to insulin by human adipose tissue in spontaneous and experimental obesity: Effects of dietary composition and adipose cell size. J. Clin. Invest., 53:848–856, 1974.

Salans, L. B., Knittle, J. L. and Hirsch, J.: The role of adipose cell size and adipose tissue insulin sensitivity in the carbohydrate intolerance of human obesity. J. Clin. Invest., 47:153–165, 1968.

Salans, L. B. and Dougherty, J. W.: The effect of insulin upon glucose metabolism by adipose cells of different size. Influence of cell lipid and protein content, age and nutritional state. J. Clin. Invest., 50:1399–1410, 1971.

Salans, L. B., Horton, E. S., and Sims, E. A. H.: Experimental obesity in man: Cellular character of the adipose tissue. J. Clin. Invest., 50:1005–1011, 1971b.

Samols, E., Marri, G. and Marks, V.: Promotion of insulin secretion by glucagon. Lancet, 2:415–416, 1965.

Saudek, C. D., Boulter, P. R. and Arky, R. A.: The natriuretic effect of glucagon and its role in starvation. J. Clin. Endocrinol. Metab., 36:761–765, 1973.

Schachner, S. H., Wieland, R. G., Maynard, D. E., Kruger, F. A. and Hamwi, G. J.: Alterations in adrenal cortical function in fasting obese subjects. Metabolism, 14:1051–1058, 1965.

Schade, D. S. and Eaton, R. P.: Role of insulin and glucagon in obesity. Diabetes, 23:657–661, 1974.

Schloeder, F. X. and Stinebaugh, B. J.: Studies on the natriuresis of fasting. Metabolism, 15:838–846, 1966.

Schteingart, D. E., Gregerman, R. I. and Conn, J. W.: A comparison of the characteristics of increased adrenocortical function in obesity and in Cushing's Syndrome. Metabolism, 12:484–497, 1963.

Schultz, A. L., Kerlow, A. and Ulstrom, R. A.: Effect of starvation on adrenal cortical function in obese subjects. J. Clin. Endocrinol., 24:1253–1257, 1964.

Schwarz, F., der Kinderen, P. J., van Riet, J. G., Thijssen, J. H. H. and van Wayjen, R. G. A.: Influence of exogenous human growth hormone on the metabolism of fasting obese patients. Metabolism, 21:297–303, 1972.

Schwarz, F., ter Haar, D. J., van Riet, H. G. and Thijssen, J. H. H.: Response of growth hormone (GH) FFA, blood sugar and insulin to exercise in obese patients and normal subjects. Metabolism, 18:1013–1020, 1969.

Shen, S. W., Reaven, G. M. and Farquhar, J. W.: Comparison of impedance to insulin-mediated glucose uptake in normal subjects and in subjects with latent diabetes. J. Clin. Invest., 49:2151–2159, 1970.

Sherman, B. M. and Korenman, S. G.: Measurement of serum LH, FSH, estradiol and progesterone in disorders of the human menstrual cycle: The inadequate luteal phase. J. Clin. Endocrinol. Metab., 39:145–149, 1974.

Sims, E. A. H., Goldman, R. F., Gluck, C. M., Horton, E. S., Kelleher, D. C. and Rowe, D. W.: Experimental obesity in Man. Trans. Assoc. Am. Physicians, 81:153–170, 1968.

Sims, E. A. H., Danforth, E. H., Jr., Horton, E. S., Bray, G. A., Glennon, J. A. and Salans, L. B.: Endocrine and metabolic effects of experimental obesity in man. Recent. Prog. Horm. Res., 29:457–487, 1973.

terests such as impending engagement or marriage are often a most potent factor in inducing them to seek help with weight loss. The most dramatic examples of weight loss which I have witnessed are in young women with upcoming marriages. In the premarital period, weight losses of more than 100 pounds can be readily achieved. Certain other situations can also induce women to lose weight. One woman successfully dieted and became the winner of a competition to be a candidate for "Miss America," only to find that following the national competition her weight gradually reaccumulated to reach its original level. In other instances, weight loss for women is a matter of personal pride and vanity augmented in many instances by the dictates of fashion, to say nothing of fears of sexual inadequacy. Very short skirts and the tendency towards maximal body exposure provide a strong stimulus towards having an attractive figure for display. A small degree of excess weight for many otherwise attractive women can be the basis for seeking help with slimming.

For men, medical illness seems to be the most important factor in efforts to lose weight. Many men will successfully lose weight after a myocardial infarction or other severe medical illness. Whatever the factors leading patients to seek medical help, however, it is important to realize that motivation in therapy is of prime importance if the therapeutic regimen is to be successful.

Traditional Techniques for Decreasing Caloric Intake

The word "diet" means many things. In the present connection, it is used primarily to describe the techniques for modifying food intake which will achieve weight loss. The popularity of diets is like the popularity of fashion—they come and they go (Harrop, 1934). If any of the numerous diets which have been recommended to the public by one or another expert had indeed been truly and lastingly successful, there would be no need for the remainder of the diets. There are presently available a variety of low calorie diets, low carbohydrate diets, high protein diets, high fat diets, and diets which emphasize only one food. This list could no doubt be supplemented by others, but the fact remains that the variety of diets suggests that none of them has unique properties that are successful in the long run. The low success rate achieved by many diets does not, however, negate the importance of caloric restriction in treating obesity. It indicates rather the chronicity of the problem and the weakness of the individual whose problem it is. Consumer Guide has recently published a very useful and readable critique of these diets. For a more detailed discussion the reader may wish to consult Berland (1974).

Several principles underlie all diets. They are: (1) selection of the quantity of calories (or carbohydrates) to be recommended; (2) selection of the components of which that caloric intake is to be comprised;

and (3) selection of the frequency with which the calories are to be eaten.

ESTIMATES OF CALORIC NEED

Figure 8–3 shows a simplified approach for examining the role of calories in maintaining stored energy (see Chapter 2). The stores of energy are augmented by food intake and depleted by basal metabolism, work, energy excretion and thermic losses after a meal (see Chapter 4). In Figure 8–3 the change in body energy stores is the difference between energy intake (E_F) and energy output ($E_F - E_W)\alpha + Q_L$ + work (Antonetti, 1973). If food intake stops, then body needs must be met from the stores of energy in the body. The rate of caloric utilization during starvation is thus a measure of minimal needs to maintain weight. In all of the adult patients we have studied, this minimal figure is greater than 1000 kCal. Thus any patient adhering strictly to a 1000 kCal diet will lose weight.

Figure 8–4 has been designed to help in assessing the patient's caloric needs (Rynearson and Gastineau, 1949). It is based on the determination of surface area derived from the measurement of height and weight. The first step is to find the patient's surface area by connecting the weight in Column I with the patient's height in Column II; the surface area in square meters can be read from the third column. If this point on Column III is then connected to the appropriate point for age and sex (Column IV), basal or resting calories are found

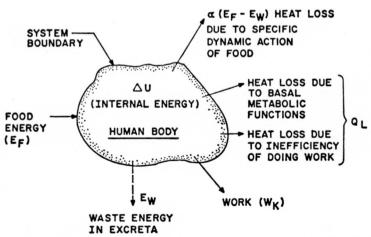

Figure 8–3.   Energy stores in the body. Intake of food energy is indicated on the left by E_F. Loss of energy shown on the right occurs by four routes: basal metabolism (Q_L); work (W_R); thermic losses (specific dynamic action $=\alpha$); and excreted energy (E_W). (Reprinted from Antonetti: Am. J. Clin. Nutr., 26:64, 1973, with permission.)

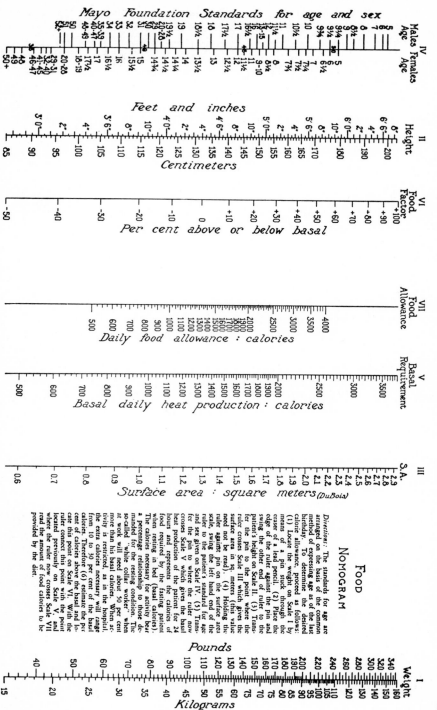

Figure 8–4. Nomogram for estimating caloric needs. (From Rynearson, E. H. and Gashineau, C. P.: Obesity, 1949. Courtesy of Charles C Thomas, Publisher, Springfield, Illinois.)

by referring to Column V. An "activity factor" must then be added to the basal caloric need to provide an assessment of total caloric need.

An alternative approach is to use the estimation of surface area from Figure 8–4 and refer to the appropriate age and level of activity in Tables 8–1 and 8–2. These figures are for adults in their middle years (aged 24–30 and 35–39) and show that even the least active person requires more than 1000 kCal/day. It is obvious that additional calories are required for physical activity. A sedentary individual requires fewer calories than an active one.

After establishing the caloric requirements to maintain body weight, it is easy to decide on the appropriate level of caloric restriction. Since 1 kg (2.2 lbs) of human fat stores about 7700 calories (see Chapter 4), this is the number of calories that must be burned to lose a pound of fat. A net deficit of 500 calories daily will produce a loss of 3500 calories in one week. Thus a caloric intake which is 500 calories less than intake each day will produce a loss of one pound or 454 g of fat tissue in a week. It is important to keep in mind that this catabolism of fat may not register immediately as a loss of weight. Each 100 g of fat which is oxidized produces 112 g of water. Excretion of this water is essential before weight loss occurs (see Chapter 7).

For most people, food intake in the range of 1000 to 1200 calories/day is generally most appropriate, but more severe restriction, including total starvation (see below), has been used. If caloric expenditure is high, a higher caloric intake may be desirable. If the patient has a small surface area, a somewhat lower intake of calories may be selected. The question naturally arises—why not use diets of 400 to 800 calories? If a little caloric restriction is good, wouldn't severe caloric restriction be better?

The studies with diets containing less than 800 calories suggest that little extra fat is catabolized (Buskirk et al., 1963; Blondheim et al., 1965). Severe caloric restriction appears to produce an adaptation which conserves energy (Bray, 1970). Measurements of oxygen consumption of obese patients during severe caloric restriction show that basal metabolism declines (see Chapter 4). Thus with severe caloric restriction, the number of calories required for basal metabolism is reduced. This reduction can amount to 15 to 20 percent of pre-diet caloric needs, and for an individual requiring 2000 calories, the reduction could amount to 400 calories. The mechanism for this conservation of energy is unknown, but it could provide a reason why reducing caloric intake below 800 Cal/day may produce little extra weight loss (Bray, 1970).

COMPOSITION OF WEIGHT LOSS DURING CALORIC RESTRICTION

Caloric restriction is associated with weight reduction, and a number of studies have focused on the body constituents which are

TABLE 8–1. *Energy Requirements for Various Levels of Physical Activity**
At Ages 24 to 30

Surface Area	MALE					FEMALE				
	Sedentary	Light	Moderate kCal	Active	Heavy	Sedentary	Light	Moderate kCal	Active	Heavy
1.40	1507	1781	2055	2329	2603	1401	1656	1911	2165	2420
1.45	1562	1846	2130	2414	2698	1452	1716	1980	2245	2509
1.50	1617	1911	2205	2499	2793	1503	1777	2050	2324	2597
1.55	1672	1976	2280	2584	2888	1554	1837	2120	2403	2685
1.60	1749	2067	2385	2703	3021	1626	1922	2218	2513	2809
1.65	1782	2106	2430	2754	3078	1657	1958	2259	2561	2862
1.70	1826	2158	2490	2822	3154	1698	2006	2315	2624	2933
1.75	1881	2223	2565	2907	3249	1749	2067	2385	2703	3021
1.80	1936	2288	2640	2992	3344	1800	2127	2455	2782	3109
1.85	1999	2363	2727	3090	3454	1859	2197	2536	2874	3212
1.90	2046	2418	2790	3162	3534	1902	2248	2594	2940	3286
1.95	2095	2476	2857	3238	3619	1948	2303	2657	3011	3366
2.00	2156	2548	2940	3332	3724	2005	2369	2734	3098	3463
2.05	2203	2603	3004	3405	3805	2049	2421	2794	3166	3539
2.10	2266	2678	3090	3502	3914	2107	2490	2873	3256	3640
2.15	2310	2730	3150	3570	3990	2148	2538	2929	3320	3710
2.20	2365	2795	3225	3655	4085	2199	2599	2999	3399	3799
2.25	2420	2860	3300	3740	4180	2250	2659	3069	3478	3887
2.30	2497	2951	3405	3859	4313	2322	2744	3166	3588	4011
2.35	2530	2990	3450	3910	4370	2352	2780	3208	3636	4064
2.40	2585	3055	3525	3995	4465	2404	2841	3278	3715	4152
2.45	2662	3146	3630	4114	4598	2475	2925	3375	3826	4276
2.50	2695	3185	3675	4165	4655	2506	2962	3417	3873	4329

*Sedentary—10 percent above basal.
Light—30 percent above basal
Moderate—50 percent above basal
Active—70 percent above basal
Heavy—90 percent above basal

TABLE 8–2. Energy Requirements for Various Levels of Physical Activity*
at Ages 35 to 39

Surface Area	MALE					FEMALE				
	Sedentary	Light	Moderate kCal	Active	Heavy	Sedentary	Light	Moderate kCal	Active	Heavy
1.40	1408	1664	1920	2176	2432	1309	1547	1785	2023	2261
1.45	1455	1719	1984	2249	2513	1353	1599	1845	2091	2337
1.50	1501	1774	2047	2320	2593	1396	1650	1904	2158	2411
1.55	1562	1846	2130	2414	2698	1452	1716	1980	2245	2509
1.60	1607	1899	2191	2483	2775	1494	1766	2038	2309	2581
1.65	1661	1963	2265	2567	2869	1544	1825	2106	2387	2668
1.70	1699	2008	2317	2626	2935	1580	1867	2155	2442	2730
1.75	1760	2080	2400	2720	3040	1636	1934	2232	2529	2827
1.80	1806	2134	2463	2791	3119	1679	1985	2290	2596	2901
1.85	1870	2210	2550	2890	3230	1739	2055	2371	2687	3003
1.90	1897	2242	2587	2932	3277	1764	2085	2406	2727	3048
1.95	1963	2320	2677	3034	3391	1826	2158	2490	2822	3154
2.00	2002	2366	2730	3094	3458	1861	2200	2538	2877	3215
2.05	2062	2437	2812	3187	3562	1918	2266	2615	2964	3313
2.10	2101	2483	2865	3247	3629	1953	2309	2664	3019	3374
2.15	2145	2535	2925	3315	3705	1994	2357	2720	3082	3445
2.20	2227	2632	3037	3442	3847	2071	2448	2824	3201	3578
2.25	2255	2665	3075	3485	3895	2097	2478	2859	3241	3622
2.30	2315	2736	3157	3578	3999	2153	2544	2936	3328	3799
2.40	2420	2860	3300	3740	4180	2250	2659	3069	3478	3887
2.45	2475	2925	3375	3825	4275	2301	2720	3138	3557	3975
2.50	2508	2964	3420	3876	4332	2332	2756	3180	3604	4028

*Sedentary—10 percent above basal
Light—30 percent above basal
Moderate—50 percent above basal
Active—70 percent above basal
Heavy—90 percent above basal

lost (Cederquist et al., 1952). Strang et al. (1930, 1931) measured the excretion of nitrogen by obese patients fed a calorically restricted diet. During the early weeks of rigid dieting, the obese patients lost between 3 and 6 g of nitrogen per day (18 to 36 g of protein) but thereafter equilibrium was re-established. This new equilibrium state usually occurred with a loss of less than 4 percent of the total nitrogen in the body. When nitrogen intake was maintained at 1 g/kg of ideal weight, nitrogen could be retained even with caloric intakes of 250 to 450 calories per day. Thus the major source of the energy for these patients was the catabolism of fat.

The composition of the fuels used to supply energy during caloric restriction has been analyzed in detail by several other groups (Passmore et al., 1958, 1959; Strong et al., 1958; Young et al., 1957; Leverton and Gram, 1951; Buskirk et al., 1963). The results of studies by Passmore et al. (1958) are shown in Figure 8–5. The diet contained 400 kCal/day and provided about 40 g of carbohydrate, 25 g of protein, and 15 g of fat. The upper half of each panel shows the cumulative caloric expenditure and the lower half the source of that caloric expenditure. The loss of calories each week was similar to that of the previous week, with only a slight decrease toward the end of the study. During the first week nearly half of the weight lost was water.

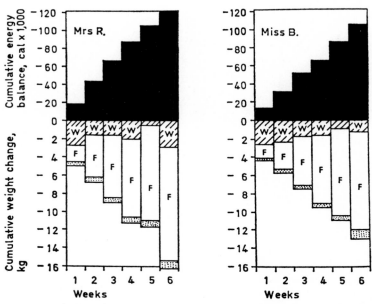

Figure 8–5. Energy balance and weight loss in 6 weeks. The cumulative energy deficit is shown above the zero line. The cumulative weight loss and relative amounts of water (W), fat (F), and protein (stippled) are shown below the zero line. (Reprinted from Passmore et al.: Brit. J. Nutr., *12*:113-122, 1958, with permission.)

Fat represented the other half of the weight lost but provided almost all of the energy. The protein loss was small and increased only slightly from week to week. This small increase in protein is consistent with the findings of Strang et al. (1931) noted above. The variation in cumulative water excretion indicates that during some weeks water was actually retained and that the major losses occurred during the first week of the study.

Buskirk et al. (1963) performed a careful analysis of the energy balance of several obese patients at three levels of caloric intake. Fat was the major source of fuel when the diet was deficient in calories. Basal energy expenditure declined when caloric intake was restricted. The most impressive long term study of weight loss, however, is the patient reported by Bortz (1969). This individual, who weighed close to 700 pounds at the time the study began, lost 500 pounds. Almost all of the triglyceride stored in his adipose tissue was used during the study, but he was able to conserve most of his nitrogen stores.

Studies on the size and number of adipose cells from obese patients during weight loss have shown that the decrease in body weight occurs almost entirely by a decrease in the size of the fat cells (with no change in their number). The data from one patient studied at the New England Medical Center is presented in Figure 8–6 (Bray, 1970).

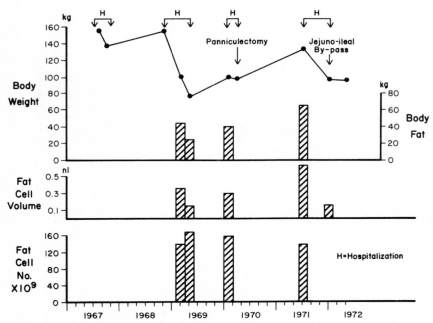

Figure 8–6. Effect of weight loss on body fat and number of fat cells. Body weight, body fat and size of individual fat cells changed in parallel. There was, however, no significant change in the estimated number of fat cells, although body fat decreased by 50 percent.

The fat from this patient was biopsied on four occasions during the loss of 100 kg of body weight (which was subsequently regained). There was no change in lean body mass as measured by body water (^3H_2O), but there was a proportional decrease in the size of her total body fat and in the size of the individual fat cells (see Chapter 3). The number of fat cells showed no significant change.

In summary, all of the data indicates that during weight reduction there is catabolism of body tissues to provide for the metabolic needs of the body. Essentially all of the energy comes from the triglyceride stored in adipose tissue. Water losses are significant during the first week but contribute little to the weight loss thereafter. Protein catabolism is most active at the beginning of the diet, but thereafter little further protein is lost, providing that protein intake is at least 0.5 to 1 g/kg of ideal body weight. There have as yet been few careful studies on the losses of vitamins and minerals.

COMPOSITION OF THE DIET

The use of low carbohydrate, high fat diets for the treatment of obesity is a recurring theme in medical circles (Dole et al., 1954; Berland, 1974). In the English language this type of diet was first popularized by Banting (1863) in his "Letter on Corpulence." His concept has been revived intermittently since that time, in books with such notable titles as *Calories Don't Count* by Dr. H. Taller and *Dr. Atkins' Diet Revolution* by Dr. R. Atkins. Pennington (1951, 1953) published a rationale for this diet based on his belief that obesity was associated with a defect in pyruvate metabolism. He claimed that fat circumvented this block and could thus be metabolized by an obese patient, but there has been no substantiation of this claim. Several medical reports have claimed, however, that a low carbohydrate diet may be associated with extra weight loss during short term dietary periods (Lyon and Dunlop, 1932; Keeton and Bone, 1935; Kekwick and Pawan, 1956; Yudkin and Carey, 1960; Young et al., 1971a). Kekwick and Pawan (1956) fed 1000 kCal diets containing 90 percent fat, 90 percent carbohydrate or 90 percent protein to obese patients for periods of up to 11 days. The weight loss was greater on the high protein or high fat diet than on a corresponding caloric intake when the diet was 90 percent carbohydrate. These experiments suggested that all calories were not equal, a concept which has received little subsequent support.

The short duration of the dietary periods was the major limitation of the studies by Kekwick and Pawan. It is well known that water balance is significantly influenced by the carbohydrate content of the diet. To achieve water balance may require more than 10 days on a diet (Worthington and Taylor, 1974a,b). Russell (1962), for example, found that the carbohydrate content of the diet had a major influence on weight loss in short term studies. There was a highly significant correlation between urine volume and weight loss, suggesting that this was the major reason for short term fluctuations in body weight.

Other authors, using longer dietary periods, have also examined the role of carbohydrate and fat and have failed to find any effect on the rate of weight loss (Werner, 1955; Olesen and Quaade, 1960; Pilkington et al., 1960; Kinsell et al., 1964; Bortz et al., 1966; Hood et al., 1970). Werner compared the effect of a diet containing 2878 kCal/day (of which 287 g was carbohydrate) with a diet containing the same number of calories but only 52 g of carbohydrate. These diets had, respectively, 146 g and 242 g of fat. The changes in body weight during feeding of these diets were identical. Pilkington et al. compared diets containing 86 percent of the calories as carbohydrate with a diet containing 91 percent of calories as fat. The rates of weight loss were similar on the same caloric intake regardless of dietary composition.

Kinsell et al. have obtained similar data (Fig. 8–7). While on con-

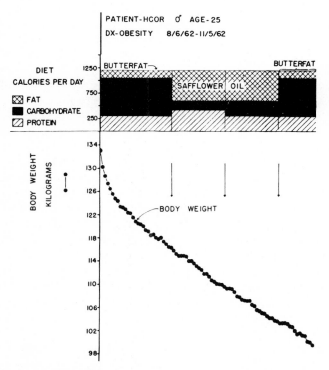

Figure 8–7. Composition of the diet, and the rate of weight loss. Protein, carbohydrate and fat were varied while total caloric intake remained constant. The caloric level, not the composition of the diet, influenced the rate of weight loss. (Reproduced from Kinsell et al.: Metabolism, *13*:195-204, 1964, with permission.)

stant caloric intakes which were below the level required to maintain body weight, the rate of weight loss was not influenced by increasing or decreasing the quantity of carbohydrate, protein or fat. The major reason for the apparent differences in weight loss is the variation in the sodium and water excreted in the urine (Hood et al., 1970).

The only exception to the group of studies cited above is the one published by Young et al. (1971a). Nine college men were fed one of 3 diets for a period of 9 weeks. One diet contained 30 g, the second 60 g, and the third 104 g of carbohydrate. The total caloric intake was 1800 kCal/day, or about half of the number of calories required for weight maintenance in these active young men. Weight losses were greater on the lowest carbohydrate intake. Measurements of body composition using densitometry (see Chapter 1) suggested that the extra weight loss was fat. However, the small number of subjects in each group did not provide statistically significant differences. Nonetheless, the data are suggestive and require careful replication with larger groups of individuals.

Yudkin and Carey (1960) (Stock and Yudkin, 1970) have pointed out one value of a moderately low carbohydrate diet. They showed that when carbohydrate is restricted, fat intake is voluntarily reduced. This observation may result from the fact that most people do not eat fat without carbohydrate. One rarely sees an individual eating butter without bread, crackers or potatoes. If these sources of carbohydrate are reduced, the quantities of fat would be reduced pari passu. Thus moderate restriction of carbohydrate may facilitate restriction in calories.

FREQUENCY OF EATING

The role of altered patterns of eating on the development of obesity has been examined in both experimental and clinical studies. The classic experimental studies on meal eating versus nibbling were conducted by Cohn and his collaborators (1965). Rats in one group were fed the same amount of food by stomach tube as was eaten spontaneously by normal rats. At the end of the experiment the animals which received their food twice daily by stomach tube had nearly twice as much body fat as did the rats allowed to eat ad libitum. (This phenomenon is discussed in more detail in Chapter 5.)

Clinical studies on the effects of the frequency of food intake on metabolism and the development of obesity are not as extensive as those on experimental animals. There are, however, several important studies on this subject. Using epidemiologic methods, Fabry and his collaborators (1964) found that obesity was associated with the frequency of eating. Individuals who ate one to two meals a day tended to be more overweight and to have higher cholesterol levels than individuals who ate three or more meals per day. These findings are entirely consistent with the clinical observation that most overweight patients tend to eat most of their food in one meal, usually in the late afternoon and evening (Huenemann, 1972).

The adverse effect on glucose metabolism and serum cholesterol of eating only one or two meals per day has been verified in careful clinical studies by Young et al. (1971b, 1972). In this study, college students were fed isocaloric diets containing the same foods in one, three or six meals. The serum cholesterol on the single feeding program was 306 mg/dl compared to 260 or 267 mg/dl for the same subjects fed three or six meals (Table 8–3). The rise in cholesterol when eating one meal per day has been observed repeatedly in studies on the frequency of feeding (Gwinup et al., 1963b; Jagannathan et al., 1964; Irwin and Feeley, 1967; Cohn, 1964). Frequent, small meals also tend to improve glucose tolerance (Young et al., 1972; Debry et al., 1973; Fabry, 1973; Gwinup, 1963a). Although the pattern of food intake significantly affects cholesterol and glucose metabolism, it has no effect on accelerating or retarding weight loss in subjects on the hypocaloric diet (Bortz et al., 1966; Finkelstein and Fryer, 1971; Swindells et al., 1968). In spite of this, the fact that eating 3 or more meals each day reduces cholesterol and improves glucose tolerance makes frequent meal plans desirable.

MEAL PLANNING

Two approaches can be used in formulating an eating plan for the obese patient. The first of these uses meal plans constructed around the caloric value of individual foods. A total calorie intake is selected as described above and a diet with this number of calories is provided for and discussed with the patient. One variant of this approach is a point system. With this method, each unit has a value of 75 calories.

TABLE 8–3. *The Effect of Frequency of Feeding on Serum Cholesterol and Triglycerides*°

FREQUENCY OF MEALS	NUMBER OF SUBJECTS	CHOLESTEROL MG/DL	TRIGLYCERIDE
1	8	306±46*†	167±55*‡
3	6	267±30	123±54
6	8	260±58	124±46

°Adapted from Young et al.: J. Am. Diet. Assoc., 59:466–472, 1971.
*Mean ± SD
†p <.001
‡p <.05

Such a modification reduces the complexity of large numbers when calories are used.

An alternative approach is to ignore calories altogether and focus on the carbohydrate content of foods. With this method, the maximim intake of carbohydrate is fixed. The restriction of carbohydrate tends to reduce total caloric intake as described above (for details see Allan, 1974).

Appendix 1 (Chapter 8) groups fruits and vegetables according to the caloric value of the one half cup measure. The goal of any meal plan is to reduce the intake of high calorie fruits and vegetables and increase the intake of those with fewer calories. The same is true for the meats which are eaten. Calorie values for meats are listed in Appendix 8–2.

Pork has more fat and thus more calories per gram than other meats. Chicken and most fish, on the other hand, are relatively low in calories and are to be preferred.

Appendix 8–3 shows the caloric value for dairy and cereal products. For additional information on calorie composition, the reader may refer to specialized publications (Pearson, 1970; Watt and Merrill, 1963). Careful instruction in nutrition is important because Ley et al. (1974) have shown that knowledge about the content of the diet is significantly associated with success in weight loss.

Based on the kinds of calorie values shown in Appendices 8–1—8–3, a 1200 calorie meal plan is presented in Appendix 8–4. For meal plans with other calorie values and for a more detailed discussion, the reader is referred to Jolliffe (1963) (Bennett and Simon, 1973).

The use of formula diets is still another approach to calorie counting. This method of dieting was popularized by Feinstein et al. (1958). There are several commercial products which have a specified calorie value on each can or package. These include Metrecal and Sego, which are two formulations which contain 225 calories in each can. In addition, there are a number of products sold in a dry form to which milk is added. The advantage of these pre-packaged products is the ease with which calorie content is determined. The major drawback is their monotony. After an initial rapid growth in popularity, these products fell into disuse (Wyden, 1965).

EFFECTIVENESS OF DIETARY TREATMENT

The effectiveness of dietary treatment for obesity has been evaluated in a number of studies; many of those prior to 1960 have been reviewed by Bauman (1928), Feinstein (1960) and Stunkard and McLaren-Hume (1959).

Several different criteria have been used in assessing the effectiveness of treatment. The simplest of these is the method devised by Stunkard and McLaren-Hume (1959). They evaluated only those studies in which the percentage of patients losing 20 and 40 pounds could be ascertained.

Trulson et al. (1947) introduced a somewhat more sophisticated approach in which both initial body weight and an appropriate weight loss for the degree of overweight were used (Trulson, 1954). This is shown in Table 8–4. The performance index introduced by Jolliffe and Alpert (1957) measures the loss of weight relative to predicted weight loss:

$$\text{Performance Index} = \frac{\text{Actual weight loss}}{\text{Anticipated weight loss}} \times (100)$$

Its major limitation is the need to compute or evaluate the appropriate rate of weight loss. Feinstein devised two approaches. The simplest was the one which measured weight loss in grams per day for the duration of the study (Feinstein, 1960). The more sophisticated approach is called the "reduction index" (Feinstein, 1959).

$$\text{Reduction Index} = W_L \left(\frac{W_I}{W_S \times W_T} \right) \times 100$$

W_I = Initial weight
W_T = Target weight
W_S = Surplus weight = $W_I - W_T$
W_L = Weight loss = $W_I - W_E$
W_E = End of treatment weight

This index considers both degree of excess weight and actual weight loss. The number for this index ranges from 0 to 200. The higher the index the greater the weight loss. Although a valuable approach, this index has not been widely used.

TABLE 8–4. *Criteria for Weight Loss Recommended by Trulson et al. (1947)*

INITIAL BODY WEIGHT		MINIMUM WEIGHT LOSS FOR SUCCESS	
LB	KG	LB	KG
less than 150	less than 70	10	–
151 to 175	70 to 80	15	5
176 to 200	81 to 90	20	7
201 to 225	91 to 100	25	9
226 to 250	101 to 110	30	11
over 250	111 to 125	35	14
	over 125		17

In a study of 523 patients, Dunlop and Lyon (1931) found an average weight loss of 1.9 pounds per week in out-patients treated with a weight reducing diet. The weekly weight loss was highest in the patients who were most overweight. Of interest was the fact that the same patients who lost most weight during treatment were the ones who tended to regain it most easily when treatment ended. Fellows (1931) followed a large number of obese patients who were treated for overweight in the Metropolitan Life Insurance Company home office. Of the initial 294 patients, 19 percent showed no weight loss, 28 percent lost between 1 and 9 pounds, and 27 percent lost between 10 and 19 pounds. Smaller amounts of weight were lost by the remaining patients. When 224 of these patients were re-evaluated one year later, 32 percent had continued to lose weight. During the initial course of treatment, this group had lost 10.2 pounds, and during the ensuing year lost an additional 3.8 pounds. Those who gained weight during the first year of follow-up had initially lost more weight (16.9 pounds) and had regained an average of 9.7.

This supports the conclusion of Dunlop and Lyon that those who lose most tend to regain it most rapidly. When followed to 5 years, Fellows (1931) found that 21 percent of the patients had continued to lose weight; on the other hand, 33 percent had regained between 1 and 14 pounds. The group who continued to lose weight over the 5 years had an initial weight loss of 10.2 pounds, and during the 5 years they lost an additional 8.9 pounds. Considering all of the patients, however, Fellows found that 85 percent of the initial weight loss had been regained.

Stunkard and McLaren-Hume (1959) evaluated weight loss in a number of studies using as a criterion the percentage of patients who had lost 20 or more pounds, and the percentage of patients who lost 40 or more pounds. These results are presented graphically in Figure 8–8 (Bray, 1970). Overall, 25 percent of the patients lost 20 pounds or more and 4 percent lost more than 40 pounds. In another study, Glennon (1966) followed 199 patients for more than one year after they were discharged from the hospital where they had been admitted for a weight loss program. He found that 12 percent of those followed over one year and 14 percent of those followed over two years had lost more than 20 pounds. Six percent had lost more than 40 pounds, and four had continued to lose weight so that they were no longer 50 percent or more overweight. Only one patient, however, had reached ideal weight.

A final long term study reported by Sohar and Sneh (1973) (Sohar, 1959) provided data on body weights obtained 14 years after the initial dietary study. Of 33 patients originally treated, 27 could be located and reweighed. These patients have been divided into three groups as shown in Table 8–5. The largest group of 17 patients lost weight initially but regained nearly all of it, and weighed almost what they had

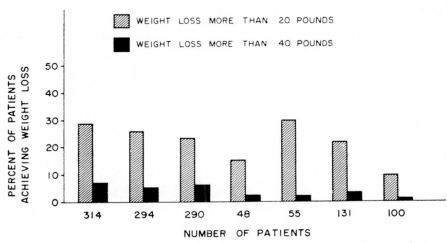

Figure 8–8. Weight loss in several nutrition clinics. The percentage of patients losing 20 or 40 pounds in each clinic is shown by a pair of bars. The number of patients in each clinic is shown below the bars. (Reprinted from Bray, G.A.: Am. J. Clin. Nutr., 23:1141, 1970, with permission.)

14 years earlier. A second group of 5 patients, however, maintained the initial weight loss and added a small increment to it. The third subgroup who were heavier at the start lost more weight but regained all of it and continued to increase in body weight. Some of the patients in this latter group had undergone an operation for obesity (see Chapter 10). From these studies on the long term results of dietary treatment, we can conclude that between 10 and 20 percent of patients who lose weight in any program will maintain or increase their weight loss with the passage of time, and a few patients will actually reach their desirable weight. The remainder of the patients will return toward their initial weight, and some will gain additional weight above this point.

There should be gratification for the physician in the fact that some patients can achieve and maintain a significant weight loss by following a dietary program. The advantages of losing weight are clear. Blood pressure may be significantly reduced, glucose tolerance and the need for insulin in the treatment of diabetes may be diminished, and abnormal blood lipids may revert to normal. Yet viewed realistically, treatment of the obese patient is a frustrating problem (Beck and Hubbard, 1939; Green and Beckman, 1947).

From this review two questions emerge. First, why do most patients fail to maintain a weight loss after participating in a weight reduction program? Second, what distinguishes the successful patients from those who fail? This latter question can be divided into two subsidiary questions: (1) what happens to the patients who drop out of treatment, and (2) what are the factors producing differing rates of weight loss among those who stay in the program?

TABLE 8-5. *Long Term Weight Loss**

GROUP	NUMBER OF PATIENTS	INITIAL WEIGHT KG	WEIGHT AFTER DIETING KG	WEIGHT 14 YEARS LATER KG	CHANGE OVER 14 YEARS KG
I	17	85	73.5	85.5	+0.5
II	5	85.8	74.5	72.5	−13.3
III	5	100.5	80.5	120.4	+19.9

*Adapted from Sohar and Sneh: Am. J. Clin. Nutr., 26:845, 1973, with permission.

In any weight reduction clinic a substantial number of patients who are seen do not return for subsequent visits. Christakis (1967) noted that 558 out of 2603 patients (20 percent) failed to return to clinic within the first 2 weeks. Seaton and Rose (1965) evaluated 1000 consecutive records of obese patients in an effort to distinguish between those who defaulted and those who continued to attend the weight reducing clinic. Nearly 25 percent (239 patients) of the total did not return after the first visit. There were no differences in age, sex, degree of obesity or occupation between patients who returned and those who did not. There was a significantly greater frequency of defaulters among the lighter patients than among the heavier patients (29 percent of the defaulters were less than 20 pounds overweight, compared with 22 percent for those who were more than 20 percent overweight). The lowest incidence of dropouts was among the diabetic patients. The source of referral was also an important factor in whether patients returned to the clinic. Of the patients referred from the hospital, 31 percent defaulted, compared with 22 percent of those referred from the outpatient clinics and 14 percent of those referred by general practitioners.

Several studies have examined the factors which lead to success among those who stay in a treatment program. Darling and Summerskill (1953) observed that success in weight reduction was highest among the patients who were emotionally adjusted as estimated by the Bell Emotional Adjustment Scale. A similar conclusion was reached by Young, Moore, Berresford and Einset (1955) who observed a high degree of success among the adult dieters who were classified as emotionally stable, and a much lower success rate among those who had significant emotional problems or who were anxious and tense.

Shipman and Plesset (1963a, b) reached similar conclusions. They showed that the individuals who were most anxious at the beginning of treatment were worse after weight loss, while those patients with a relatively low degree of anxiety and depression became even calmer during treatment. Successful dieters were thus characterized as having a low level of anxiety. Ley et al. (1974) showed that most personality measures did not correlate with successful weight loss. However, one test which measures the locus of control over one's actions on an internal-external axis was correlated with weight loss. Those patients who viewed control over their actions as "internal" were more successful than those who viewed the control of their actions as largely "external" or outside their control.

Several investigators have observed that depression may develop during dieting (Stunkard, 1957; Silverstone and Lascelles, 1966; Robinson and Winnik, 1973). In a recent review of this problem, Stunkard and Rush (1974) examined the relation between depression and dieting. First, they found that when obesity began in childhood, patients were more vulnerable to developing depression during treatment than when obesity began in adult life (Grinker, Hirsch, and Levin, 1973b). This finding is in harmony with the distorted body image which is present in most patients with juvenile onset obesity (Stunkard and Mendelson, 1967) (see Chapter 5).

Obesity beginning after puberty shows no aberrations in body image, whereas juvenile onset obesity is almost always associated with a distorted body image. Morever, estimates of body size progressively increase during weight loss in patients with childhood onset obesity, but no such change occurs in the adult onset form (Glucksman and Hirsch, 1969). Similarly, patients with juvenile onset obesity significantly underestimated one and three second time intervals following weight loss. Patients with onset of obesity in adult life show no such alterations in estimating times (Grinker, Glucksman, Hirsch and Viseltear, 1973a; Grinker, Hirsch and Levin, 1973b; Grinker, 1973), and there is no distortion before weight loss.

Stunkard and Rush noted that the degree and duration of caloric restriction were related to the appearance of symptoms. Short term fasts lasting no more than 2 weeks rarely produced depression. Longer fasts were associated with increasing emotional instability; with low calorie diets, emotional symptoms are usually delayed until the patient has lost 7 to 9 kg.

Finally, outpatient treatment may be more stressful than inpatient treatment. Although dieting frequently leads to nervousness and depression, this is not observed in most patients who lose weight after intestinal bypass (see Chapter 10).

BEHAVIOR MODIFICATION

The frequent failure of traditional methods for treating obesity has led to the search for new approaches. Several of these will be discussed below. The first of these are the techniques of behavior modification. The focus of our discussion to this point has been on the decision about the quantity and types of food to be eaten, but many other factors are involved in the eating situation, including the time and place of eating, the persons who are sharing the meal, and the mood in which it is eaten. Since any effective treatment for obesity must modify the quantity of food calories eaten or the quantity of calories expended (exercise), they must modify some of these behavioral aspects of eating. The use of various techniques from clinical psychology, broadly called behavior modification, is directed towards this purpose. For a more extensive discussion of this approach, the reader is referred to recent publications by Stuart and Davis (1972), Stuart (1975), Stunkard (1972b), and Jordan and Levitz (1973, 1975).

Trends in body weight in the American population illustrate the operation of environmental and behavioral factors in our daily life.

There has been a divergence in weight trends for men and women over the past several decades. Women at any given height tend to be lighter at comparable age if born later in this century (see Chapter 1). In the Framingham Study women have shown a gradual downward trend in weight with successive examinations since 1948, but men have grown heavier (Fig. 8–9) (Gordon and Kannel, 1973). The inductees into the Army in 1942, for example, were heavier on average than men of the same height inducted in 1918. These differing trends may well reflect social modification of eating patterns. As more and more of the female body becomes exposed to view, it is ever more difficult to hide excess body fat. The factors controlling food intake which we have previously labeled "environmental" must modify eating (or exercise) in some fashion. The large difference in body weight of some pairs of identical twins is a case in point. Since these individuals presumably have the same genetic constitution, differences in body weight and fat must reflect differences in eating behavior (i.e., environmental factors). These factors operating in large populations represent the results of social pressures.

The use of more formal techniques of behavior modification are

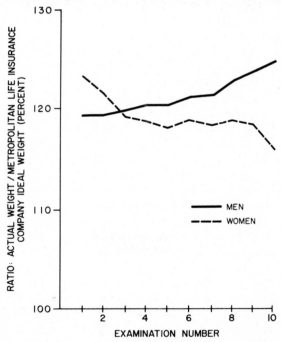

Figure 8–9. Changes in body weight of men and women in the Framingham study since its inception. The 1st examination occurred between 1948 and 1950 and subsequent examinations occurred at 2 year intervals. The average weight of the women has declined and that for the men increased over the 18 years of this study. (Reprinted with permission of the authors from Geriatrics, Volume 28, No. 8, pp. 80–83, Copyright The New York Times Media Company, Inc.)

based on the experimental work of Pavlov on conditioned reflexes, and the studies of Skinner and others on operant conditioning. A rationale for applying these principles to the treatment of obesity is provided by the concept that obese people are more responsive to external signals for eating than are lean subjects (Schachter and Rodin, 1974) (see Chapter 2). However, it was Stuart (1967) who first applied these ideas to the behavioral control of overeating. In his first study, 8 subjects were instructed over a period of weeks in methods of gaining conscious control over food intake (Fig. 8–10 shows data on 4 of these patients). These patients lost an average of 13.2 pounds during the 12 weeks of treatment and continued to lose weight afterwards. One year after beginning treatment the average weight loss was 32 pounds. This striking result has been the cornerstone for many trials which have confirmed the value of these techniques and suggested their widespread application to obese humans (see Stuart, 1975; Jordan and Levitz, 1975).

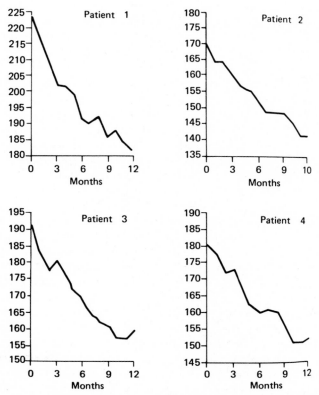

Figure 8–10. Weight curves of four patients treated by behavior modification. Weight loss occurred during the 3 months of active treatment and for the ensuing 9 months. (Reprinted from Stuart: Behav. Res. Ther., 5:357–365, 1967, with permission of the Pergamon Press.)

Broadly speaking, two different approaches have been used in behavior modification: (1) classical avoidance conditioning, and (2) operant conditioning. The attempt to use classical (Pavlovian) conditioning has taken several forms. One group has attempted to produce an aversion to food by introducing an electrical shock or obnoxious odor every time the food is eaten (Meyer and Crisp, 1964; Fureyt and Kennedy, 1971). Other investigators have attempted to produce a generalized state of tension in association with the ingestion of food. Ley et al. (1974) found that two classical aversion techniques produced significantly more weight loss in the short term but not in the long term. These techniques have in general suffered from a high dropout rate during treatment. However, weight loss is rapid among those who remain in treatment.

The second broad approach has been the use of operant conditioning. Two general tacks have been taken. Some investigators have used contracts in which patients give money or other valuables to the doctor who returns them to the patient as a "reward" for successful weight loss (Harris and Bruner, 1971). The second operant method involves reconditioning the environment rather than the subject (Bernard, 1968). Basically this technique is a set of rules designed to reprogram troublesome features of the environment.

A general scheme is shown in Table 8–6 (Stuart, 1971, 1975). The first step is to identify the time and place of eating, as well as the quantity and quality of food eaten and the circumstances which surround the act of eating. To do this a diary of food intake and activity is kept which serves two functions. (For a detailed program see *Obesity in Perspective*, Appendix V.) First, it provides a record from which the patient and physician can identify the problematic foods and difficult situations in which food is often eaten. Second, this technique focuses the patient's attention on a number of "behavioral" components of eating. The next steps involve reprogramming the environment to reduce, eliminate or suppress the cues to eat. Additional steps involve strengthening the rewards and enhancing the conditions for eating less. The results of a study by Stuart (1971) are shown in Figure 8–11. In this study, behavior modification and standard forms of treatment were compared. The beneficial effect of behavior modification in this study is clear.

Although promising, the place of behavior modification is still uncertain. Most of the more than 50 studies of behavior modification as treatment for obesity were conducted with college students or other academic personnel (Stuart, 1975; Jordan and Levitz, 1975). Whether these same approaches will produce similar results with patients from other social and economic groups is not known. Yet it is these other groups that have the greatest frequency of "overweight."

Only a few clinical studies have been reported so far. Penick et al. (1971) reported on 32 patients, of whom 2 (13 percent) lost more than

TABLE 8-6. *Sample Procedures Used to Strengthen Appropriate Eating and to Weaken Inappropriate Eating**

Cue elimination	Cue suppression	Cue strengthening
1. Eat in one room only.	1. Have company while eating.	1. Keep food weight chart.
2. Do nothing while eating.	2. Prepare and serve small quantities only.	2. Use food exchange diet.
3. Make available proper foods only:	3. Eat slowly.	3. Allow extra money for proper foods.
(a) shop from a list;	4. Save one item from meal to eat later.	4. Experiment with attractive preparation of diet foods.
(b) shop only after full meal.	5. If high calorie foods are eaten, they must require preparation.	5. Keep available pictures of desired clothes, list of desirable activities.
4. Clear dishes directly into garbage.		
5. Allow children to take own sweets.		

Reduce strength of undesirable responses:		Increase strength of desirable responses:
1. Swallow food already in mouth before adding more.		1. Introduce planned delays during meal.
2. Eat with utensils.		2. Chew food slowly, thoroughly.
3. Drink as little as possible during meals.		3. Concentrate on what is being eaten.

Provide decelerating consequences:		Provide accelerating consequences:
1. Develop means for display of caloric value of food eaten daily and weight changes.		1. Develop means for display of caloric value of food eaten daily and weight changes.
2. Arrange to have deviations from program ignored by others except professionals.		2. Develop means of providing social feedback for all success by: (a) family; (b) friends; (c) co-workers; (d) other weight losers; and (e) professionals.
3. Arrange to have overeater re-read program when items have not been followed and to write techniques which might have succeeded.		3. Program material and social consequences to follow: (a) the attainment of weight loss subgoals; (b) completion of specific daily behavioral control objectives.

*From Stuart: Behav. Res. Ther., 9:177–186, 1971.

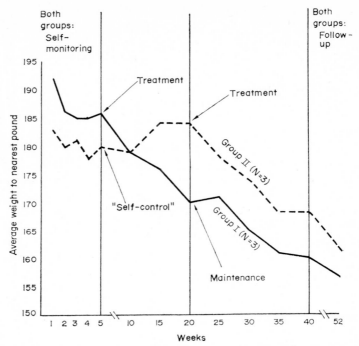

Figure 8–11. Behavior modification as a treatment for obesity. Subjects were actively assisted or passively observed. The benefits of treatment are shown by the increased weight loss. (Reprinted from Stuart: Behav. Res. Ther., 9:177–186, 1971, with permission of the Pergamon Press.)

40 pounds, and 8 (53 percent) lost more than 20 pounds in 12 weeks. The weight loss continued after 52 weeks. Five subjects had lost 40 pounds, and 4 had lost over 20 pounds. The weight loss expected from a review of the literature was 5 percent losing 40 pounds or more and 25 percent losing 20 pounds or more. In a study by Jordan and Levitz (Levitz, 1973 and unpublished), 28 of 92 patients (31 percent) had lost or kept off more than 20 pounds for one year. During their 20 week program, the average weight loss was 21 pounds in 59 women and 36 pounds in 30 men. The dropout rates were 9 and 27 percent respectively. These two clinical trials are very encouraging indeed.

Weisenberg and Fray (1974), however, are more cautious. They compared three groups using behavior modification, a group approach and individual counseling. Although the 3 groups had significantly different starting weights, they each had a comparable percent weight loss. Blacks, Caucasians and Orientals were in all three groups. Weight loss among the blacks was smaller and behavior modification seemed ineffective. Ley et al. also voiced caution after finding that a set of instructions on how to develop self control in treating obesity had no greater effect on weight loss than placebo instructions or diet alone.

The second problem in assessing results with behavior modification is the "flush of enthusiasm" which has followed the initial reports with this technique (Stunkard, 1972; Stuart, 1967; Stuart and Davis, 1972). This is a common response to any new therapeutic approach. Only with the passage of time and more experience can the true value of this technique be assessed.

The third problem in assessing the currently available data is the necessity of having "new" methods and data to pass editorial review by a scientific journal. Thus variations in technique with positive results are easy to publish. Negative, unfavorable or repetitious work is much more difficult to get into print. Stuart (1975) has reviewed these and other of the clinical aspects of trials of behavior modification and cautions against a stampede to this approach.

At the present time it is my belief that, whatever nutritional approach is taken with the obese patient, it should be accompanied by behavioral modification in some form. It is widely recognized that patients drop out of all treatment programs, and that many patients who are initially "successful" will eventually regain some or all of the weight they lost. Only modification of eating patterns will be likely to lead to long term success.

GROUP THERAPY FOR OBESITY

Obese patients have been treated in groups as well as individually. Studies by Harvey and Simmons (1954) showed that group therapy could be effective. The experiences with group therapy reported by Goodman, Schwartz and Frankel (1953), Kalb (1956), and Chapman (1953) also demonstrated the effectiveness of groups in the treatment of obese patients. Two good studies have compared treatment in groups with treatment by individual therapists.

Bowser, Trulson, Bowling and Stare (1953) compared body weights one and two years after treatment by one of three methods: individual instruction, group therapy and no treatment. It was clear in the long term that individual therapy was comparable to group therapy, and that either was slightly but not impressively better than no therapy at all. This is shown in Figure 8–12, which plots the percent overweight at one and two year follow-up with the initial percent overweight. There are a few patients above the broken line, indicating individuals who weighed more two years after treatment. In addition, there are a number of patients, some from each group, whose body weight at follow-up was less than at the beginning of therapy. In another study, Munves (1953) evaluated 48 subjects who were divided into two groups. Each group was followed for 8 months; 4 months

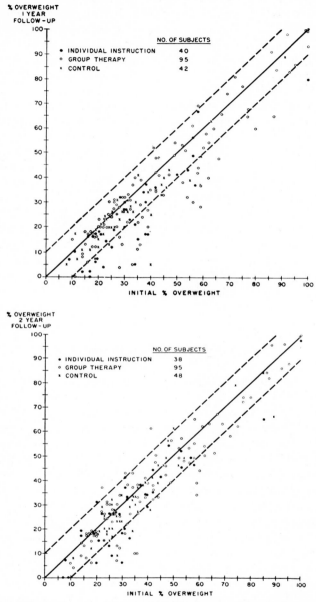

Figure 8–12. Effects of group therapy, individual counselling and no treatment on body weight one and 2 years later. There was no consistent advantage to one treatment over another at these intervals after terminating therapy. (Copyright the American Dietetic Association. Reprinted by permission from the Journal of The American Dietetic Association, 53:1193, 1953.)

during therapy for weight loss and four months during maintenance of body weight. During weight loss there was no significant difference between the two groups. But in the 4 months of maintenance, the patients receiving individual instruction appeared to do somewhat better.

These lukewarm results are in contrast to the data of Howard (1969) who has reported on the positive aspects of group therapy. Others have been similarly impressed (Simmons, 1954; Kurlander, 1953; Jenkins, 1956; Kotkov, 1953), though without adequate controls. Since group therapy is probably no worse than individual therapy, the use of groups may prove an effective way of extending the use of skilled personnel. Ley and his collaborators (1974) have evaluated several approaches to improving the success of nutritional treatment in obesity. Allowing patients to participate as a group in decisions about the techniques of treatment for obesity produced no more weight loss than using a lecture. The degree of fear aroused about the complications of obesity did not affect weight loss. Similarly, a point system for successful dieting leading to "diet holidays" as a reward had no effect on weight loss and, if anything, tended to decrease compliance with the diet.

SELF HELP GROUPS

The meeting of obese patients in groups has been highly touted as an effective technique for helping some people lose weight. The best known of these groups is Weight Watchers, Inc., a privately owned company with regional franchises around the world. The story of the origin and growth of Weight Watchers has been told by its founder Jean Nidetch (1970) and by Peter Wyden (1965). There is no concrete data on the success in combating obesity, however, since no figures have ever been published. In our obesity clinic, 118 of 267 women have been to Weight Watchers; the average duration was 25 weeks; the average weight loss was 21 pounds; but almost all regained weight. Similar findings have been reported recently by Garrow (1975).

Other self help groups include Overeaters Anonymous, Diet Kitchen, Diet Workshop and TOPS (Take Off Pounds Sensibly). The founding and development of TOPS has been told in a delightful chapter by Wyden (1965). Stunkard (1972, 1976) has examined the operation of TOPS chapters in the Philadelphia area. In the 1968 survey, the average member was 42 years old and had a desirable weight of 119 pounds, but actually weighed 188 pounds. The average membership in TOPS lasted 16½ months. The dropout rate was highest for those who were least overweight on joining. To test whether effectiveness in weight loss might be increased, behavior modification was introduced into a few chapters (Fig. 8–13). Both the amount of weight loss and the length of membership increased by this maneuver. This finding suggests that application of behavior modification to already existing self help groups might significantly improve the degree of weight loss.

HYPNOSIS

Hypnosis has been tried as a treatment for obesity (Winkelstein, 1959), but its effectiveness has rarely been assessed by objective means. In one study, Winkelstein studied 42 patients who had two characteristics in common: (1) they could enter a deep trance; (2) they had a normal history and physical examination. This group of patients was, on an average, 32 pounds overweight and between 16 and 52 years of age. The average weight loss during the 14 weeks of treatment was 1.66 pounds per week, and during the 6 months after the end of treatment the patient lost on average another one pound per week. Thus the initial weight loss which began during the period of hypnosis was continued at rates which would be quite acceptable. Thus it appears that for some individuals hypnosis can be valuable in achieveing weight loss.

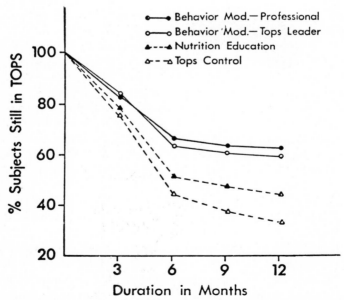

Figure 8–13. Effectiveness of behavior modification in the self-help group TOPS. The use of professional therapists increased weight loss and duration of membership in the TOPS chapter. (Reprinted from Stunkard, A. J.: *In: Obesity in Perspective.* Washington, D.C., U.S. Government Printing Office, Vol. II, II, 1976.)

FASTING

The adaptation to prolonged fasting has been studied in normal (Benedict, 1915; Keys et al., 1950; Cahill et al., 1966) and obese subjects (Cahill, 1970; Bray et al., 1972; Drenick et al., 1964; Bloom, 1959; Duncan et al., 1962, 1963; Ball et al., 1967). In 1915, Benedict reported the results of a 28 day fast in an otherwise healthy man. By measuring nitrogen excretion and metabolic rate, Benedict could estimate body fuels being used to sustain life during this period. Glycogen stores were exhausted within 36 hours. The excretion of nitrogen gradually fell, and respiratory quotient (RQ) reached 0.7, indicating that fat had become the principal metabolic fuel. Metabolic rate also declined slightly.

Our understanding of the adaptation to fasting has been extended by the study of obese patients who can tolerate food deprivation for many weeks. The changes in circulating substrate concentrations have been well documented. Fatty acids from adipose tissue rise and supply the liver with the substrate to form ketone bodies. The peak levels of beta hydroxybutyrate are reached in 8 to 10 days. The rising levels of ketones surpass the renal mechanisms for reabsorption and ketonuria develops. Appearance of ketones in the urine can be used to assess the continuation of fasting. However, as little as 30 to 50 g of carbohydrate will abolish the ketosis and ketonuria. Increased uric acid in the plasma is one consequence of the high plasma ketones. Short chain organic acids such as lactic, acetoacetic, and beta hydroxybutyric acid compete with uric acid for excretion by the renal tubule. Thus the rise in ketoacids during fasting reduces the excretion of uric acid and hyperuricemia develops; in some individuals this can precipitate gout or kidney stones (Cheifetz, 1965; Lloyd-Mostyn et al., 1970). Drenick (1975) has reported three patients who developed renal stones during fasting, and we have seen one such patient. This can be prevented by treatment with allopurinol (Drenick, Fisler and Dennin, 1971).

The metabolic response to a short term fast differs from the response to more prolonged fasting (Cahill et al., 1970). Some of these relationships are depicted schematically in Figure 8–14. During the first week or so the body excretes 10 to 14 g of nitrogen per day. This is equivalent to the catabolism of 75 g of protein each day. After 4 to 5 weeks of fasting, however, nitrogen excretion has fallen to 3 to 5 g/day. The breakdown of protein and release of amino acids provides the major source of carbon for glucose synthesis by the liver, yet the concentration of glucose which initially falls reaches a plateau and does not continue to decline. Maintenance of plasma glucose results primarily from a decrease in metabolic demands for glucose by peripheral tissues.

Owen et al. (1967), in a classic study, showed that after adaptation

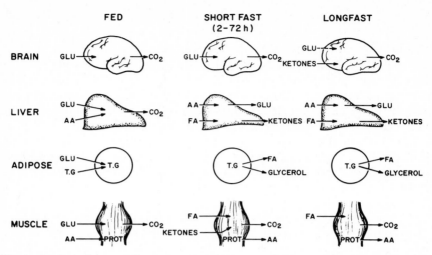

Figure 8–14. Schematic diagram of short and long term fasting on metabolism. The principal difference between a short and long term fast is the decreased gluconeogenesis and decreased utilization of protein with long term fasting. (Adapted from Cahill, G. F. and Owen, O. E.: International Psychiatry Clinics, Vol. 7., No. 1, 1970, pp. 25—36.)

to a long term fast, circulating ketoacids were supplying the brain with its major source of metabolic fuel. The recycling of lactate, pyruvate and glycerol, along with the catabolism of small quantities of protein, provides sufficient substrate to maintain glucose production by the liver (Cahill, 1970). Thus with prolonged fasting there is a reduced need for amino acids from tissue protein, and this is reflected in the concentration of various amino acids in the plasma. The gluco-neogenic amino acids such as alanine decline steadily and this is paralleled by the fall in the concentration of glucose to low normal levels. The concentration of glycine rises and then falls. The other essential amino acids decline.

The pattern of hormonal change during fasting is shown in Figure 8–15 (Marliss et al., 1970). There is a decline in insulin and a rise in glucagon. Growth hormone, which is low in obese patients, shows little change with fasting (Beck et al., 1964). Corticosteroid excretion may fall slightly, but gonadal hormones apparently do not change (see Chapter 7).

The overall metabolic rate declines with starvation (Drenick, 1975) and with marked caloric restriction (Bray, 1969). Before starvation, the basal metabolism rate in a group of obese men ranged between 62 and 160 kCal/hour. After a 21 day fast it had dropped to 45 to 95 kCal/hour (Drenick, 1975). This decline is faster than the decrease in body weight. A decline in metabolic rate was also observed during starvation of normal volunteers (see Chapter 4). Although the decline in metabolic rate reduces the metabolic demand for most vitamins, some deficiencies still occur. Folic acid and thiamine both drop, and Drenick has reported the development of Wernicke's syndrome in one patient who fasted for more than four weeks.

A number of other metabolic adaptations occur during fasting (Benoit et al., 1965; Bolinger et al., 1966; Smith and Drenick, 1966; Forbes, 1970). The excretion of sodium, potassium, calcium and magnesium falls. After the initial loss of sodium, this ion is retained by the kidney and only small additional quantities are lost. Conservation of potassium is less complete. The losses of potassium average 41 mEq/ day for the first 10 days, and are between 480 and 820 mEq in the first month. Most of the potassium comes from cellular stores and reflects

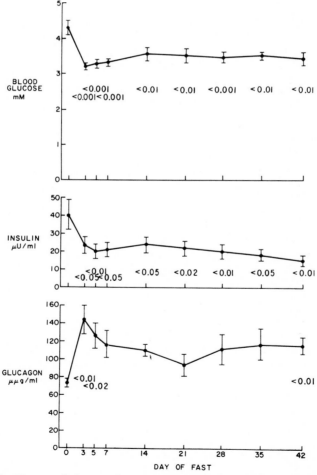

Figure 8–15. Hormonal changes during prolonged fasting. Glucose drops, insulin declines, and glucagon rises and then falls toward control level. (From Marliss et al.: J. Clin. Invest., *49:*2256-2270, 1970, reprinted with permission.)

protein breakdown. The loss of potassium can also be detected by the decline in ^{40}K (see Chapter 1).

The loss of intracellular and extracellular cations is associated with a contraction of body water which declines by an average of 11.8 liters in the first month of fasting (Drenick, 1975). Plasma volume also decreases by 400 to 600 ml. The hypotension and occasional episodes of fainting may in part be due to this loss of vascular and extracellular fluid volume. A decline in the glomerular filtration rate and in urine volume may also reflect the contraction of extracellular fluid volumes.

The production of ketoacids and the catabolism of tissue proteins provide an acid load for excretion by the kidney. During the first two weeks of fasting, there is a rise of 40 to 70 mEq/day in the excretion of titratable acid. Ammonia production by the kidney increases rapidly to a peak of 150 mEq/day by the 15th day of the fast. This is the time of maximal excretion of phosphate and sulfate. As protein catabolism declines because the body reduces its need for glucose, the load of sulfate and phosphate falls, and the excretion of ammonia and titratable acid by the kidney drops to lower levels.

Fasting as a mode of treatment for obesity has been widely used since the initial report by Bloom (1959) on 9 patients who had fasted for a short period in the hospital with rapid weight loss and no ill effects (Forbes, 1970). It has been shown subsequently that weight loss is predictable and ranges between 7 and 13 pounds per week after the first 10 days (Drenick et al., 1964). Patients are not troubled by hunger. Indeed after the first few days appetite is generally much reduced, although hunger ratings may not change (Silverstone, Stark and Buckle, 1966). Fasts of nearly a year in duration have been reported by several groups of investigators (Table 8–7). With these prolonged fasts large amounts of weight were lost, the largest amount being 276 pounds (Rooth and Carlstrom, 1970; Runcie and Thompson, 1970; Collison, 1967; Stewart and Fleming, 1973; Thomson et al., 1966).

TABLE 8–7.   *Fasts Lasting More Than 200 Days*

Author	Year	Age	Sex	Duration of Fast	Weights (lb) Initial	Weights (lb) Final	Weights (lb) Loss
Thomas et al.	1966	28	F	236	281	184	97
		54	F	249	264	189	75
Collison	1967	20	F	234	322	168	154
Garnett et al.	1969	20	F	210	260	*	
Runcie and Thomas	1970	–	–	210	420	280	140
Stewart and Fleming	1970	27	M	382	456	180	276

*No final weight given. Patient died during first week of refeeding after weight returned to "ideal" level.

Studies on the psychological response to prolonged fasting have been reported from several clinics (Rowland, 1968; Kollar and Atkinson, 1966; Swanson and Dinello, 1970). During short term fasts little emotional difficulty occurs, but with more prolonged fasting significant aberrations occur. Depression and anxiety occurred in all 7 patients studied by Kollar and Atkinson (1966). Rowland also observed marked emotional fluctuations with near psychotic episodes in two of the six patients he studied.

Several physiological changes characterize the clinical response to fasting. The skin uniformly becomes thinner and hair may fall out. The fatty liver which is almost uniformly present in obese patients improves. Fat decreases and there is no evidence of fibrotic or cirrhotic changes (Drenick, 1975). The hematocrit and leucocyte count both decline. After 3 months of fasting the hematocrit in one patient had declined from 46.2 percent to 41.0 percent (Drenick, 1975). With rehydration it dropped to 36.1, indicating the decrease in red cell mass.

Although several complications have resulted from fasting, it has in general been safe and rewarding to the patient. Hypotension is a common complaint, and fainting can occur. Kidney stones composed of uric acid have been reported on several occasions. One man developed Wernicke's syndrome, a manifestation of thiamine deficiency (Drenick, 1975). Several deaths have also been reported (Herrmann and Iverson, 1968; Spencer, 1968; Berger, 1967; Cubberly et al., 1965; Garnett et al., 1969). In most of them the patient had been receiving medications, such as phenforminhydrochloride, which may have been partially responsible.

The most distressing feature of the studies with fasting is the poor long term results (Harrison and Harden, 1966; Maage and Mogensen, 1970; Hunscher, 1966; Hollifield et al., 1964; Maccuish et al., 1968). Three studies are now available on the long term evaluation of weight loss in patients who were admitted to the hospital for fasting Campbell et al. (1974) has followed 75 patients. Five patients discharged themselves from the hospital within a week or so after initiating the program. During the fast which averaged 14 weeks, the 70 remaining patients lost an average of 29.6 kg (2.1 kg/week). Only 39 of the 70 patients were starved until they were less than 25 percent overweight.

The follow-up period averaged 28.2 months (12 to 64 months). During this period the percentage of excess weight rose from 28.2 percent at discharge to 62.7 percent at maximal follow-up. As noted in most studies, the incidence of failure increases with the length of the period of follow-up. Even among the failures, however, this method of treatment, like most others, has its good side. In the report by Campbell et al. (1974), 10 patients have had 12 elective operations, 9 have married and 6 have become pregnant. Eleven patients had obtained jobs for which they had not previously been eligible.

PROTEIN SUPPLEMENTED FASTING

The effectiveness of fasting as a technique for reducing body fat is now accepted. Its major disadvantage is the need for hospitalization, since the risk of hypotension and syncope makes it undesirable to use this technique at home. Because the hypotension reflects loss of lean body tissue and fluid, several groups have evaluated the possibility of giving enough protein and electrolytes to prevent protein loss and fluid contraction (Apfelbaum et al., 1970; Blackburn et al., 1973; Baird et al., 1974; Genuth, Castro and Vertes, 1974). Strang, McCluggage and Evans (1930, 1931) originally showed that 1 g of protein/kg body weight would almost completely prevent the loss of body protein during severe caloric restriction, but Apfelbaum and his collaborators were the first to apply this to the outpatient treatment of obese patients. When protein was given, nitrogen losses were reduced or abolished, yet weight loss was gratifying (Evans and Strang, 1929, 1931; Evans, 1938).

Three groups have adapted this technique to outpatient treatment of obesity. Blackburn and Bistrian (unpublished data) carefully screen patients before initiating this program. The successful patients begin a fast supplemented by 1.3 to 1.5 g of protein per kilogram of ideal body weight. The protein is provided as lean meat, fish or fowl. The caloric intake on this program ranges between 400 and 700 kCal/day depending on the fat content of the meat.

Genuth, Castro and Vertes (1974) have used a different approach for protein supplementation. All patients are hospitalized for one week and then treated on an outpatient basis. The dietary supplement contains 45 g of casein, 30 g of glucose and 0.25 mEq of potassium. In addition, each patient receives a multivitamin tablet and folic acid. With this program, nitrogen equilibrium is nearly achieved and losses of potassium and phosphate are minimal. Between September, 1971 and June, 1974, 141 patients were begun on this program, and 70 percent lost more than 40 pounds. The data are summarized in Figure 8–16. One man lost 305 pounds during one year. These authors noted no difficulty with wound healing. No psychiatric, hematologic, renal or hepatic problems were noted. The .only difficulties were temporary hair loss, transient dryness to the skin, cold intolerance, muscle cramps and constipation. These seem minor indeed compared with the success of this program.

EXERCISE

In his review published in 1960, Feinstein made the following comment about exercise. "There has been ample demonstration that exercise is an *in*effective method of increasing energy output, since it takes far too much activity to burn up calories for a significant weight

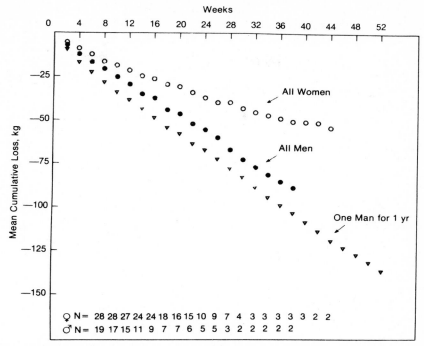

Figure 8–16. Effect of protein-supplemented fasting on weight loss. (From Genuth, J.A.M.A., *230*:987–992, Copyright 1974, American Medical Association, reprinted with permission.)

loss." In addition, he says "no clinical results have been cited to indicate its (exercise's) therapeutic effectiveness in weight reduction." Since this dismal statement was authored 15 years ago, several studies have been published which suggest that an exercise program can be helpful for some patients. First, it is important to point out that exercise is accompanied by reduction in food intake (Edholm, Fletcher, Widdowson and McCance, 1955; Crews, Fuge, Oscai, Holloszy and Shank, 1969). In animal studies, chronic exercise was accompanied by long term continuing reduction in food intake.

Not only can exercise decrease food intake, but it can also decrease body fat. Several studies in college age students showed that during periods of exercise consisting of mild walking and jogging, obese women showed a reduction in body weight and a decrease in skinfold thickness (Moody et al., 1969; 1972). Boileau, Buskirk, Horstman, Mendez and Nicholas (1971) showed that a program with exercise carried on during weekdays by obese college men reduced body fat and produced a small reduction in body weight. Thus for college age students it is clear that a program of mild to moderate physical activity consisting of jogging or walking on a treadmill can reduce body fat content, increase lean body mass, and decrease body weight without other dietary control.

Appendix 8–5 shows the exercise equivalents for a number of foods (Konishi, 1965). It shows that, with grossly obese patients, it is more difficult to achieve effective levels of exercise, but when successful more weight is lost (Wunderlich et al., 1973). In a study of 12 massively obese patients, 6 of whom had an exercise program and 6 of whom did not, Kenrick, Ball and Canary (1972) demonstrated that exercise increased the rate of fat loss and weight loss by obese subjects maintained on a liquid formula diet. In commenting about these studies, however, the physical therapists noted the psychological barriers that these obese patients had to overcome in order to exercise. It became increasingly difficult to get them to participate in this program. Thus the evidence that exercise will work in reducing body fat content and decreasing body weight without restriction of dietary intake is clear (Mayer and Stare, 1953). The difficulty in getting obese patients to participate in such a program, however, probably accounts for the relative dislike for this form of therapeutic approach.

MASSAGE AND SPOT REDUCING

Many obese patients would like to lose fat selectively from one spot but not another. This desire has led to the introduction of many approaches including massage and sauna belts. The early study by Cuthbertson (1932) and by Short and Carnegie (1939) suggested that massage might have metabolic effect. Kalb (1944), however, demonstrated unequivocally that massage was not effective in spot reducing. One group of 40 patients were placed on an 800 calorie diet, 20 of which received a massage twice a week. There was a loss of weight in all patients, and the sizes of the arm and thigh were smaller. The group receiving massage showed no greater reduction than the control group. In a second study, massage was without effect when there was no dietary restriction and no weight loss. Similarly, there is no demonstrated effectiveness of other methods of spot reducing.

APPENDICES TO CHAPTER 8

(8–1—8–4 adapted from Jolliffe, 1963)*

APPENDIX 8–1. *Caloric Value of Fruits and Vegetables*

One standard portion is ½ cup in the form eaten. When feasible, other indications of standard portions will be given.

Syrup packed fruits or fruits with added sugar are not listed.

Calorie Count may be substituted for any other vegetable or fruit or combination thereof of like Calorie Count.

Vegetables   Fruits

12½ Calorie Count

Beans: snap, green, wax
Cabbage: celery, Chinese
Cauliflower
Celery
Chard
Cucumber
Endive
Lettuce
Mushrooms
Parsley
Peppers
Pickles: sour, dill
Radishes
Scallions
Squash: summer

25 Calorie Count

Vegetables	Fruits
Artichokes: French, medium	Cranberries
Asparagus (6 spears)	Currants
Beet greens	Gooseberries
Beets	Honeydew melon (cubes or balls)**
Broccoli	Lemon (1 medium)
Brussels sprouts	Lemon juice
Carrots	Lime (1 medium)
Eggplant	Lime juice
Kohlrabi	Plum (1)
Mustard greens	Raisins (1 tbsp.)
Rutabagas	Rhubarb
Sauerkraut	Tomato
Spinach	Tomato juice

---

*Copyright 1952, 1957 by Simon and Schuster, Inc. Reprinted by permission.

**Honeydew melon is included in both the 25 and 50 Calorie Count groups, depending on how it is served. One half cup is given 25 Calorie Count, while a 2 inch wedge is given in a Calorie Count of 50.

Table continued on the following page.

APPENDIX 8–1. *Caloric Value of Fruits and Vegetables (continued)*

Turnip greens	Strawberries
Turnips	Watermelon (cubes or balls)†

50 Calorie Count

Dandelion greens	Applesauce
Leeks	Apricots, raw or canned (3 medium)
Onions (1 medium)	Blackberries, raw or canned
Parsnips	Blueberries, raw or canned
Pumpkin	Cantaloupe (½ medium)
Squash, winter	Cherries, canned
	Grapefruit sections, raw or canned
	Grapefruit juice, fresh, canned or frozen
	Grapefruit and orange juice blend
	Grapes
	Honeydew melon (2″ wedge)*
	Loganberries
	Nectarine (2 small)
	Orange sections
	Orange juice: fresh, frozen, or canned
	Papayas
	Peaches, raw or canned
	Pear, canned
	Pineapple: raw or canned,
	Juice: canned or frozen
	Raspberries, raw or canned
	Tangerine (1 large or 2 small)

75 Calorie Count

Beans, lima	Apple juice
Peas: green, canned, frozen	Apple (1 medium)
	Grape juice
	Grapefruit (½ medium)
	Guava
	Mango
	Orange (1)
	Plums, canned
	Persimmons, Japanese

100 Calorie Count

Artichokes: raw, Jerusalem	Apricots: dried, cooked
(five 1½″ diam.)	Banana (1 medium)
Corn: on cob, raw, frozen (1)	Cherries, sweet (20 to 30)
Potato (1 medium)	Dates: raw, dried (4)
Succotash	figs: raw, dried (2 medium or 3 small)
Sweet potato (1 small)	Pear, raw
	Pomegranate
	Prune juice, canned
	Prunes: dried, cooked, raw (4 medium)
	Watermelon (1 slice ¾″ × 6″ diam.)†

†Watermelon is included in both the 25 and 50 Calorie Count groups. In ½ cup portion it counts as 25 calories. It is usually eaten in large amounts, so a small slice should be counted as 100 calories. The traditional large 2/3 pound slice will give nearly 250 calories. Be very careful with size of portion of this food.

APPENDIX 8–2 *Caloric Value of Meats*

50 Calories in 1 ounce

Lean meats with fat trimmed	Kidney
Dried or chipped beef	Liver
Game	Poultry
Heart	Veal

Abalone	Pike, lake
Bluefish	Pollack
Bonito	Salmon, canned, pink or red, fresh
Butterfish	Shad
Cod	Shad roe
Eels, raw	Sturgeon
Finnan haddie	Swordfish
Flounder	Tilefish
Haddock	Tuna, fresh or canned, water pack
Halibut	Weakfish
Herring, raw	Whitefish
Ocean perch	

50 Calories in 2 ounces

Clams	Oysters
Crabmeat	Scallops
Lobster	Shrimp
Mussels	

75 Calories in 1 ounce

Lean cut meat—visible fat trimmed

Beef	Bologna
Ham	Frankfurters
Lamb	Tongue
Pork	

Bass, average	Sardines
Herring, pickled	Trout, brook
Mackerel	Tuna, canned in oil

90 Calories in 1 ounce

Sweetbreads, beef	Liverwurst
Duck	Luncheon meats
Goose	
Eel, smoked	Trout, lake

APPENDIX 8–3 *Calorie Count of Dairy Foods, Breads and Cereals*

FOOD	AMOUNT	CALORIES
Cheese, cottage (including "creamed" cottage, and pot cheese)	2 oz. (¼ cup)	60
all others (including cream cheese)	1 oz.	100
Egg	1	75
Milk, cow, fluid, whole	1 cup	165
nonfat (skim)	1 cup	85
nonfat, fortified or modified	1 cup	100
nonfat (skim) dry solids	3 tbsp.	85
canned, evaporated	½ cup	175
	2 tbsp.	50
condensed, sweetened	½ cup	500
	1 tbsp.	75

Table continued on the following page.

APPENDIX 8–3. *Calorie Count of Dairy Foods, Breads and Cereals*

buttermilk, cultured from skim milk	1 cup	85
cultured from whole milk	1 cup	100
malted, dry	1 oz.	125
Bread (including white, rye, wholewheat, cracked-wheat, protein, etc.)	1 slice	65
Special varieties:		
Boston brown bread	1 slice	75
Corn bread	2″ square	150
Melba toast	1 piece	25
Rusk, Holland	1 rusk	50
Ry-Krisp	1 piece	25
Zwieback	1 piece	35
Biscuits, baking powder	1 2″	100
Muffins, all varieties	1	125
Rolls, average	1	100
Cereals, cooked	½ to ¾ cup	75
dry, flaked (as Corn Flakes, Rice-Krispies, Wheaties, Rice-toasties)	1 cup	75
puffed	1 cup	50
shredded	1 large biscuit	100
Grape nuts	¼ cup	100
Crackers and cookies		
Arrowroot biscuit	1 biscuit	25
Butter Thins	3 crackers	50
Cheese Tid-Bits	12 1″	25
Chocolate Chip	1 cookie	50
Fig Newtons	1 bar	50
Gingersnaps	1 cookie	15
Graham crackers	3 crackers	100
Macaroons	1 large or 2 small	100

APPENDIX 8–4. *Recommended 1200 Calorie Meal Plans*

FOOD ITEM	HOUSEHOLD MEASURE	CALORIE COUNT
Fruit, citrus group	Fruit or juice, ½ cup	50
other	2 portions	
	1 of 50 calories	50
	1 of 75 calories	75
Vegetables, cooked	1 portion	25
12½ Calorie Count	all you want	50
Bread and cereal	3 portions	195
Meat, fish or poultry[1]	6 ounces	360
Cottage cheese[2]	3 ounces	90
Skim milk	2 cups	170
Optional Calorie Budget	2 cups	135
	Total	1200

[1]The meat, fish or poultry must be chosen from the lean and moderately fat groups with equal frequency. Four oz. of lean fish (25 Calorie Count) may be substituted for 3 oz. of cottage cheese.

[2]Egg may be substituted for 3 oz. of cottage cheese up to 4 times a week.

Suggested distribution of optional calorie budget:

I
1 75 Calorie Count egg
1 50 Calorie Count fruit

II
1 50 Calorie Count fruit
1 100 Calorie Count vegetable

III
1 65 Calorie Count bread
1 75 Calorie Count fruit

Suggested Menu Plans

I	II	III
Breakfast	Breakfast	Breakfast
Orange juice, ½ cup	Strawberries, 1 cup	Grapefruit sections,
Egg, cooked or	Corn flakes, ⅔ cup	½ cup
poached, 1	Skim milk, 1 cup	Cottage cheese, 3 oz.
Toasted roll, ½	Beverage	Toast, 1 slice
Beverage		Beverage
Lunch	Lunch	Lunch
Sardine sandwich	Cottage cheese and	Tomato stuffed with shrimp,
sardines, 2 oz.	chives, 3 oz.	seafood cocktail sauce,
bread, 2 slices	Celery hearts	4 oz.
Cottage cheese, 3 oz.	Whole wheat bread,	Green bean salad
with mixed green	2 slices	vinegar dressing
vegetables	Apple, 1	Roll, 1
Peach, 1	Beverage	Plums, raw, 3
Beverage		Beverage
Dinner	Dinner	Dinner
Tomato juice, 8 oz.	Salmon, broiled or	Broiled chicken, 4 oz.
Ham steak, 4 oz.	poached, 6 oz.	Steamed carrots, ½ cup
Brussels sprouts, ½ cup	Baked potato	Romaine lettuce, lemon
Mixed green salad	Broiled tomato	dressing
with lemon or	Tossed green salad with	Pineapple, 1 slice
vinegar dressing	spiced vinegar dressing	Beverage
Grapefruit, ½	Cantaloupe, ½	
Beverage	Beverage	
Snack	Snack	Snack
Skim milk, 2 cups	Skim milk, 1 cup	Skim milk, 2 cups
	Berries, ½ cup	Puffed wheat, ⅔ cup
		Orange, 1

APPENDIX 8-5. *Energy Equivalents of Food Calories*
Expressed in Minutes of Activity (Konishi, 1965)

FOOD	CALORIES	WALKING*	RIDING BICYCLE†	SWIMMING±	RUNNING#	RECLINING¶
		min.	min.	min.	min.	min.
Apple, large	101	19	12	9	5	78
Bacon, 2 strips	96	18	12	9	5	74
Banana, small	88	17	11	8	4	68
Beans, green, 1 cup	27	5	3	2	1	21
Beer, 1 glass	114	22	14	10	6	88
Bread and butter	78	15	10	7	4	60
Cake, 1/12, 2 layer	356	68	43	32	18	274
Carbonated beverage, 1 glass	106	20	13	9	5	82
Carrot, raw	42	8	5	4	2	32
Cereal, dry, ½ c., with milk and sugar	200	38	24	18	10	154
Cheese, cottage, 1 tbsp.	27	5	3	2	1	21
Cheese, Cheddar, 1 oz.	111	21	14	10	6	85
Chicken, fried, ½ breast	232	45	28	21	12	178
Chicken, "TV" dinner	542	104	66	48	28	417
Cookie, plain, 148/lb.	15	3	2	1	1	12
Cookie, chocolate chip	51	10	6	5	3	39
Doughnut	151	29	18	13	8	116
Egg, fried	110	21	13	10	6	85
Egg, boiled	77	15	9	7	4	59
French dressing, 1 tbsp.	59	11	7	5	3	45
Halibut steak, ¼ lb.	205	39	25	18	11	158
Ham, 2 slices	167	32	20	15	9	128
Ice cream, 1/6 qt.	193	37	24	17	10	148
Ice cream soda	255	49	31	23	13	196
Ice milk, 1/6 qt.	144	28	18	13	7	111

Food	Calories	Walking*	Riding bicycle†	Swimming±	Running#	Reclining¶
Gelatin, with cream	117	23	14	10	6	90
Malted milk shake	502	97	61	45	26	386
Mayonnaise, 1 tbsp.	92	18	11	8	5	71
Milk, whole, 1 glass	166	32	20	15	9	128
Milk, skim, 1 glass	81	16	10	7	4	62
Milk shake	421	81	51	38	22	324
Orange, medium	68	13	8	6	4	52
Orange juice, 1 glass	120	23	15	11	6	92
Pancake with syrup	124	24	15	11	6	95
Peach, medium	46	9	6	4	2	35
Peas, green, ½ cup	56	11	7	5	3	43
Pie, apple, 1/6	377	73	46	34	19	290
Pie, raisin, 1/6	437	84	53	39	23	336
Pizza, cheese, 1/8	180	35	22	16	9	138
Pork chop, loin	314	60	38	28	16	242
Potato chips, 1 serving	108	21	13	10	6	83
Sandwiches						
Club	590	113	72	53	30	454
Hamburger	350	67	43	31	18	269
Roast beef with gravy	430	83	52	38	22	331
Tuna fish salad	278	53	34	25	14	214
Sherbet, 1/6 qt.	177	34	22	16	9	136
Shrimp, French fried	180	35	22	16	9	138
Spaghetti, 1 serving	396	76	48	35	20	305
Steak, T-bone	235	45	29	21	12	181
Strawberry shortcake	400	77	49	36	21	308

*Energy cost of walking for 70-kg. individual=5.2 calories per minute at 3.5 m.p.h.

†Energy cost of riding bicycle=8.2 calories per minute.

±Energy cost of swimming=11.2 calories per minute.

#Energy cost of running=19.4 calories per minute.

¶Energy cost of reclining=1.3 calories per minute.

REFERENCES

Allan, M.: The joy of slimming. London, Wolfe Publishing, 1974.

Antonetti, V. W.: The equations governing weight change in human beings. Am. J. Clin. Nutr., 26:64, 1973.

Apfelbaum, M., Boudon, P. and Lacatis, D.: Effets métaboliques de la diète protidique chez 41 sujets obeses. Presse Med., 78:1917–1920, 1970.

Baird, I. M., Parsons, R. L. and Howard, A. N.: Clinical and metabolic studies of chemically defined diets in the management of obesity. Metabolism, 23:645–657, 1974.

Ball, M. F., Canary, J. J. and Kyle, L. H.: Comparative effect of caloric restriction and total starvation on body composition in obesity. Ann. Intern. Med., 67:60–67, 1967.

Banting, W.: Letter on corpulence. Addressed to the public. John Ebers, London, Harrison, 1863.

Bauman, L.: Obesity: Recent reports in the literature and results of treatment. J.A.M.A., 90:22–24, 1928.

Beck, P., Koumans, J. H., Winterling, C. A., Stein, M. F., Daughaday, W. H. and Kipnis, D. M.: Studies of insulin and growth hormone secretion in human obesity. J. Lab. Clin. Med., 64:654–667, 1964.

Beck, E. C. and Hubbard, R. S.: A study of 63 patients before and after weight reduction. N.Y. State J. Med., 39:1102–1105, 1939.

Benedict, F. G.: A study of prolonged fasting. Washington, D.C., Carnegie Inst., Publ. 203, 1915.

Bennett, I. and Simon, M.: The prudent diet. New York, David White, Inc., 1973.

Benoit, F. L., Martin, R. L. and Watten, R. H.: Changes in body composition during weight reduction in obesity: Balance studies comparing the effect of fasting and a ketogenic diet. Ann. Intern. Med., 63:604–612, 1965.

Berger, H.: Fatal lactic acidosis during "crash" reducing diet. N.Y. State J. Med., 67:2258–2263, 1967.

Berland, T.: Rating the diets. Consumer Guide, 1974.

Bernard, J. L.: Rapid treatment of gross obesity by operant techniques. Psychol. Rep., 23:663–666, 1968.

Blackburn, G. L., Flatt, J. P. and Clowes, G. H., Jr.: Protein-sparing therapy during periods of starvation with sepsis or trauma. Ann. Surg., 177:588–594, 1973.

Blondheim, S. H., Kaufman, N. A. and Stein, M.: Comparison of fasting and 800–1000 calorie diet in obesity. Lancet, 1:250–252, 1965.

Bloom, W. L.: Fasting as an introduction to the treatment of obesity. Metabolism, 8:214–220, 1959.

Boileau, R. A., Buskirk, E. R., Horstman, D. H., Mendez, J. and Nicholas, W. C.: Body composition changes in obese and lean men during physical conditioning. Med. Sci. Sports, 3:183–189, 1971.

Bolinger, R. E., Lukert, B. P., Brown, R. W., Guevera, L. and Steinberg, R.: Metabolic balance of obese patients during fasting. Arch. Intern. Med., 118:3–8, 1966.

Bortz, W. M., Wroldsen, A., Issekutz, B. and Rodahl, K.: Weight loss and frequency of feeding. N. Engl. J. Med., 274:376–379, 1966.

Bortz, W. M.: A 500 pound weight loss. Am. J. Med., 47:325–331, 1969.

Bowser, L. J., Trulson, M. F., Bowling, R. C. and Stare, F. J.: Methods of reducing. Group therapy vs. individual clinic interview. J. Am. Diet. Assoc., 29:1193–1196, 1953.

Braunstein, J. J.: Management of the obese patient. Med. Clin. North Am., 55:391–401, 1971.

Bray, G. A.: Effect of caloric restriction on energy expenditure in obese patients. Lancet, 2:397–398, 1969.

Bray, G. A.: The myth of diet in the management of obesity. Am. J. Clin. Nutr., 23:1141–1148, 1970.

Bray, G. A., Davidson, M. B. and Drenick, E. J.: Obesity: A serious symptom. Ann. Intern. Med., 77:779–795, 1972.

Bray, G. A.: Clinical management of the obese adult. Postgrad. Med., 51:125–130, 1972.

Bray, G. A., Jordan, H. A. and Sims, E. A. H.: Evaluation of the obese patient. J.A.M.A., (in press) 1976a.

Bray, G. A., Atkinson, R. L., Dahms, W., Frey, C., Greenway, F. L., Holbrook, I.,

Marriott, M. and Molitch, M.: Clinical evaluation of the obese patient using an algorithm. J.A.M.A. (in press) 1976b.

Buskirk, E. R., Thompson, R. H., Lutwak, L. and Whedon, G. D.: Energy balance of obese patients during weight reduction: Influence of diet restriction and exercise. Ann. N.Y. Acad. Sci., *110*:918–940, 1963.

Cahill, G. F., Jr., Herrera, M. G., Morgan, A. P., Soeldner, J. S., Steinke, J., Levy, P. L., Reichard, G. A., Jr. and Kipnis, D. M.: Hormone-fuel interrelationships during fasting. J. Clin. Invest., *45*:1751–1769, 1966.

Cahill, G. F., Jr. and Owen, O. E.: Body Fuels and Starvation. *In:* Anorexia and Obesity. (Rowland, C. V., Jr. ed.) International Psychiatry Clinics, Vol. 7, No. 1. Boston, Little, Brown and Co., 1970, pp. 25–36.

Cahill, G. F. Jr.: Starvation in man. N. Engl. J. Med., *282*:668–675, 1970.

Campbell, C. J., Campbell, I. W., Innes, J. A., Munro, J. F. and Needle, A. L.: Further follow-up experience after prolonged therapeutic starvation. *In:* Obesity (Burland, W. L., Samuel, P. and Yudkin, J. eds.) London, Churchill Livingstone, 1974, pp. 281–292.

Cederquist, D. C., Brewer, W. D., Beegle, R. M., Wagoner, A. N., Dunsing, D. and Ohlson, M. A.: Weight reduction on low-fat and low-carbohydrate diets. I. Clinical results and energy metabolism. J. Am. Diet. Assoc., *28*:113–116, 1952.

Chapman, A. L.: An experiment with group conferences for weight reduction. Pub. Health Rep., *68*:439–440, 1953.

Cheifetz, P. N.: Uric acid excretion and ketosis in fasting. Metabolism, *14*:1267–1272, 1965.

Christakis, G.: Community programs for weight reduction: Experience of the Bureau of Nutrition, New York City. Can. J. Public Health, *58*:499–504, 1967.

Cohn, C.: Feeding patterns and some aspects of cholesterol metabolism. Fed. Proc., *23*:76–81, 1964.

Cohn, C., Joseph, D., Bell, L. and Allweiss, M. D.: Studies on the effects of feeding frequency and dietary composition on fat deposition. Ann. N.Y. Acad. Sci., *131*:507–518, 1965.

Collison, D. R.: Total fasting for up to 249 days. Lancet, *1*:112, 1967. (letter)

Craddock, D.: Obesity and its management. Edinburgh and London, E & S Livingstone Ltd., 2nd Ed., 1974.

Crews, E. L., III., Fuge, K. W., Oscai, L. B., Holloszy, J. O. and Shank, R. E.: Weight food intake and body composition: Effects of exercise and protein deficiency. Am. J. Physiol., *216*:359–363, 1969.

Cubberley, P. T., Polster, S. A. and Schulman, C. L.: Lactic acidosis and death after the treatment of obesity by fasting. N. Engl. J. Med., *272*:628–630, 1965.

Cuthbertson, D. P.: The effect of massage on the metabolism of normal individuals. Q. J. Med., *1*:387–400, 1932.

Cutting, W. C.: The treatment of obesity. J. Clin. Endocrinol., *3*:85–88, 1943.

Danowski, T. S. and Winker, A. W.: Obesity as a clinical problem. Am. J. Med. Sci., *208*:622, 1944.

Darling, C. D. and Summerskill, J.: Emotional factors in obesity and weight reduction. J. Am. Diet. Assoc., *29*:1204–1207, 1953.

Debry, G., Rohr, R., Azouaou, R. and Vassilitch, I.: Ponderal losses in obese subjects submitted to restricted diets differing by nibbling and by lipid carbohydrate composition. *In:* Energy Balance in Man. (Apfelbaum, M., ed.) Paris, Masson et Cie, 1973, pp. 305–310.

Dole, V. P., Schwartz, I. L., Thaysen, J. H., Thorn, N. A. and Silver, L.: Treatment of obesity with a low protein calorically unrestricted diet. Am. J. Clin. Nutr., *2*:381–390, 1954.

Drenick, E. J., Fisler, J. L. and Dennin, H. F.: The effect of allopurinol on the hyperuricemia of fasting. Clin. Pharmacol. Ther., *12*:68–72, 1971.

Drenick, E. J., Swendseid, M. E., Blahd, W. H. and Tuttle, S. G.: Prolonged starvation as treatment for severe obesity. J.A.M.A., *187*:100–105, 1964.

Drenick, E. J.: Weight reduction by prolonged fasting. *In:* Obesity in Perspective. Fogarty International Center Series on Preventive Medicine, Vol. II, Part II. (Bray, G. A. ed.) Washington, D.C., U.S. Government Printing Office. 1976.

Duncan, G. G., Jenson, W. K., Fraser, R. I. and Cristofori, F. C.: Correction and control of intractable obesity. J.A.M.A., *181*:309–312, 1962.

Duncan, G. G., Jenson, W. K., Cristofori, F. C. and Schless, G. L.: Intermittent fasts in the correction and control of intractable obesity. Am. J. Med. Sci., 245:515–520, 1963.

Dunlop, D. M. and Lyon, R. M. M.: A study of 523 cases of obesity. Edinburgh, M. J., 38:561–577, 1931.

Dwyer, J. T. and Mayer, J.: Potential dieters: Who are they? Attitudes towards body weight and dieting behavior. J. Am. Diet. Assoc., 56:510–514, 1970.

Dwyer, J. T., Feldman, J. J. and Mayer, J.: The social psychology of dieting. J. Health Soc. Behav., 11:269–287, 1970.

Edholm, O. G., Fletcher, J. G., Widdowson, E. M. and McCance, R. A.: The energy expenditure and food intake of individual men. Br. J. Nutr., 9:286–300, 1955.

Evans, F. A. and Strang, J. M.: A departure from the usual methods of treating obesity. Am. J. Med. Sci., 177:339–348, 1929.

Evans, F. A. and Strang, J. M.: The treatment of obesity with low calorie diets. J.A.M.A., 97:1063–1068, 1931.

Evans, F. A.: Treatment of obesity with low calorie diets: Report of 121 additional cases. Internat. Clin., 3:19–23, 1938.

Fabry, P., Fodor, J., Hejl, Z., Braun, T. and Zvolankova, K.: The frequency of meals: Its relationship to overweight, hypercholesterolemia, and decreased glucose-tolerance. Lancet, 2:614–615, 1964.

Fabry, P.: Food intake pattern and energy balance. In: Energy Balance in Man. (Apfelbaum, M. ed.) Paris, Masson et Cie, pp. 297–303, 1973.

Feinstein, A. R., Dole, V. P. and Schwartz, I. L.: The use of a formula diet for weight reduction of obese out-patients. Ann. Intern. Med., 48:330–343, 1958.

Feinstein, A. R.: The measurement of success in weight reduction: An analysis of methods and a new index. J. Chronic Dis., 10:439–456, 1959.

Feinstein, A. R.: The treatment of obesity. An analysis of methods, results and factors which influence success. J. Chronic Dis., 11:349–393, 1960.

Fellows, H. H.: Studies of relatively normal obese individuals during and after weight reduction. Am. J. Med. Sci., 181:301–312, 1931.

Finkelstein, B. and Fryer, B. A.: Meal frequency and weight reduction in young women. Am. J. Clin. Nutr., 24:465–468, 1971.

Forbes, G. B.: Weight loss during fasting: Implications for the obese. Am. J. Clin. Nutr., 23:1212–1219, 1970.

Foreyt, J. P. and Kennedy, W. A.: Treatment of overweight by aversion therapy. Behav. Res. Ther., 9:29–34, 1971.

Garnett, E. S., Barnard, D. L., Ford, J., Goodbody, R. A. and Woodhouse, M. A.: Gross fragmentation of cardiac myofibrils after therapeutic starvation for obesity. Lancet, 1:914–916, 1969.

Garrow, J. S.: A survey of three slimming and weight control organizations in the U.K. In (Howard, A. ed.) Recent Advances in Obesity Research: I. Proceedings of the First International Congress on Obesity. London, Newman Publishing Ltd., 1975, pp. 301–304.

Genuth, S. M., Castro, J. H. and Vertes, V.: Weight reduction in obesity by outpatient semistarvation. J.A.M.A., 230:987–992, 1974.

Glennon, J. A.: Weight reduction—An enigma. Arch. Intern. Med., 118:1–2, 1966.

Glucksman, M. L. and Hirsch, J.: The response of obese patients to weight reduction. 3. The perception of body size. Psychosomat. Med., 31:1–7, 1969.

Goodman, J. I., Schwartz, E. D. and Frankel, L.: Group therapy of obese diabetic patients. Diabetes, 2:280, 1953.

Gordon, T. and Kannel, W. B.: The effects of overweight on cardiovascular diseases. Geriatrics, 28:80–88, 1973.

Green, M. B. and Beckman, M.: Obesity and its management. A survey of 671 patients. Med. Rec., 160:223–228, 1947.

Grinker, J.: Behavioral and metabolic consequences of weight reduction. J. Am. Diet. Assoc., 62:30–34, 1973.

Grinker, J., Hirsch, J. and Levin, B.: The afffective responses of obese patients to weight reduction: A differentiation based on age at onset of obesity. Psychosom. Med., 35:57–63, 1973b.

Grinker, J., Glucksman, M. L., Hirsch, J. and Viseltear, G.: Time perception as a function of weight reduction: A differentiation based on age at onset of obesity. Psychosom. Med., 35:104–111, 1973a.

Gwinup, G., Byron, R. C., Roush, W. H., Kruger, F. A. and Hamwi, G. J.: Effect of nibbling versus gorging on glucose tolerance. Lancet, 2:165–167, 1963a.

Gwinup, G. R., Byron, R. C., Roush, W. H., Kruger, F. A. and Hamwi, G. J.: Effect of nibbling versus gorging on serum lipids in man. Am. J. Clin. Nutr., 13:209–213, 1963b.

Harris, M. B., and Bruner, C. G.: A comparison of a self-control and a contract procedure for weight control. Behav. Res. Ther., 9:347–354, 1971.

Harrison, R. and Harden, R. M.: The long term value of fasting in the treatment of obesity. Lancet, 2:1340–1342, 1966.

Harrop, G. A.: A milk and banana diet for the treatment of obesity. J.A.M.A., 102:2003–2005, 1934.

Harvey, H. I. and Simmons, W. D.: Weight reduction: A study of the group method. Report of Progress. Am. J. Med. Sci., 227:521–525, 1954.

Hermann, L. S. and Iverson, M.: Death during therapeutic starvation. Lancet, 2:217, 1968.

Hollifield, G., Owen, J. A., Jr., Lindsay, R. W. and Parson, W.: Effects of prolonged fasting on subsequent food intake in obese humans. South. Med. J., 57:1012–1016, 1964.

Hood, C. E. A., Goodhart, J. M., Fletcher, R. F.: Observations on obese patients eating isocaloric reducing diets with varying proportions of carbohydrate. Br. J. Nutr., 24:39–44, 1970.

Howard, A. N.: Dietary treatment of obesity. In: Obesity: Medical and Scientific Aspects. (McLean-Baird, I., and Howard, A. N., eds.) Edinburgh, E. and S. Livingston Ltd., 1969, pp. 96–111.

Huenemann, R. L.: Food habits of obese and non-obese adolescents. Postgrad. Med., 51:99–105, 1972.

Hunscher, M. A.: A posthospitalization study of patients treated for obesity by a total fast regimen. Metabolism, 15:383–393, 1966.

Irwin, I. M. and Feeley, R. M.: Frequency and size of meals and serum lipids, nitrogen and mineral retention, fat digestibility and urinary thiamine and riboflavin in young women. Am. J. Clin. Nutr., 20:816–824, 1967.

Jagannathan, S. N., Connell, W. F. and Beveridge, J. M. R.: Effects of gourmandizing and semicontinuous eating of equicaloric amounts of formula-type high fat diets on plasma cholesterol and triglyceride levels in human volunteer subjects. Am. J. Clin. Nutr., 15:90–94, 1964.

Jenkins, B. W.: Group therapy for obesity—without the group. G.P., 14:110–112, 1956.

Jolliffe, N. and Alpert, E.: The "performance index" as a method for estimating the effectiveness of reducing regimens. Postgrad. Med., 9:106–115, 1957.

Jolliffe, N.: Reduce and stay reduced on the prudent diet. New York, Simon and Schuster, 1963.

Jordan, H. A. and Levitz, L. S.: Behavior modification in a self-help group. J. Am. Diet. Assoc., 62:27–29, 1973.

Jordan, H. A. and Levitz, L. S.: A behavioral approach to the problem of obesity. Obesity and Bariatric Med., 4:58–69, 1975.

Kalb, S. W.: The fallacy of massage in the treatment of obesity. J. Med. Soc. N.J., 41:406—407, 1944.

Kalb, S. W.: A review of group therapy in weight reduction. Am. J. Gastroenterol., 26:75–80, 1956.

Keeton, R. W. and Bone, D. D.: Diets low in calories containing varying amounts of fat, their effect on loss in weight and on the metabolic rate in obese patients. Arch. Intern. Med., 55:262–270, 1935.

Kekwick, A. and Pawan, G. L. S.: Calorie intake in relation to body-weight changes in the obese. Lancet, 2:155–161, 1956.

Kenrick, M. M., Ball, M. F, and Canary, J. J.: Exercise and weight reduction in obesity. Arch. Phys. Med. Rehabil., 53:323–327, 1972.

Keys, A., Anderson, J. T. and Brozek, J.: The biology of human starvation. Minneapolis, University of Minnesota Press, 1950, p. 1385.

Kinsell, L. W., Gunning, B., Michaels, G. D., Richardson, J., Cox, S. E. and Lemon, C.: Calories do count. Metabolism, 13:195–204, 1964.

Kollar, E. J. and Atkinson, R. M.: Responses of extremely obese patients to starvation. Psychosom. Med., 28:227–245, 1966.

Konishi, F.: Food energy equivalents of various activities. J. Am. Diet. Assoc., 46:186–188, 1965.

Kotkov, B.: Experiences in group psychotherapy with the obese. Psychosom. Med., 15:243–251, 1953.

Kurlander, A. B.: Group therapy in reducing. J. Am. Diet. Assoc., 29:337–339, 1953.

Leverton, R. M. and Gram, M. R.: Further studies of obese young women during weight reduction: Calcium, phosphorus, and nitrogen metabolism. J. Am. Diet. Assoc., 27:480–484, 1951.

Levitz, L. S.: Behavior therapy in treating obesity. J. Am. Diet. Assoc., 62:22–26, 1973.

Ley, P., Bradshaw, P. W., Kincey, J. A., Couper-Smartt, J. and Wilson, M.: Psychological variables in the control of obesity. In: Obesity Symposium (Burland, W. L., Samuel, P. D. and Yudkin, J. eds.) Edinburgh, Churchill Livingstone, 1974, pp. 316–337.

Lloyd-Mostyn, R. H., Lord, P. S. and Glover, R.: Uric acid metabolism in starvation. Ann. Rheum. Dis., 29:553–555, 1970.

Lyon, D. M. and Dunlop, D. M.: The treatment of obesity. A comparison of the effects of diet and of thyroid extract. Quart. J. Med., 1:331–352, 1932.

Maage, H. and Mogensen, E. F.: Effect of treatment on obesity: A follow-up of material treated with complete starvation. Dan. Med. Bull., 17:206–209, 1970.

Maccuish, A. C., Munro, J. F. and Duncan, L. J. P.: Follow-up study of refractory obesity treated by fasting. Br. Med. J., 1:91–92, 1968.

Marliss, E. B., Aoki, T. T., Unger, R. H., Soeldner, J. S. and Cahill, G. F., Jr.: Glucagon levels and metabolic effects in fasting man. J. Clin. Invest., 49:2256–2270, 1970.

Mayer, J. and Stare, F. J.: Exercise and weight control; frequent misconceptions. J. Am. Diet. Assoc., 29:340–343, 1953.

Meyer, V. and Crisp, A. H.: Aversion therapy in two cases of obesity. Behav. Res. Ther., 2:143–147, 1964.

Moody, D. L., Kollias, J. and Buskirk, E. R.: The effect of a moderate exercise program on body weight and skinfold thickness in overweight college women. Med. Sci. Sports, 1:75–80, 1969.

Moody, D. L., Wilmore, J. H., Girandola, R. N. and Reyce, J. P.: The effects of a jogging program on the body composition of normal and obese high school girls. Med. Sci. Sports, 4:210–213, 1972.

Munves, E. D.: Dietetic interview or group discussion-decision in reducing. J. Am. Diet. Assoc., 29:1197–1203, 1953.

Nidetch, J.: The story of Weight Watchers. New York, W/W Twentyfirst Corporation, 1970.

Olesen, E. S. and Quaade, F.: Fatty foods and obesity. Lancet, 1:1048–1051, 1960.

Owen, O. E., Morgan, A. P., Kemp, H. G., Sullivan, J. M., Herrera, M. G. and Cahill, G. F., Jr.: Brain metabolism during fasting. J. Clin. Invest., 46:1589–1595, 1967.

Passmore, R., Strong, J. A. and Ritchie, F. J.: Water and electrolyte analysis of obese patients on a reducing regimen. Br. J. Nutr., 13:17–25, 1959.

Passmore, R., Strong, J. A. and Ritchie, F. J.: The chemical composition of the tissue lost by obese patients on a reducing regimen. Br. J. Nutr., 12:113–122, 1958.

Pearson, D.: The chemical analysis of food. 6th Ed. London, Churchill, 1970, p. 16.

Penick, S. B., Filion, R., Fox, S. and Stunkard, A. J.: Behavior modification in the treatment of obesity. Psychosom. Med., 33:49–55, 1971.

Pennington, A. W.: Use of fat in weight-reducing diet. Del. Med. J., 23:79–86, 1951.

Pennington, A. W.: An alternate approach to the problem of obesity. Am. J. Clin. Nutr., 1:100–106, 1953.

Pilkington, T. R. E., Gainsborough, H., Rosenoer, V. M. and Carey, M.: Diet and weight reduction in the obese. Lancet, 1:856–858, 1960.

Robinson, S. and Winnik, H. Z.: Severe psychotic disturbances following crash diet weight loss. Arch. Gen. Psychiatry, 29:559–562, 1973.

Rooth, G. and Carlstrom, S.: Therapeutic fasting. Acta Med. Scand., 187:455–463, 1970.

Rowland, C. V., Jr.: Psychotherapy of six hyperobese adults during total starvation. Arch. Gen. Psychiatry, 18:541–548, 1968.

Runcie, J. and Thomson, T. J.: Prolonged starvation: A dangerous procedure? Br. Med. J., 3:432–435, 1970.

Russell, G. F. M.: The effect of diets of different composition on weight loss and sodium balance in obese patients. Clin. Sci., 22:269–277, 1962.

Rynearson, E. H. and Gastineau, C. P.: Obesity. Springfield, Illinois. Charles C Thomas, 1949.

Schachter, S. and Rodin, J.: Obese humans and rats. Washington: Erlbaum/Halsted, 1974.

Seaton, D. A. and Rose, K.: Defaulters from a weight reduction clinic. J. Chronic Dis., 18:1007–1011, 1965.

Shipman, W. G. and Plesset, M. R.: Anxiety and depression in obese dieters. Arch. Gen. Psychiatry, 8:530–535, 1963a.

Shipman, W. G. and Plesset, M. R.: Predicting the outcome for obese dieters. J. Am. Diet. Assoc., 42:383–386, 1963b.

Short, J. J. and Carnegie, J. D.: An attempt to mobilize lipoids from storage depots by deep massage and increased tissue temperatures. J. Lab. Clin. Med., 24:395–397, 1939.

Silverstone, J. T. and Lascelles, B. D.: Dieting and depression. Br. J. Psychiatry, 112:513–519, 1966.

Silverstone, J. T., Stark, J. E. and Buckle, R. M.: Hunger during total starvation. Lancet, 1:1343–1344, 1666.

Simmons, W. D.: The group approach to weight reduction. I. A review of the project. J. Am. Diet. Assoc., 30:437–441, 1954.

Smith, R. and Drenick, E. J.: Changes in body water and sodium during prolonged starvation for extreme obesity. Clin. Sci., 31:437–447, 1966.

Sohar, E.: A forty day 550 calorie diet in the treatment of obese outpatients. Am. J. Clin. Nutr., 7:514–518, 1959.

Sohar, E. and Sneh, E.: Follow-up of obese patients: 14 years after a successful reducing diet. Am. J. Clin. Nutr., 26:845–848, 1973.

Spencer, I. O. B.: Death during therapeutic starvation for obesity. Lancet, 1:1288–1290, 1968.

Stewart, W. K. and Fleming, L. W.: Features of a successful therapeutic fast of 382 days' duration. Postgrad. Med. J., 49:203–209, 1973.

Stock, A. L. and Yudkin, J.: Nutrient intake of subjects on low carbohydrate diet used in treatment of obesity. Am. J. Clin. Nutr., 23:948–952, 1970.

Strang, J. M., McClugage, H. B. and Evans, F. A.: Further studies in the dietary correction of obesity. Am. J. Med. Sci., 179:687–694, 1930.

Strang, J. M., McClugage, H. B. and Evans, F. A.: The nitrogen balance during dietary correction of obesity. Am. J. Med. Sci., 181:336–349, 1931.

Strong, J. A., Passmore, R. and Ritchie, F. J.: Clinical observations on obese patients during a strict reducing regimen. Br. J. Nutr., 12:105–112, 1958.

Stuart, R. B.: Behavioral control overeating. Behav. Res. Ther., 5:357–365, 1967.

Stuart, R. B.: A three dimensional program for the treatment of obesity. Behav. Res. Ther., 9:177–186, 1971.

Stuart, R. B. and Davis, B.: Slim chance in a fat world: Behavioral control of obesity. Champaign, Illinois, Research Press Co., 1972.

Stuart, R. B.: Behavioral control of overeating: A status report. In: Obesity in Perspective. Fogarty International Center Series on Preventive Medicine, Vol. II, Part II. (Bray, G. A. ed.) Washington, D.C., U.S. Government Printing Office. 1976.

Stunkard, A. J.: Dieting-depression: Incidence and clinical characteristics of untoward responses to weight reduction regimens. Am. J. Med., 23:77–86, 1957.

Stunkard, A. J. and McLaren-Hume, M.: The results of treatment for obesity. Arch. Intern. Med., 103:79–85, 1959.

Stunkard, A. J. and Mendelsen, M.: Obesity and the body image. I. Characteristics of disturbances in the body image of some obese persons. Am. J. Psychiatr., 123:1296–1300, 1967.

Stunkard, A. J.: The success of TOPS: A self-help group. Postgrad. Med., 51:143–147, 1972.

Stunkard, A. J.: Studies on TOPS: A self-help group for obesity. In: Obesity in Perspective. Fogarty International Center Series on Preventive Medicine, Vol. II, Part II. (Bray, G. A. ed.) Washington, D.C., U.S. Government Printing Office. 1976.

Stunkard, A. J.: New therapies for the eating disorders: Behavior modification of obesity and anorexia nervosa. Arch. Gen. Psychiatry, 26:391–398, 1972b.

Stunkard, A. J. and Rush, J.: Dieting and depression reexamined. A critical review of reports of untoward responses during weight reduction for obesity. Ann. Intern. Med., 81:526–533, 1974.

Swanson, D. W. and Dinello, F. A.: Follow-up of patients starved for obesity. Psychosom. Med., 32:209–214, 1970.

Swindells, Y. E., Holmes, S. A. and Robinson, M. F.: The metabolic responses of young women to changes in the frequency of meals. Br. J. Nutr. 22:667–680, 1968.

Thomson, T. J., Runcie, J. and Miller, V.: Treatment of obesity by total fasting up to 249 days. Lancet, 2:992–996, 1966.

Trulson, J., Walsh, E. D. and Caso, E. K.: A study of obese patients in a nutrition clinic. J. Am. Diet. Assoc., 23:941–946, 1947.

Trulson, M. F.: Assessment of dietary study methods. I. Comparison of methods for obtaining data for clinical work. J. Am. Diet. Assoc., 30:991–995, 1954.

Tullis, I. F.: Rational diet for mild and grand obesity. J. Am. Med. Assoc., 226:70–73, 1973.

Watt, B. K. and Merrill, A. L.: Composition of foods. Agriculture Handbook No. 8. Agriculture Research Service, United States Department of Agriculture, 1963.

Weisenberg, M. and Fray, E.: What's missing in the treatment of obesity by behavior modification? J. Am. Diet. Assoc., 64:410–414, 1974.

Werner, S. C.: Comparison between weight reduction on a high-calorie, high-fat diet and on an isocaloric regimen high in carbohydrate. N. Engl. J. Med., 252:661–665, 1955.

Winkelstein, L. B.: Hypnosis, diet and weight reduction. N.Y. State J. Med., 59:1751–1756, 1959.

Worthington, B. S. and Taylor, L. E.: Balanced low-calorie vs. low-protein-low-carbohydrate reducing diets. II. Biochemical changes. J. Am. Diet. Assoc., 64:52–55, 1974a.

Worthington, B. S. and Taylor, L. E.: Balanced low-calorie vs. high-protein-low-carbohydrate reducing diets. 1. Weight loss, nutrient intake, and subjective evaluation. J. Am. Diet. Assoc., 64:47–51, 1974b.

Wunderlich, R. A., Kenrick, M., Pearce, M., Lozes, J. and Ball, M. F.: Psychologic considerations in physical therapy for obese patients. Phys. Ther., 53:757–761, 1973.

Wyden, P.: The overweight Society: An authoritative entertaining investigation into the facts and follies of girth control. New York, William Morrow and Company, 1965.

Young, C. M., Moore, N. S., Berresford, K. K. and Einset, B. M.: What can be done for the obese patient? A report of a study in an experimental clinic. Am. Pract. Digest Treat., 6:685–695, 1955.

Young, C. M., Empey, E. L., Serraon, V. U. and Pierce, Z. H.: Weight reduction in obese young men. Metabolic studies. J. Nutr., 61:437–456, 1957.

Young, C. M., Scanlan, S. S., Im, H. S., and Lutwak, L.: Effect on body composition and other parameters in obese young men of carbohydrate level of reduction diet. Am. J. Clin. Nutr., 24:290–296, 1971a.

Young, C. M., Scanlan, S. S., Topping, C. M., Simko, V. and Lutwak, L.: Frequency of feeding, weight reduction and body composition. J. Am. Diet. Assoc., 59:466–472, 1971b.

Young, C. M., Hutter, L. F., Scanlan, S. S., and Rand, C. E., Lutwak, L. and Simko, V.: Metabolic effects of meal frequency on normal young men. J. Am. Diet. Assoc., 61:391–398, 1972.

Yudkin, J. and Carey, M.: The treatment of obesity by the "high fat" diet. The inevitability of calories. Lancet, 2:939–941, 1960.

CHAPTER 9

DRUG THERAPY FOR THE OBESE PATIENT

The frustration confronting many obese patients in their quest for a lean body is evident from the low success rate of most nutritional clinics which treat obesity (see Chapter 8). This frustration has prompted the search for other methods of treatment. Among these methods are various drugs which are reviewed in this chapter, and the surgical approaches which are reviewed in Chapter 10.

Pharmacologic agents can facilitate the process of "reducing." Since there are hazards associated with being 20 to 30 percent overweight (Chapter 6), any pharmacologic agent which is to be used in treating such patients must have very little risk. The ideal agent for this purpose ought to be free of long and short term toxicity, be well tolerated, allow titration of body weight to a desired level, have no deleterious metabolic effects and be inexpensive. Obviously no agent currently available meets these criteria. In this chapter we will examine some of the agents which are now in use as adjuncts for the treatment of the obese patient. We will also discuss some of the drugs which have been considered for this purpose but have been abandoned, and some newer approaches which might be fruitful in the future.

CLASSIFICATION OF PHARMACOLOGIC AGENTS

The drugs which have been used to treat obesity fall into several categories. The first group are the drugs which suppress the appetite. Dextroamphetamine was the first member of this group, which now numbers an even dozen. The potential for habituation and drug abuse by the parent compound has led to a controversy both inside and outside of the medical profession as to the relative value of any of the drugs in this group. It is this author's view that some of the agents do indeed have a useful place in the treatment of some overweight patients.

The second group of drugs that we will examine are the thyroid hormones. Although even more ancient as a treatment for obesity than the appetite-suppressing drugs, the use of thyroid is also controversial. The original justification for its use was the observation that many obese patients were "hypometabolic" as measured by their basal metabolism rate, and that they were probably hypothyroid. As we have learned more about the function of the thyroid gland in obesity and have acquired ever more sophisticated tests, we know that this original premise is usually not true. Therefore, the rationale for use of thyroid hormones in obesity is unclear, and their place in the armamentarium of the physician treating obesity must be re-examined.

The remaining group of agents are on even less secure ground. Human chorionic gonadotropin is currently in wide use in clinics which specialize in treating obesity, but whether this preparation itself has any intrinsic effect on weight loss is uncertain. Other hormones, however, such as glucagon and growth hormones can clearly modify food intake or metabolic rate and possess theoretical potential in treating obesity. The drugs which modify intestinal absorption have received little use although one of them, cholestyramine, has been tried. This field may be one of great potential in the future. Dinitrophenol and digitalis have no place in the therapy of obesity.

It is clear from this brief summary that the potential and actual usefulness of the various agents to be discussed below is highly variable. The concept of a pharmacologic adjunct for use in treating the overweight patient remains an important avenue to improving our ability to deal with this problem as it affects the national health.

APPETITE SUPPRESSING OR ANOREXIGENIC DRUGS

Historical Background

The anorexigenic drugs are in most instances derivatives of phenethylamine. They possess many of the pharmacologic properties of the naturally occurring adrenergic hormones epinephrine and norepinephrine.

Amphetamine was first synthesized in 1887 by Edeleano. It was not until 1927, however, that Alles described the psychopharmacologic properties of amphetamine. These included: decreased fatigue, wakefulness, alertness, euphoria and increased energy. In 1937 during clinical tests of amphetamine as a treatment for depression and narcolepsy, three separate groups of scientists observed al-

most simultaneously that patients receiving this drug lost weight
(Nathanson, 1937; Ulrich, 1937). It was less than a year later that
Lesses and Myerson (1938) demonstrated that this drug could be used
for treatment of obesity (Ersner, 1940; Kalb, 1942a). In subsequent
clinical trials this agent was shown to be effective in decreasing
weight in adults as well as in children.

The physiological basis for this effect, however, was unclear until
Harris et al. (1947) demonstrated that the major action was to decrease
food intake. They performed two series of studies: one with dogs and
the other with human subjects. For the canine experiments, 8 dogs
were trained to eat their entire daily food intake in a 45 minute period.
The quantity of the food eaten in this period was carefully weighed
each day. The animals were treated with doses of amphetamine ranging from 2.5 to 20 milligrams. When 10 or 20 mg were given one hour
before meal time, food intake was practically abolished. When the
drug was given over a period of two weeks, these animals lost up to 26
percent of their initial body weight. When injections of saline were
given instead of amphetamine, however, food intake was not impaired.

Two studies were carried out with human subjects. In the first
experiment, 7 obese and 2 nonobese individuals ate as much as they
wanted during three meals each day and the actual intake was recorded. This procedure was continued over two 8 week periods separated by a 4 week vacation. During one of these periods they received
amphetamine, and during the other a placebo. Two conclusions were
apparent from these studies: first, the obese subjects, when allowed to
eat all of the food they wanted, actually lost weight. Part of this may
have been due to the fact that they did not eat between meals. Second,
the administration of d,l-amphetamine sulfate, 10 milligrams, before
each meal decreased the intake of food and increased the rate of
weight loss. The placebo capsules given during half of each of the
treatment periods had no effect on the average weight loss.

In the final study, amphetamine was administered to subjects who
ate the same quantity of food whether or not they took the drug. Under
these circumstances, amphetamine had no effect on body weight, indicating that the primary action of the drug was to decrease food intake and not to increase combustion of calories (i.e., energy expenditure did not increase). Following the introduction of this drug into
clinical practice (Albrecht, 1944), a number of additional agents have
been developed in an effort to modify the unwanted stimulation of the
central nervous system observed with amphetamines.

Chemical Structure

Table 9–1 shows the chemical structure of the adrenergic trans-
mitters (dopamine, norepinephrine and epinephrine) and the cur-

TABLE 9–1. *Catecholamines and Related Anorectic Drugs*

COMPOUND	TRADE NAME	STRUCTURE					
		R_1	R_2	R_3	β	α	R_4
Dopamine		OH	OH	H	H	H	H
Norepinephrine	Levophed	OH	OH	H	OH	—H	H
Epinephrine	Adrenalin	OH	OH	H	OH	—H	CH₃
d,l-Amphetamine	Benzedrine	H	H	H	H	—CH₃	H
d-Amphetamine	Dexedrine	H	H	H	H	—CH₃	H
Methamphetamine	Desoxyn	H	H	H	H	—CH₃	CH₃
Phenmetrazine	Preludin	H	H	H	(see structure)		
Phendimetrazine	Plegine	H	H	H	(see structure)		
Benzphetamine	Didrex	H	H	H	H	CH₃	—CH₃ / —CH₂ φ
Phentermine resin	Ionamin	H	H	H	H	(CH₃)₂	H
Chlorphentermine	Presate	Cl	H	H	H	(CH₃)₂	H
Clortermine hydrochloride	Voranil	H	H	Cl	H	(CH₃)₂	H
Mazindol	Sanorex	Cl	H	H	—OH	see structure p. 379	
Diethylpropion	Tenuate	H	H	H	=O	CH₃	(C₂H₅)₂
Fenfluramine hydrochloride	Pondimin	H	CH₃	H	H	CH₃	C₂H₅
Phenylpropanolamine	Propadrine	H	H	H	OH	CH₃	H

Phenethylamine base structure:

$$R_1 \text{—(ring with } R_2, R_3 \text{)—CH}_\beta\text{—CH}_\alpha\text{—NH—}R_4$$

Phenmetrazine: ring–CH₂–O–CH₂–CH₂–N (morpholine ring)

Phendimetrazine: ring–CH(CH₃)–O–CH(CH₃)–CH–N—CH₃

rently available appetite suppressing drugs. All members of this group contain a phenyl ring and a side chain. In all but mazindol there are two carbons between the phenyl group and the aminonitrogen. Four types of chemical modification have been useful in dissociating the cardiovascular effects and the effects of these drugs on the excitability of the central nervous system from their effects as appetite suppressants.

1. *Hydroxylation of the side chain.* The addition of a keto group onto the beta carbon (as in diethylpropion) decreases stimulatory effects on the central nervous system more than it reduces the anorectic properties.

2. *Substitution of the alpha carbon.* The addition of a methyl group on the alpha carbon of the phenethylamine nucleus serves to protect the compound from oxidation by monamine oxidase. Chemical substitution in this position is also responsible for the high affinity of amphetamine for the membranes of the central nervous system and for its ability to decrease the uptake or norepinephrine by these neurons.

3. *N-terminal substitutions.* The introduction of methyl, ethyl or benzyl groups on the amino group serves to reduce the central stimulatory effects of the phenethylamine nucleus without destroying the appetite suppressing properties. Cyclization of the amphetamine side chain as exists in phenmetrazine, phendimetrazine and aminoxaphen preserves anorectic properties but diminishes the cardiovascular and stimulatory effects on the central nervous system.

4. *Substitution on the phenyl ring.* Modification on the phenyl ring can completely abolish or significantly enhance the effects of phenethylamine. Substitution of a hydroxyl or methoxy group on the phenyl ring markedly reduces the anorexigenic activity of the compound. Introduction of an electro-negative group such as $Cl-$ or CF_3- markedly decreases the central nervous system stimulatory effects of these compounds, but only moderately reduces the anorectic properties.

Further chemical modification of these structures will produce many interesting compounds. For more details the reader should consult recent reviews (Biel, 1970; Beckett and Brookes 1970; Beregi et al., 1970; Heil and Ross, 1975).

Mechanism of Action

Our recent knowledge of the formation, release and action of central noradrenergic mechanisms is depicted in Fig. 9–1 (Anden, 1970; Carlsson, 1970). This figure is a schematic representation of the terminal axon and receptor neuron of the central adrenergic nervous system. Within the axon tyrosine is converted to dihydroxyphenylalanine dopa by the addition of a hydroxyl to the phenyl ring. Tyrosine hydroxylase, the enzyme which performs this transformation, limits the rate at which this process can occur. In the presence of the enzyme dopa decarboxylase, dopa is converted to dopamine,

TYR – Tyrosine NE – Norepinephrine
DOPA– Dihydroxyphenylalanine ATP– Adenosinetriphosphate
DA Dopamine MAO– Monoamine Oxidase

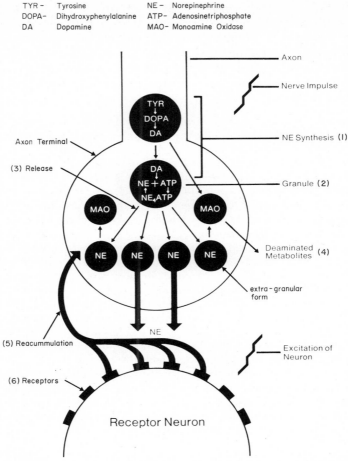

Figure 9–1. Synaptic junction. The adrenergic nerve ending is adjacent to its receptor neuron. (1) Represents the sites of norepinephrine synthesis from tyrosine; (2) represents the storage granule in which the active catecholamines are stored; (3) shows the intracellular release of catecholamines; (4) is the mitochondrial focus of monoamine oxidase which destroys excess intracellular catecholamines; (5) and (6) shows the site of reaccumulation of catecholamines by the neuron and the sites of action on the receptor neuron. (Reprinted from the Sandoz Manual on Sanorex, 1974, with permission.)

which can be stored in the granule. Dopamine may also be converted to norepinephrine by dopamine hydroxylase.

The dense storage granule in which dopamine and norepinephrine are stored is located primarily in the nerve ending. The active neurotransmitters are released in small amounts into the nerve ending from the storage granules. This extragranular norepinephrine may be oxidized by monoamine oxidase, reaccumulated by the storage granule or released into the interneuronal space. Once released from the nerve ending the norepinephrine can either act on receptors, be o-methylated by an enzyme called catechol-o-methyltransferase (COMT), or be reaccumulated into the cytoplasm of the neuronal axon.

A drug such as amphetamine might interfere with this process in a number of ways. It might reduce synthesis of norepinephrine, modify storage or enhance release of norepinephrine from the granule. The metabolism within the terminal axon might be accelerated, or the release and reaccumulation of norepinephrine into the receptor neuron might be blocked. More than 30 years ago it was proposed that amphetamine might act by inhibiting monoamine oxidase, an enzyme which is located in the mitochondria of the axonal ending and which destroys norepinephrine. This concept was undermined, however, when potent inhibitors of monamine oxidase were found which did not decrease food intake. In spite of these negative studies, the concept that amphetamines acted on the central nervous system led to further studies on the effect of this drug on the formation, release and action of norepinephrine in the central nervous system.

AMPHETAMINES

Our understanding of the mechanism of the action of amphetamines has been aided by improved neuropharmacologic techniques which have made it possible to separate the effects of high and low doses of this drug (Table 9–2). Amphetamines produce both immediate and long term effects. The immediate effects include: hyperthermia, increased motor activity and loss of appetite. With con-

TABLE 9–2. *Comparison of Low and High Doses of d-Amphetamine on Brain Metabolism in Rats**

METABOLIC FACTOR	LOW DOSE (5 mg/kg)	HIGH DOSE (20 mg/kg)
Accumulation ^{3}H-Norepinephrine by brain	Unaffected	Inhibited
Metabolites in brain	Unchanged	↑ Methylation ↑ Normetanephrine ↓ Deamination
Enzymatic activity of monoamine oxidase	None	Inhibited
Norepinephrine content in brain	Unchanged	↓ 25–30%
Turnover of ^{3}H-Norepinephrine	↑	↑

*Adapted from Glowinski, J.: *In* Amphetamines and Related Compounds, (E. Costa and S. Garattini, eds.), New York, Raven Press, 1970.

tinued treatment at high dose levels, there is a gradual depletion of norepinephrine in both heart and brain, but low doses do not deplete brain norepinephrine. The accumulation of radioactive norepinephrine by the brain tissue following its injection into the intraventricular system of the central nervous system is inhibited by high doses of amphetamine, but not by low doses (Glowinski, 1970).

Similarly the metabolites formed within the brains of rats treated with high doses of amphetamine are different from those of rats receiving low doses. Deamination is decreased and methylation is increased (Table 9–2). This suggests that amphetamine is inhibiting monamine oxidase (MAO) to cause the decrease in deamination and that the increased quantity of methylated metabolites results from increased release of norepinephrine. In contrast, low doses of amphetamine do not affect the metabolites of norepinephrine in the brain. The release of norepinephrine from the storage granules is more rapid from the brains of rats treated with low doses of amphetamine. With high doses there is no change in the turnover of norepinephrine. Since both high and low doses of amphetamines produce the same characteristic alterations in behavior, one must conclude that the mechanism involved in the central activity of amphetamine does not involve the inhibition of monamine oxidase or the depletion of norepinephrine.

There is also convincing evidence that amphetamines do not act directly on the axonal receptors. This can be demonstrated in experiments where norepinephrine synthesis is totally blocked by administering alpha-methyltyrosine, a blocker of tyrosine-hydroxylase. This drug prevents the conversion of tyrosine to dopa and thus prevents the synthesis of dopamine and norepinephrine. In animals simultaneously treated with reserpine and alpha-methyltyrosine, the storage granules can be totally depleted of norepinephrine and further synthesis of norepinephrine is inhibited. When these animals are then treated with amphetamines, the drug produces no central effects. This implies that at least some norepinephrine must be present for the action of amphetamine, and that amphetamine does not act directly to inhibit the receptors at which norepinephrine act (Fig. 9–2). Amphetamine may also have a weak inhibitory effect of the reaccumulation of norepinephrine by the nerve membrane, but this seems to be a relatively minor component of its action.

The present data are most easily interpreted in the following way (Fig. 9–2): The primary action of amphetamines is to increase the release from the neuron of the small store of norepinephrine, which is located outside of the major storage granules. The increased release of norepinephrine increases the effective concentration of this compound at the receptor neuron. Other possible sites of action do not appear to be of importance for the primary action of this drug.

In summary, amphetamine in high doses can release and deplete

TYR— Tyrosine
DOPA— Dihydroxyphenylalanine
DA— Dopamine

NE— Norepinephrine
ATP— Adenosinetriphosphate
MOA— Monoamine Oxidase

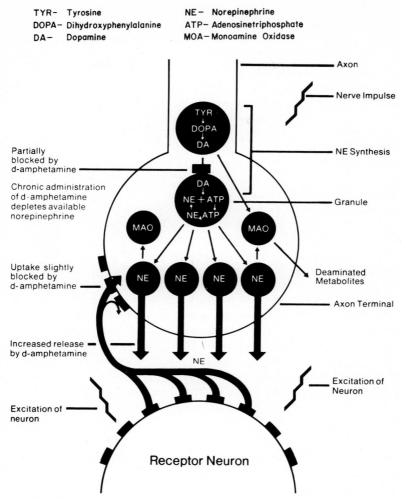

Figure 9–2. The site of action of amphetamine at the synaptic junction. Amphetamine acts by enhancing the release of norenephrine from the axon and by slightly reducing its reaccumulation. (Reprinted from the Sandoz Manual on Sanorex, 1974, with permission.)

brain norepinephrine and alter the storage and metabolism of this drug. In low doses, however, it increases the turnover of dopamine and norepinephrine and facilitates their release from the extragranular sites. The anorexia produced by amphetamine can be inhibited by complete blockade of norepinephrine synthesis, or by pretreatment with p-cholorphenylalanine or cyproheptadine. The anorexia induced by amphetamine is enhanced by desmethylimipramine, a drug which blocks the reuptake of norepinehrine by the nerve ending.

MAZINDOL

The basic mechanism for the action of mazindol differs significantly from the one described for amphetamine. The major evidence for this point of view comes from two kinds of experiments. First, the effects of mazindol on metabolism of catecholamines in the central nervous system differ from those of amphetamine. Mazindol increases the availability of norepinephrine at the axonal receptor sites largely by inhibiting the reaccumulation of norepinephrine by the axonal membrane (step 5, Fig. 9–1). In this respect it differs significantly from the action of amphetamine. Second, mazindol has an additional effect on rats with an instinct for killing mice; an effect which amphetamine does not have.

Mazindol abolished the mouse killing behavior of these rats. However, after destroying the septal region of the brain with electrolytic lesions, the dose of mazindol required to reduce the mouse killing behavior of killer rats was greater than 25 mg/kg, while there was no change in the dose required for methamphetamine or chlorphentermine. This strongly suggests that mazindol has an important action on the septal region of the brain. Further support for an action of mazindol on the septal region was provided by experiments in which changes in the evoked potentials in the hypothalamus were recorded following stimulation in the septum pellucidum. Norepinephrine potentiates the positive wave form elicited in the hypothalamus by stimulation of the septum, whereas mazindol appears to abolish these effects mediated through the septum. In summary, the differences between the mechanism of action of mazindol and amphetamine provide additional tools for exploring hypothalamic control of food intake.

FENFLURAMINE

Studies on fenfluramine also suggest a mechanism of action which differs from that of amphetamine. A number of these differences have been summarized in Table 9–3 (Bizzi et al., 1970; Garattini et al., 1974, 1975). Fenfluramine reduces the brain concentration of serotonin and its metabolite, 5-hydroxy-indolacetic acid, but has little or no effect on the concentration of norepinephrine or dopamine. As seen in Table 9–3, the action of fenfluramine is inhibited by drugs which antagonize the action of dopamine and serotonin. The action of amphetamine, on the other hand, is not affected by such antagonists. The high concentration of hydroxyvanillic acid found in the brain after treatment with either drug indicates increased dopamine metabolism. Amphetamine is thought to produce this effect by directly releasing dopamine. Fenfluramine, on the other hand, may block the action of

TABLE 9–3. *Comparison of the Action of d-Amphetamine and Fenfluramine* *

	D-AMPHETAMINE	FENFLURAMINE
Brain		
Norepinephrine	↓	→
Serotonin	→	↓
5-hydroxy-indoleacetic acid	→	↓
Dopamine	→	→
Hydroxyvanillic acid	↑	↑
Acetylcholine	↑	↑
Antagonists of dopamine	No effect	Inhibited
Antagonists of serotonin	No effect	Inhibited
Dihydroxytryptamine	No effect	Inhibited
Alpha-methyl-p-tyrosine	Antagonized	No effect
6-hydroxy-dopamine	Antagonized	No effect
Brain lesions in		
Ventromedial hypothalamus	Enhanced	No effect
Lateral hypothalamus	Antagonized	Enhanced
Midbrain raphe	No effect	Antagonized

↓ = Decreased; → = No Change; ↑ = Increased
*Adapted from Garattini et al.: *In* Obesity: Causes, Consequences and Treatment, (Lasagna, L., ed.), Medcom Press, 1974.

dopamine at its receptors and thus indirectly increase dopamine metabolism.

The important differences in mechanism of action can be summarized as follows: Fenfluramine has a major action through neurons that involve serotonin; amphetamine has little effect on serotonin metabolism but has a major influence on brain norepinephrine and dopamine. Morever, fenfluramine antagonizes some of the effects of amphetamine, such as the toxicity of mice to amphetamine when the animals are maintained in groups. Similarly, fenfluramine can antagonize the hyperthermia and vasoconstriction elicited by amphetamine in the isolated artery of the mouse. Finally, in man, fenfluramine has an effect on the brain (electroencephalogram) which resembles that observed with barbiturates, and which differs sharply from that observed with amphetamines. For these reasons it would appear that the mechanism of central action of fenfluramine is substantially different from that observed with amphetamine (Groppetti et al., 1972).

PHARMACOLOGY

Effects on the Central Nervous System

All of the drugs listed in Table 9–1 can increase locomotor activity and stimulate the central nervous system, but the relative potency differs greatly (Domino et al., 1972; Smart et al., 1967). Amphetamine and methamphetamine are the most potent, and fenfluramine is the least potent. The latter drug has a mixed stimulant and depressant effect. In rats, food intake was suppressed 50 to 96 percent by a variety of doses (Table 9–4). Benzphetamine and d-amphetamine produced the greatest increase in spontaneous activity. Fenfluramine and chlorphentermine had almost no effect on activity (Von Rossum and Simons, 1969).

In monkeys the pattern is similar (Table 9–5). The food intake was suppressed by 40 to 60 percent with all of the drugs except methamphetamine and benzphetamine (Tang and Kirch, 1971). Methamphetamine (Table 9–5) was the most potent stimulator of spontaneous activity, with phenmetrazine only a little behind. At the other extreme were cholorphentermine, diethylpropion, and fenfluramine, which had little effect on spontaneous activity. Chlorphentermine and diethylpropion likewise produced almost no delay in the onset or duration of sleep, whereas diethylpropion was more like the other drugs. Aggregate toxicity in groups of mice has been observed with the amphetamines and methamphetamine. This means that these drugs are more toxic when given to mice living in groups than when given to mice housed in individual cages.

Fenfluramine antagonizes this effect of amphetamines. Diethylpropion and phentermine are less toxic when given to mice in groups than is amphetamine itself. An assessment of the anorexigenic effect of amphetamine and its derivatives is shown in Tables 9–4 and 9–5. Amphetamine and methamphetamine are the most potent and the other drugs are only a third to a tenth as active (Lawlor et al., 1969). These reductions in activity are a result of adding various substitutions (Table 9–1).

TABLE 9–4. *Effect of Several Anorexigenic Drugs on Spontaneous Activity and Food Intake in Rats*

DRUG	DOSE $\frac{\mu mol}{kg}$	FOOD INTAKE % of control	SPONTANEOUS ACTIVITY % of control
None	—	100	100
d-Amphetamine	3.16	57	400
Methamphetamine	1.00	86	208
Phenmetrazine	17.8	96	234
Phendimetrazine	31.6	76	234
Phentermine	17.8	52	257
Chlorphentermine	10.0	50	106
Benzphetamine	31.6	51	389
Fenfluramine	10.0	61	116

*Adapted from von Rossum and Simons: Psychopharmacologia, *14*:248–254, 1969.

TABLE 9–5. *Comparison of Several Anorexigenic Drugs on Food Intake, Spontaneous Activity and Sleep in the Rhesus Monkey**

DRUG	DOSE	FOOD INTAKE	SPONTANEOUS ACTIVITY	SLEEP PATTERN	
	mg/kg	Percent of control	Percent of control	Delay in onset (hours)	Decrease in duration (hours)
Placebo	–	100	100	0	0
d-Amphetamine	0.3	44	352	3.62	4.10
Methamphetamine	0.3	90	754	2.19	2.12
Phenmetrazine	10	42	673	4.19	3.90
Benzphetamine	3	75	266	3.81	3.50
Chlorphentermine	10	57	83	0.06	0.19
Diethylpropion	10	55	115	1.88	2.85
Fenfluramine	3	49	101	0.06	0.44

*Adapted from Tang and Kirch: Psychopharmacologia, 24:139–146, 1971.

Cardiovascular Effects

Cardiovascular effects are frequently observed with these drugs. An increase in heart rate and an increase in blood pressure are the most common responses. However, the effect on blood pressure can be paradoxical. With amphetamine the acute administration will increase the sensitivity of the animal to the hypertensive effect of tyramine and norepinephrine. After chronic administration of amphetamine, however, the hypertensive effect of tyramine is reduced but the hypertensive effect of infusing norepinephrine is unchanged. Tachycardia is produced by many of these drugs, but is minimal with mazindol and fenfluramine.

One careful comparative study of several amphetamines has been conducted at the Addiction Research Center. In this study amphetamine, methamphetamine, ephedrine, phenmetrazine and methylphenidate were compared in man (Martin et al., 1971). All drugs produced a dose related increase in blood pressure. The potency estimates were similar for all drugs, and both systolic and diastolic blood pressure were increased. Respiratory rate was similarly increased by all of the drugs.

The effect on pulse rate was quite complex. Although all of the drugs produced tachycardia, there was an overall negative correlation between pulse rate and the rise in blood pressure when amphetamine, methamphetamine, ephedrine and phenmetrazine were studied. The relative bradycardia seen during the increased pressor responses was probably of reflex origin. This suggests that the pressor response was increasing the carotid body output and inhibiting heart rate by stimulating the vagus nerve.

These drugs also increased body temperature, dilated the pupils, reduced food intake, and reduced the duration of time spent in sleeping. Amphetamine and methamphetamine were nearly identical on all parameters studied. Phenmetrazine was generally only one third to one fourth as potent as the other two amphetamines on most of the cardiovascular and central nervous system responses which were examined.

Metabolic Effect

Some of these drugs produce metabolic effects. Amphetamine, methamphetamine, phenmetrazine and fenfluramine all increase the concentration of free fatty acids and glycerol concentrations in the plasma (Laurian et al., 1968). Depletion of catecholamines by prolonged administration of reserpine almost completely abolished the rise of plasma free fatty acids produced by amphetamine (Pinter and Pattee, 1968). These data suggest that amphetamines were acting by releasing endogenous norepinephrine at or near the adipocyte membrane.

The effects of fenfluramine have been subjected to more intensive investigation (Burland, 1976; Garrow et al., 1972). Fenfluramine has no direct action on isolated adipocytes, yet in vivo it potentiates the release of free fatty acids. The mobilization of free fatty acids by these drugs has been examined further. Fenfluramine and methamphetamine have no effect on the release of free fatty acids from adipose cells in vitro at concentrations more than 200 times that of an effective dose of norepinephrine. However, methamphetamine and fenfluramine both antagonized the lipolytic effects of norepinephrine in vitro. Fenfluramine inhibits the lipolysis stimulated by ACTH, whereas methamphetamine is only a weak antagonist. Moreover, fenfluramine slightly but significantly reduced the release of free fatty acids and glycerol following the addition of dibutyl cyclic AMP to adipose tissue, while methamphetamine had no effect on this response. Fenfluramine inhibited the stimulation of lipolysis following the addition of growth hormone plus dexamethasone, but did not modify the increased lipolysis observed with adipose tissue from fasting animals. Methamphetamine had no effect on lipolysis after fasting or on the lipolytic effects of growth hormone and dexamethasone in vitro, again demonstrating an important difference between these two anorectic drugs.

When methamphetamine and fenfluramine were incubated in the presence of radioactively labeled glucose, the incorporation of radioactivity into glyceride-glycerol was unaffected, but the incorporation into long chain fatty acids was significantly reduced.

Of the anorectic drugs, only mazindol appears to be without effect on lipid metabolism, indicating its difference in mechanism of action from that of the other drugs listed in Table 9–1. The effects of fenfluramine on glucose metabolism have also been examined. Wichelow and Butterfield (1970) showed that the intraarterial injection of 0.4 μg/min of fenfluramine increased the glucose uptake and blood flow in the infused arm above that in the control arm. Following two weeks of oral fenfluramine therapy, 3 obese subjects lost weight and demonstrated increased glucose uptake and utilization by peripheral tissues. Similar effects of fenfluramine on glucose uptake by peripheral tissues have also been demonstrated by Turtle (1973) and Bliss et al., (1972). The importance of this phenomenon in the action of fenfluramine as an appetite suppressing drug, however, is unclear.

METABOLISM OF AMPHETAMINE AND ITS DERIVATIVES

Absorption

Most of the compounds shown in Table 9–1 are orally absorbed. The time for peak blood levels is 1 to 2 hours for many of these compounds. The half-time in blood varies from 4 to more than 30 hours (Table 9–6). This is undoubtedly influenced by the chemical structure of the compound, as well as by the acidity of the urine. The excretion of these compounds in the unchanged form is increased when the urine is acidic. This would be expected because the partition between acidic urine and more alkaline body fluids would favor diffusion into the acidic urine. In acidic urine, the excretion of unchanged compound varies from a low of 4 to upwards of 70 percent, but excretion is delayed if the urine is alkaline.

TABLE 9–6. *Clinical Effects of Anorexigenic Drugs*

DRUG	BLOOD LEVELS (HOURS)		PERCENT ORAL DOSE EXCRETED IN URINE	
	peak	half-time	in 24 hours	in 7 days
d-Amphetamine	1 to 2	13	60–90[+]	
Methamphetamine	1 to 2	13	45[+]	
Benzphetamine	1 to 2	4.3°(?)	–	80 to 90°
Phentermine		22	80	
Phenmetrazine				
Phendimetrazine		not available		
Chlorphentermine		38	35	
Diethylpropion	2			
sustained release	12	12	4	
Clortermine	2 to 5	9		
Mazindol	4	13	22	
Fenfluramine	5	20	20[+]	100

°Unpublished data
[+]pH dependent

The metabolism of these compounds has been studied in detail. It has been established clearly that the metabolic fate of each compound varies from one species to another, as well as between drugs. At least 4 pathways have been defined for the metabolism of these compounds. The first is hydroxylation of the aromatic phenyl ring. The second is oxidative deamination of the aminoalkyl group. The third is beta-hydroxylation of the two carbon side chains, and the fourth is dealkylation of the N-alkyl phenyl-isopropanolamine side chain.

The pathway for metabolism of amphetamine is shown in Figure 9–3 (Axelrod, 1970). The first step in metabolism is removal of the N-terminal methyl group. This is followed by two alternative pathways, one of which is the oxidation of the amino group to a keto group, and the other is hydroxylation of the phenyl ring. The unchanged amphetamine is a small percentage of the metabolites in the rabbit, but is approximately 30 to 40 percent in dog and man. The parahydroxylated derivative represents only a small fraction of the metabolites in man. The other major component in human urine is the benzoic acid derivative. In contrast, the benzomethylketone and benzoic acid

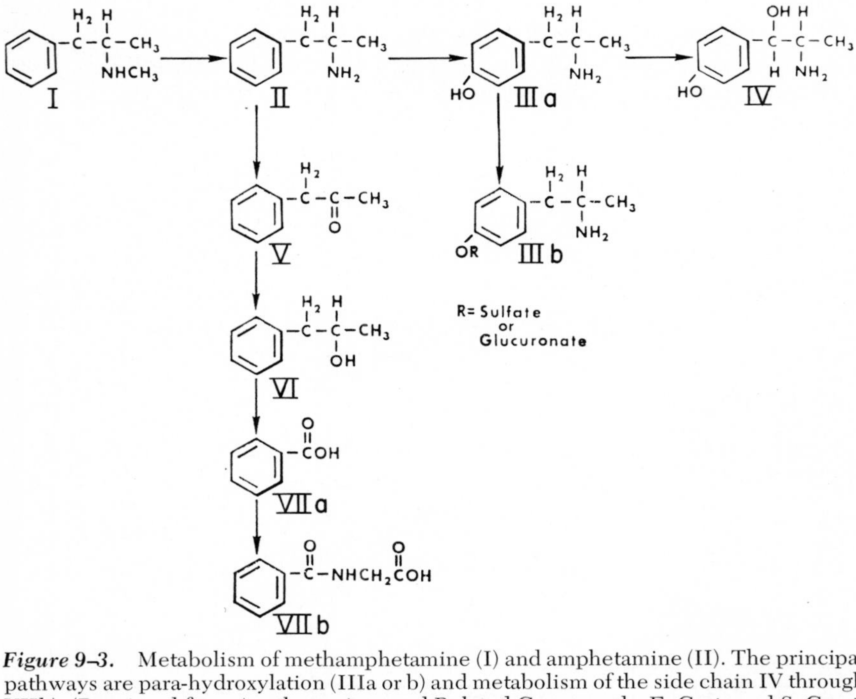

Figure 9–3. Metabolism of methamphetamine (I) and amphetamine (II). The principal pathways are para-hydroxylation (IIIa or b) and metabolism of the side chain IV through VIIb). (Reprinted from Amphetamines and Related Compounds. E. Costa and S. Garattini, eds. New York, Raven Press, 1970, with permission.)

metabolites make up the major products of metabolism in the rabbit and are also prominent metabolites in the dog (Angrist et al., 1972).

CLINICAL USE OF ANORECTIC DRUGS

In evaluating the clinical usefulness of these drugs two questions need to be answered: (1) are they effective, and (2) are they safe? After examining these two questions, the general principles for use of these agents will be enumerated, followed by a discussion of the properties of specific compounds. (Feinstein, 1960; Fineberg, 1972; Lasagna, 1973; Roberts, 1951; Samuel and Burland, 1976).

Effectiveness

The effectiveness of a compound can be established by showing that it has a significantly greater effect on weight loss than a placebo used in a double blind randomized trial. The Food and Drug Administration (FDA) has recently evaluated 105 new drug applications submitted for marketing these drugs. The applications contain 210 studies conducted by a double blind technique, and an additional 145 studies which include two active drugs. This group of applications contained data on nearly 10,000 patients and provides the most extensive body of data yet assembled on these agents (Scoville, 1975). The drugs included in this study are listed in Table 9–7, along with some of the trade names and usual dose.

TABLE 9–7. *Currently Available Drugs Which Allegedly Depress Appetite*

GENERIC NAME	TRADE NAME	SIZES OF TABLET OR CAPSULE (mg)
Schedule II*		
d-Amphetamine	Many	5, 10, 15
Methamphetamine	Many	5, 10, 15
Phenmetrazine	Preludin	25, 50, 75
Schedule III*		
Phendimetrazine	Plegine	35
Benzphetamine	Didrex	25, 50
Phentermine	Ionamin	15, 30
Chlorphentermine	Presate	65
Clortermine	Voranil	50
Diethylpropion	Tepanil Tenuate	25, 75
Mazindol	Sanorex	1, 2
Schedule IV*		
Fenfluramine	Pondimin	20

*Prescription Schedule imposed by Drug Enforcement Agency (DEA).

The data analyzed by the Food and Drug Administration reported on 4543 patients on active drugs and 3100 patients on placebo. In this group the dropout rate was approximately 18.5 percent for the patients on placebo and 24 percent for the patients with active drug in studies lasting 3, 4 or 6 weeks. At the end of the study period, whatever that duration might be (3, 4, 6, 8, 12, 20 or more), equal numbers of patients receiving placebo and active drug were retained (49 percent placebo vs 47.9 percent for active drug). The weight loss averaged 0.56 pounds per week more for patients receiving active drugs than for patients receiving placebos.

Another way of looking at these data was in terms of the percentage of patients losing one pound per week or more. A weight loss of one pound or more per week was almost twice as common in patients receiving active drug as in those on placebo (44 percent for active drug vs. 26 percent for placebo). When a weight loss of 3 pounds per week were evaluated, the group receiving active drug was again almost twice as successful as those receiving placebo (2 percent of those on active drug lost 3 pounds per week vs. 1 percent on placebo). Evaluating weight loss over 4 weeks showed that 68 percent of the patients on active drug lost 1 pound per week, compared with 46 percent on placebo. Over the same duration, 10 percent of the patients on active drug lost 3 pounds per week, whereas only 4 percent of the patients receiving placebo lost the same amount of weight.

These same data can be examined in a diagrammatic way by looking at the weight loss for patients on a placebo and those on an active drug (Fig. 9–4). In the right panel is shown the weight loss in pounds per week, and in the left panel absolute body weight for the two groups. It is clear that the patients receiving the placebo lost weight, but the patients receiving the active drug lost significantly more weight. The rate of weight loss in pounds per week was initially more rapid in the group receiving active drug than in the group receiving placebo. This difference remained greater throughout the duration of the study. An analysis of the rate of weight loss after 8 weeks of the study showed that the slope remained greater in the patients receiving active drug than in those receiving placebo.

Thus the effectiveness of amphetamine-like drugs is significantly greater than that of placebo. Analysis of the data from the 145 parallel studies, however, revealed no significant differences between any of the drugs in Table 9–7. Thus in clinically effective doses, there was little choice among these compounds in terms of effectiveness of weight loss, or in the duration over which this weight loss could be induced. That is, in studies lasting up to 20 weeks in which sufficient numbers of patients were retained, those on active drug lost significantly more weight than patients receiving placebo (Fig. 9–4).

The long term effectiveness of these drugs, however, has never been established. The longest trials in which sufficient numbers of

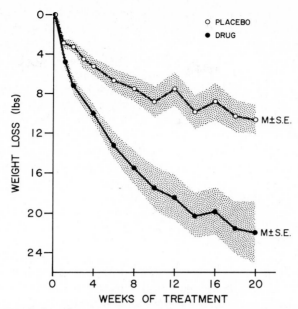

Figure 9–4. Weight loss during treatment with an appetite suppressing drug. Weight loss is most rapid initially. Patients treated with active drug lost (●) significantly more weight than those on placebo (○).

patients were retained in the placebo and drug treatment groups ranged between 20 and 24 weeks. Beyond that point, the dropout rate is too high to allow effective evaluation. However, that data up to 20 weeks suggest the possibility that these drugs might retain their ability to reset the internal control systems which regulate body fat at a lower level for a prolonged period of time. Such a trial, however, has not been conducted.

Safety

The safety of these agents has also been the subject of considerable discussion. The possibility of enhanced mortality in patients receiving diet pills was brought to public attention in reports by Henry (1967) and Jelliffe et al. (1969) of deaths in patients receiving these drugs. In these patients the agents used were amphetamine, thyroid, potassium-depleting diuretics and laxatives. In some of the patients it would appear that potassium deficiency and the ensuing hypokalemia may have been the major factors leading to death. This possibility remains a potentially serious one, although Asher and Dietz (1972), in a review of deaths using amphetamines and thyroid in "reasonable doses," could find no evidence for increased mortality.

An equally serious problem is the potential for development of tolerance and the possibility of drug abuse. Indeed, it is the latter problem of habituation and addiction to certain of these drugs which has led to the current reassessment of their relative value in the treatment of obesity. If they were not subject to widespread abuse by certain groups in our society, there would be far less concern about their use in treating obese patients. Drug abuse has been reported for amphetamine, methamphetamine and phenmetrazine. Claims of drug abuse for other members of this class are less frequent, but because all (except possibly fenfluramine) possess significant degrees of central stimulating properties the potential for drug abuse remains one of real concern.

In addition to the potential for abuse, there are a number of side effects which are summarized in Table 9–8. These data are expressed as the ratio of the side effect of the drug compared with that of the placebo (100 percent = placebo). In instances where the side effect was greater in the placebo, the percentage is less than 100. The two most prominent side effects are insomnia and dry mouth. The other effects occur in small numbers with the exception of depression and diarrhea, which occur mainly with fenfluramine.

From the previous discussion, it is clear that these agents can be effective as adjuncts in the treatment of obesity. Their usefulness depends on employing them as *part* of a total program for treatment for obesity and not relying solely on them. Several rules would appear to be applicable to their use. First, the drug abuse potential is higher for those compounds classed in Schedule II (Table 9–7). It would appear more reasonable, therefore, to select a preparation classified in Schedules III or IV. It would also appear appropriate to use drugs with a minimum number of side effects. The high frequency of depression in patients receiving fenfluramine would suggest that this drug should be avoided in patients with psychiatric or depressive tendencies. In patients with hypertension, mazindol may well be the drug of choice. In patients with diabetes who have no psychiatric problems, fenfluramine might be the first choice. For patients with essential obesity not complicated by high blood pressure or diabetes, diethylpropion or clortermine might be the agents of choice.

With most of these drugs, fenfluramine being a notable exception, the use of intermittent courses of therapy can be as effective as continuous use of the drug. Interrupted courses of therapy usually last for 3 to 6 weeks with discontinuation for a period half the length or longer than the original period of treatment. Because of the tendency toward postdrug depression in some patients, intermittent therapy with fenfluramine is inadvisable. Some of these drugs have been used with apparent effectiveness in children and during pregnancy, but for the present it would be wiser not to use these drugs in pregnant women.

TABLE 9–8. *Side Effects of Various Anorectic Drugs Compared with Placebo**

Drug	Headache	Insomnia	Nervousness	Dizziness	Weakness or Fatigue	Depression	Rise in Blood Pressure	Tachycardia	Palpitations	Dry Mouth	Nausea	Abdominal Discomfort	Constipation	Diarrhea	Edema	Polyuria or Frequency
Amphetamine	2.2	6.9	2.1	6.3	0.9	1.2	38	30	25	1.6	1.8	0.9	2.7	–	–	1.8
Methamphetamine	0.9	6.5	5.5	5.6	1.3	0.4	5	1.7	20	3.8	3.3	0.4	1.6	–	2.3	0
Phenmetrazine	0	4.6	1.4	6.6	–	a0.9	–	–	–	4.6	–	2.5	1.8	–	–	9.5
Phendimetrazine	–	2.1	7.4	2.2	0	0	–	–	0.7	1.7	2.0	3.0	–	–	–	–
Benzphetamine	–	3.2	–	1.6	–	1.0	–	–	–	–	2.7	–	–	–	–	–
Phentermine	1.6	6.2	0.9	3.1	0.8	–	–	–	–	3.7	2.3	–	2.5	–	5.0	–
Chlorphentermine	1.7	7.8	1.1	1.2	0.8	–	–	–	–	3.4	1.1	–	2.5	–	2.6	–
Clortermine	1.2	0.9	1.2	0.7	0.8	–	–	–	–	1.2	3.2	1.3	1.8	–	–	–
Diethylpropion	0.8	4.8	1.3	3.1	0.9	0.4	0	–	16	3.5	3.4	0.6	0.9	–	–	3.3
Mazindol	1.15	1.4	0.7	1.0	1.0	–	–	–	–	3.0	1.1	–	–	–	–	1.5
Fenfluramine	–	–	–	–	–	3.2	–	–	–	–	–	–	–	7.2	–	–
Placebo†	3.4	1.8	3.6	1.0	2.8	1.1	0.1	0.3	0.1	3.1	1.4	2.7	3.7	–	1.8	–

*Each drug-related side effect was correlated with the same effect in the placebo group.

$$\text{ratio} = \frac{\%\ \text{of drug treated patients with side effect}}{\%\ \text{of placebo treated patients with side effect}}$$

†Placebo treated patients also experienced: dysuria, 0.3 percent; headache, 3.4 percent; chills, 0.1 percent; and depression, 1.1 percent.

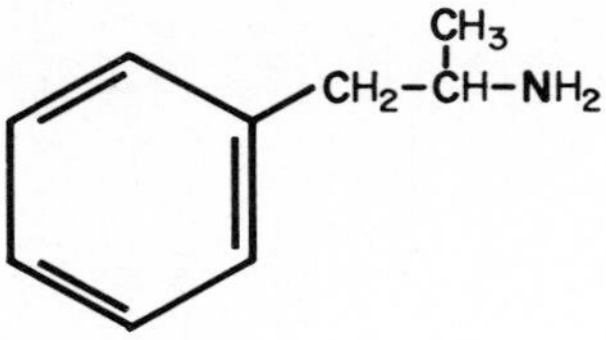

Figure 9–5.   d-Amphetamine.

DEXTROAMPHETAMINE

This drug has been prescribed alone or with various additives such as chlorperadzine, meprobamate, vitamins and barbiturates (Rosenberg, 1953). The anorectic dosage ranges from 5 to 30 mg/day (Resnick and Joubert, 1967; Silverstone and Stunkard, 1968). Insomnia and hyperactivity are present in a high percentage of patients treated with this compound. Because this compound elevates blood pressure and has a significant tendency to produce addiction, (Edison, 1971) it is doubtful that it has any present role in the treatment of obesity. This is notwithstanding the fact that it is the least expensive of the compounds on the market (Adlersberg and Mayer, 1949; Edwards and Swyer, 1950; Freed and Mizel, 1952; Gelvin and McGarack, 1949; Goodman and Housel, 1954; Rosenthal and Solomon, 1940; Schapiro and Bogran, 1960).

METHAMPHETAMINE

This compound is available under a variety of trade names in both tablet and injectable form. The side effects are similar to those observed with amphetamine, but it may have a higher tendency to stimulate the central nervous system. This tendency toward CNS stimulation has led to widespread abuse of the compound. Because of the high frequency of abuse, there would appear to be *no* indication for the use of this compound in treating obese patients.

PHENMETRAZINE

This compound is distributed in the United States under the trade name of Preludin (Fig. 9–7). It comes in tablets of 25 mg and in sustained action capsules of 50 mg. Its effects are similar to those of the

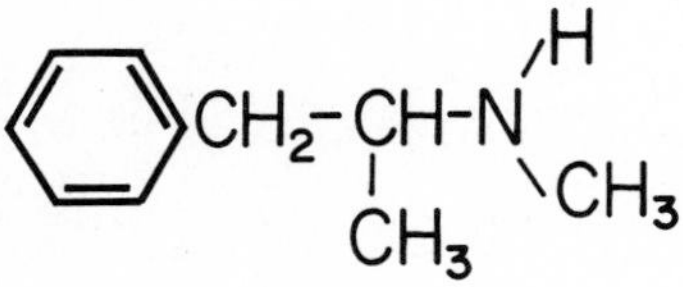

Figure 9–6.   Methamphetamine.

Figure 9–7.   Phenmetrazine (Preludin).

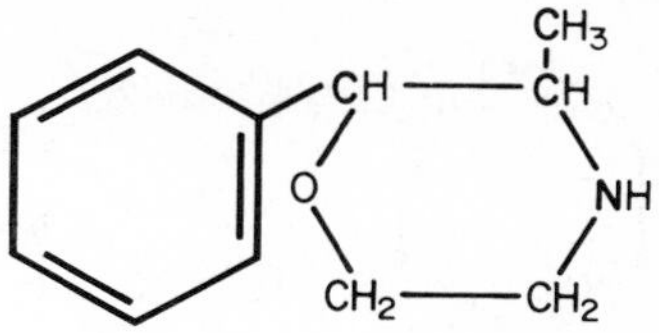

other amphetamines in producing stimulation of the central nervous system, hyperthermia, elevation in blood pressure, mydriasis and tachycardia. These side effects are less common with the long acting preparation. This drug, like amphetamine and methamphetamine, has had a significant history of drug abuse. It is significantly more effective than placebo (as demonstrated in several studies), but is not more effective than other anorectic drugs. This drug has been shown to be effective in both obese adults and obese children. One of the serious side effects with this drug is the appearance of toxic psychosis which is indistinguishable from the psychosis observed with amphetamines or from the hallucinations observed in alcoholism (Bethell, 1957; Kahan and Mullins, 1958; Silverman, 1959). Because of the frequency of abuse with this compound, it likewise has only a secondary role in the treatment of obesity. (Berneike, 1955; Boxer et al., 1961; Gelvin et al., 1956; Hadler, 1967a; Hampson, 1960; Martel, 1957; Natenshon, 1956; Ressler, 1957; Robillard, 1957).

PHENDIMETRAZINE

Phendimetrazine (Plegine) differs from phenmetrazine in having a second methyl group on the nitrogen of the ring structure. It is provided in 35 mg tablets. The effects on cardiac and respiratory systems in dogs and cats are less potent than those with phenmetrazine. Tachycardia and alterations in the electrocardiogram are not produced with phendimetrazine, although they have been observed with phenmetrazine. Like phenmetrazine, phendimetrazine produces significant weight loss. This compound may have a more important role than phenmetrazine, but its similarity must lead to caution in its use. (Cass, 1962; Hadler, 1968; LeRiche and Van Belle, 1962; Ressler and Schneider, 1961; Runyan, 1962).

Figure 9–8.   Phendimetrazine (Plegine).

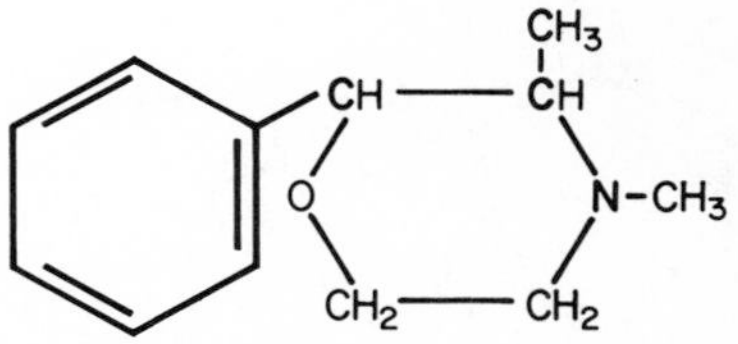

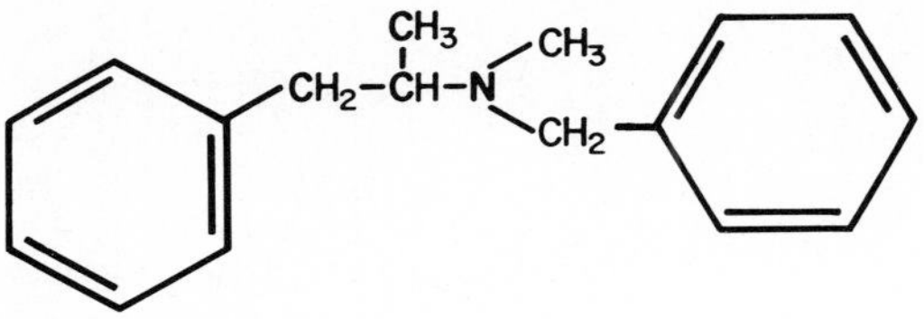

Figure 9-9. Benzphetamine (Didrex).

BENZPHETAMINE

This compound (Didrex) (Fig. 9–9) is available in 25 mg tablets and was first used in the United States in 1960. The side effects of this agent are generally similar to those observed with amphetamine. In the study by Poindexter, (1960) however, benzphetamine and phenmetrazine had fewer side effects than amphetamine. There is little to recommend this compound over the compounds described below (Patel et al., 1963; Simkin and Wallace, 1960).

PHENTERMINE

This compound is available as a resin in 15 or 30 mg capsules (Fig. 9–10). Phentermine (Ionamin) causes less stimulation of the central nervous system than amphetamine because of the alpha-methyl substitution. However, it can increase blood pressure and produce tachycardia. Insomnia is a significant side effect with this compound, occurring in 20 percent of the patients observed by Steel et al., (1973). In addition, dry mouth is a common complaint. Because this compound has fewer effects on the central nervous system, it is preferable to the group of compounds discussed previously. (LeRiche, 1960; Poindexter, 1960; Steel et al., 1973; Truant et al., 1972).

CHLORPHENTERMINE

This drug (Presate) is available in 65 mg tablets as a sustained release preparation, and was first used in Europe in 1960 and in the United States in 1965 (Fig. 9–11). The introduction of the chlorine into the phenyl ring reduces the tendency for central stimulation (Nielsen

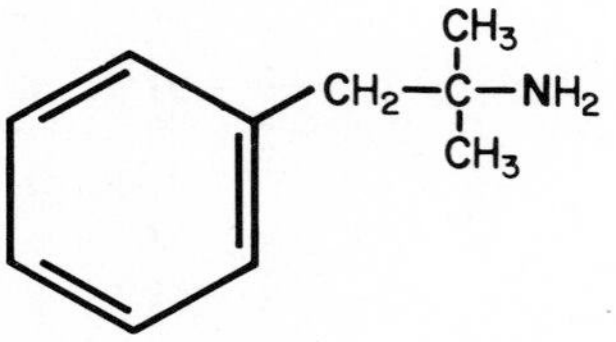

Figure 9-10. Phentermine (Ionamin).

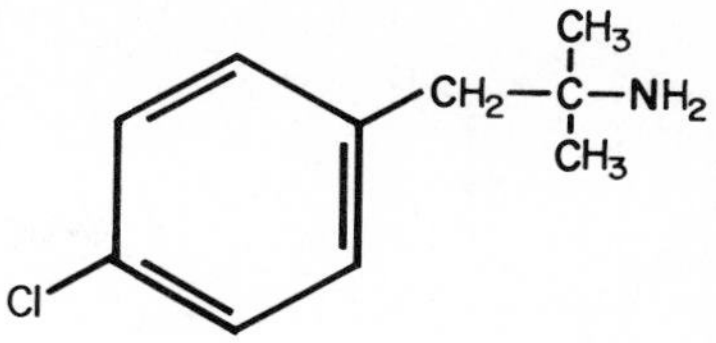

Figure 9–11. Chlorphentermine (Pre-Sate).

and Dubnick, 1970). In the early clinical trials, the drug was shown to produce significant weight loss. Its major side effects were dry mouth, nausea and vertigo. Some patients actually complained about the lack of central stimulation. In addition, restlessness and insomnia noted with many of the compounds listed above were not noted with this drug. Weight losses with this compound are comparable to that observed with amphetamine, phenmetrazine, diethylpropion and amphetamine. This drug would appear to be more useful than the agents noted above because of its reduced tendency towards central stimulation and its documented effectiveness in inducing weight loss. (Berry, 1965; Boxer et al., 1961; Duckman et al., 1968; Fineberg, 1962; Jackson and Whyte, 1965; Levin et al., 1963; Lucey and Hadden 1962; Rauh and Lipp, 1968; Seaton et al., 1964).

CLORTERMINE

This compound is available in 50 mg tablets and was released by the FDA for use in the United States in 1973 (Fig. 9–12). It seems to be similar in most respects to chlorphentermine. It reduces significant weight loss and would appear to merit consideration along with chlorphentermine (Asher, 1974).

DIETHYLPROPION

This compound (Tenuate, Tepanil) is available as 25 mg tablets and 75 mg sustained release capsules (Fig. 9–13). The introduction of a keto group on the beta carbon of the phenethylamine side chain lowers the incidence of side effects due to central nervous system

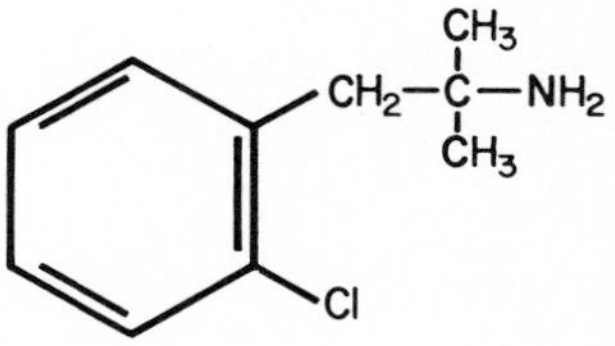

Figure 9–12. Clortermine (Voranil).

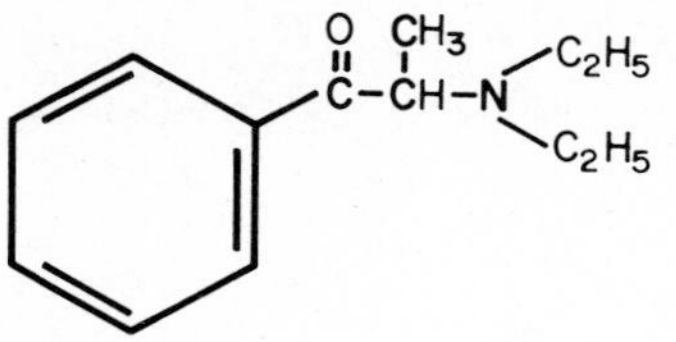

Figure 9–13. Diethylpropion (Tepanil; Tenuate).

stimulation. CNS stimulation was observed in less than 1 percent of 752 patients. It has only minimal effects on blood pressure and respiration, and it rarely alters the electrocardiogram, even after intravenous injection in patients with hypertension, early congestive failure, coronary artery disease or angina pectoris. It is clinically effective (Silverstone et al., 1968). Intermittent courses of therapy are probably the preferred mode of administration. Continuous therapy for up to 24 weeks has shown significantly greater weight loss than with patients receiving placebo. This drug has been shown effective during pregnancy (Boileau, 1968; Jordan and Bader, 1961; Silverman and Okun, 1971) in patients with cardiovascular disease, in those with diabetes mellitus, and in obese children (Stewart et al., 1970). There have been a few reports of drug abuse (Clein and Benady, 1962; Jones, 1968). Because of its wide use, relative lack of significant side effects and low tendency to habituation, this is one of the drugs with the most sound bases for recommendation for use (Alfaro et al., 1960; Bose, 1969; Cunningham, 1963; Decina and Tanyol, 1960; Rosenberg, 1961; Russek, 1966; Williams, 1968).

FENFLURAMINE

This compound (Pondimin) is available in 20 mg tablets (Fig. 9–14). It was first used in France and has received numerous trials throughout the world. It is a unique compound in that it has the trifluromethyl substitution on the meta position of the phenyl ring. This drug differs from the other members of this group in its effects on the central nervous system. In studies with the electroencephalogram (EEG), it was found to act like a barbiturate, producing sedation and slowing rather than stimulation. Numerous studies have shown it to

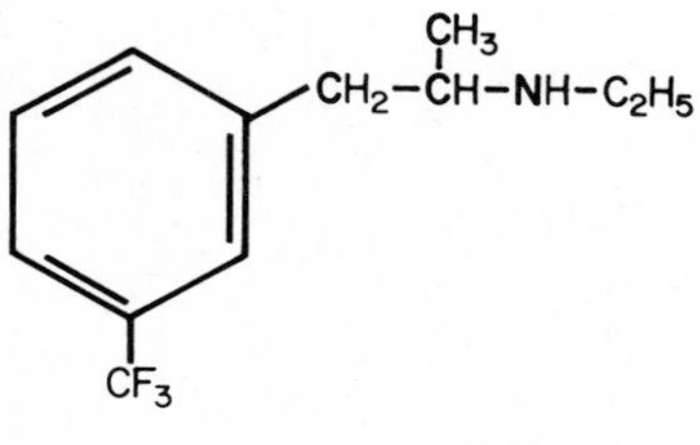

Figure 9–14. Fenfluramine (Pondimin).

be a clinically effective drug in producing more weight loss than observed with placebo. It is relatively free of additive potential (Gotestam and Gunne, 1972). Its major side effects are diarrhea and depression, observed in a significant number of patients (Steel and Briggs, 1972). It is effective in treating patients with hypertension, as well as obese diabetics and obese children (Burland, 1976; Follows, 1971; Goldrick et al.,1973; Kaufman and Blondheim, 1973; Lele et al., 1972; O'Connor and Brodkin, 1970; Pinder et al., 1975; Robins, 1973; Sedgewick, 1970; Stunkard et al., 1973; Waal-Manning and Simpson, 1969).

MAZINDOL

This compound (Sanorex) is available in 1 and 2 mg tablets, and was released by the FDA in July of 1973 (Fig. 9–15). The side effects of this drug are mild stimulation of the central nervous system, insomnia, dizziness and dry mouth. It has a lower tendency to stimulate the cardiovascular system than other amphetamine derivatives. Weight loss is significantly greater than with placebo, but there is no difference between this drug and other compounds. Potential for drug abuse has not been established (DeFelice et al., 1969; Hadler, 1972; Sandoz-Wander, 1973).

PHENYLPROPANOLAMINE

This compound (Propadrine) whose structure is shown in Table 9–1, is one of the most frequently used nasal decongestants. It has many of the same physiologic effects as epinephrine and ephedrine, but has a more prolonged duration of action. Its potency as a central nervous system stimulant is low in comparison with the other compounds in this family, and it is thus not subject to regulation by the Drug Enforcement Agency. It is available as an over-the-counter preparation.

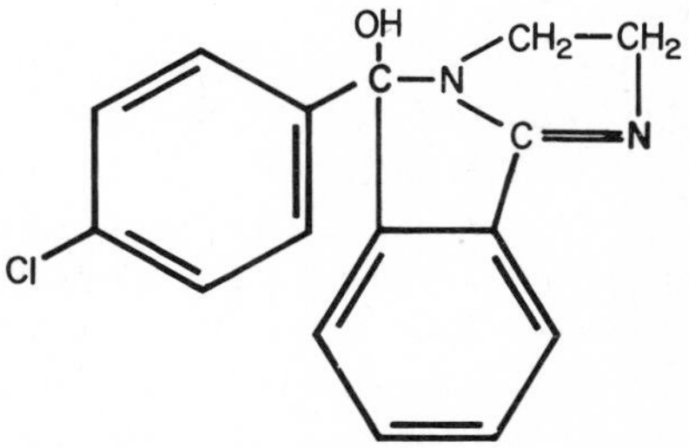

Figure 9–15. Mazindol (Sanorex).

Its clinical use was described by Hirsch (1940), but the best early study was the one of Kalb (1942b). He administered phenyl-propanolamine (propadrine) in doses of 45 or 25 mg accompanied by a topical anesthetic to 464 and 216 patients. These were compared with 1200 patients receiving dextroamphetamine in doses of 10 to 20 mg. The patients receiving propadrine and amphetamine demonstrated a decrease in appetite in 40 to 45 percent of the cases, as compared with a decrease in appetite in only 12 percent of the 100 control patients.

More recently, Hoebel (1975) has conducted a double blind, crossover trial of propadrine and placebo. During the initial phase, there was no significant difference in the rate of weight loss between subjects treated with propadrine and placebo. However, in the cross-over period there was a statistically significant increase in the weight loss experienced by the subjects receiving propadrine, as compared with the group receiving placebo. Thus it appears that this drug, which has minimal effects on the central nervous system, may be an effective agent as an adjunct to the treatment of obesity (Hoebel et al., 1975a,b).

OTHER ANORECTIC DRUGS

Aminorex differs from amphetamine in that it has a ring structure in the side chain. Early studies had demonstrated that it was an effective anorectic agent (Hadler, 1967b; Wood and Owen, 1965). However, in 1968 this drug was shown to be associated with an increased incidence of pulmonary hypertension (Follath et al., 1971) and it was withdrawn from use.

Two other drugs not currently marketed have been shown to be effective in a weight reduction program. One is pipradrol (Gelvin et al., 1955) and the other is levonor (Gadek et al., 1958). In the study with pipradrol [alpha-(2-piperidyl)-benzhydrol hydrochloride], Gelvin et al. observed significantly greater weight losses with the active drug than with placebo in double blind studies of the crossover and parallel type. The weight losses with pipradrol were 1 and 1.2 pounds per week, those with placebo 0.3 and 0.6 pounds per week. The side effects, particularly dizziness, were substantial, and no further trials have been reported. A second drug, levonor (1-phenyl-2-aminopropane) was evaluated by Gadek et al. (1958) on 80 patients. It was reported to have fewer side effects than other drugs with which they had experience, but there were no controlled studies.

In summary, among the group of compounds listed in Table 9–8, the last 5 merit initial consideration in the treatment of the obese patients. They must be used only as adjuncts in treatment, however. Diethylpropion might merit initial consideration, with clortermine, chlorphentermine, fenfluramine and mazindol in second place.

Among patients with a history of depression or mental illness, mazindol, clortermine and diethylpropion would merit first choice; fenfluramine should probably not be used. Among diabetics, fenfluramine might be the drug of choice. Among hypertensive patients, diethylpropion merits first consideration. The value of intermittent or interrupted courses of therapy should be kept in mind (Munro et al., 1968; LeRiche and Csima, 1967).

CALORIGENIC DRUGS—THYROID

The first use of thyroid hormones in the treatment of obesity is attributed to Baron in 1893 (Putnam, 1893). In the ensuing 80 years, more than 200 publications have appeared in which thyroid hormones have been administered to obese patients, but we shall focus on only three aspects of this vast literature. (1) Some of the data on thyroid function in obese patients will be reviewed, (2) some of the biologic effects of thyroid hormones will be discussed, and (3) the relative merits of treating obese patients with thyroid hormones will be evaluated.

Thyroid Status in Obese Patients

Levels of thyroid hormone have been measured in obese patients, with discordant results. Scriba et al. (1967) found the protein-bound iodine (PBI) of 61 obese patients to be significantly (p <.01) lower than that of 37 lean ones (4.47 ± 1.01 vs. 5.09 ± 0.97 m ± SD). In addition, they found that binding of radioactively labeled triiodothyronine to serum proteins was significantly increased in the obese patients. Glennon and Brech (1965), on the other hand, measured the PBI in groups of patients subdivided by the degrees of excess weight and could find no differences. Other groups have also found no differences (Hung et al., 1965; Benoit and Durrance, 1965; Nicoloff and Drenick, 1966).

We have reinvestigated this question by examining the correlation in 95 patients between measures of overweight and the concentration of thyroxine (T_4) and triiodothyronine (T_3) in the serum as determined in radioimmunoassay. Relative weight was expressed in three ways: as percentage over desirable weight, as the ratio of height/weight and as the ratio w/h^2 (the body mass index). Serum triiodothyronine had a small (r = .36) but statistically significant correlation with body weight, with percent overweight (Fig. 9–16) with w/h, and with w/h^2. Thyroxine, on the other hand, was not significantly correlated with any of these measures. Since the basal metabolism rate remains normal, we currently interpret the rise in T_3 with overweight to indicate an element of cellular resistance.

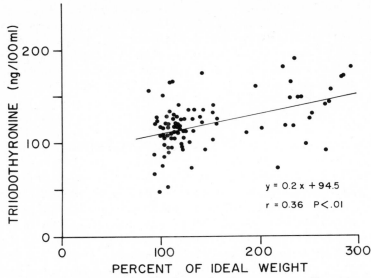

Figure 9–16. Triiodothyronine and body weight. There was a small positive and significant correlation between triiodothyronine and percent ideal weight. There was no correlation between thyroxine and body weight. (From Bray, Chopra and Fisher, unpublished observations.)

Several other abnormalities in thyroid function have also been reported. Premachandra et al. (1969) found that 5.7 percent of 599 obese patients had an abnormality in the transport system for thyroid hormones. When samples of serum were equilibrated with radioactively labeled thyroxine, the binding of the thyroxine occurred between the alpha-2 and beta-globulin rather than in the inter-alpha globulin area where it is normally bound. The significance of this alteration in transport of thryoxine is at present unclear, but it is interesting to note that it is reversed by treatment with triiodothyronine.

The rate at which thyroid hormones are removed from the circulation has been assessed in several studies. Nicoloff and Drenick (1966) have found that obese patients with long standing disease have a reduced rate of thyroxine disposal. These authors compared a control population against obese patients before weight loss, a group who had lost weight and a third group with obesity of recent onset. Only in this latter group did thyroxine disposal approach normal. There was no significant change in the PBI in any group, but the distribution and hepatic content of thyroxine were reduced.

Oddie et al. (1966) have also suggested that there is a decrease in thyroxine space in obesity. Direct measurements of the disappearance rate for thyroxine (Hung et al., 1965; Benoit and Durrance, 1965; Croughs et al., 1965) and for triiodothyronine (Rabinowitz and Myerson, 1967) have also been performed. Benoit and Durrance found that the 5.5 day biologic half-life for thyroxine in the eight normal subjects was significantly longer than the 4.3 days observed in 10 obese patients (p <.001). Moreover, there was a significant negative correlation between turnover of radiothyroxine and the ratio of actual to desired weight in this group (r = 0.745, p <.05) (i.e., turnover was more rapid in the lean subjects).

However, studies of thyroxine metabolism in adolescent males showed that the degradation of thyroxine was higher in obese boys than in the lean ones (Hung et al., 1965). In contrast with the adults, the adolescent boys showed an increase in the distribution of organic iodine but no differences in the biologic half-life. Degradation rates were 40.8 and 45.7 μg/day at two stages of puberty in lean boys, and 73.2 and 68.1 μg/day during the same stages of puberty in the obese boys. Croughs et al. (1965) found a longer half-life and slower degradation rate in 5 children, 4 of which were females. These studies of Benoit and Durrance (1965) and Hung et al. (1965) showing increased turnover of thyroxine differ from the conclusion of Nicoloff and Drenick (1966), Oddie et al. (1966), and Croughs et al. (1965); the basis for this discrepancy is at present unclear.

Measurements of triiodothyronine turnover by Rabinowitz and Myerson (1967), like those of Benoit and Durrance, have shown that obese patients have a shortened half-life for radioactive T_3 in the serum. Among 9 obese patients, the biologic half-life for T_3 was 1.6 days, but it was prolonged to 2.9 days in the three normal weight controls. After treatment with triiodothyronine, four obese patients showed a prolongation in biologic half-life toward normal (1.78 to 2.05 days). Consistent with the shortened half-life for T_3 was the increased removal of T_3 via the biliary tract.

Other tests of thyroid function are generally normal in obesity. The uptake of radioactive iodine by the thyroid is similar in lean and obese patients. Administration of 75 μg/day of triiodothyronine for one week suppresses uptake to low levels. Thyrotropin releasing hormone (TRH), a tripeptide which stimulates the release of TSH from the pituitary, has been administered to a number of obese patients. The release of TSH after this stimulus is normal or slightly exaggerated, indicating no impairment of pituitary release of TSH.

Biologic Effects

Oxygen utilization (basal metabolic rate) is a major parameter for the action of thyroid hormone and, as such, has been widely studied in obesity. Evidence from several laboratories indicates that total oxygen consumption of obese patients is higher than for lean ones. However, if the oxygen requirement is related to surface area to compensate for differences in body weight, the oxygen requirements of lean and obese people are similar. Boothby and Sandiford (1922) studied 8614 subjects (including obese patients) and found that they all had similar rates of basal metabolism. Subsequently, several groups of investigators have reached the same conclusion for obese adults (Means, 1916; Miller and Blyth, 1952; Johnston and Bernstein, 1955; Bray et al., 1970) and obese adolescents (Benoit and Durrance, 1965; Mossberg, 1948; Nelson et al., 1973).

Thyroid hormones increase the activity of the mitochondrial glycerophosphate oxidase in fat and other tissues of the experimental animal (Rivlin, 1970). In human adipose tissue, too, the activity of this enzyme can be increased by thyroid hormones (Bray, 1969b). Moreover, the resting levels of the mitochondrial glycerophosphate oxidase are lower in obese than in lean individuals under similar circumstances (Galton and Bray, 1967). The possible significance of this enzyme in obesity has been discussed previously (see Chapter 3).

Thyroid hormones can also modify the secretion of growth hormone in obesity (Londono et al., 1969). This has been shown using arginine, one of several provocative stimuli for increasing the circulating concentration of growth hormone in normal subjects. When arginine is infused into obese patients, the rise in growth hormone concentration is markedly reduced (Coppinschi et al., 1967; El-Khodary et al., 1972; Londono et al., 1969). After 14 to 21 days of pretreatment with T_3 (200 μg/day), arginine evokes a much greater release of growth hormone than before treatment, whereas weight loss of a comparable degree without T_3 produced little change in the growth hormone response to arginine (Londono et al., 1969). The increased response of growth hormone to arginine after treatment of obese patients with T_3 and the rise in the mitochondrial glycerophosphate oxidase during the same treatment have raised the possibility that these patients may be resistant to the actions of the thyroid hormones.

Clinical Uses

In 1949 Adlersberg and Mayer reported a double blind Latin square study comparing 90 mg of thyroid and 15 mg of amphetamine. The patients receiving amphetamine lost significantly more weight than those on placebo, but thyroid had no effect in this study. Following the discovery of triiodothyronine by Pitt-Rivers and Gross in (1952), interest in the use of this compound in treating obesity was renewed (Ressler, 1959; Weidenhamer, 1957).

Gelvin, Kenigsberg and Boyd (1959) reported that triiodothyronine (T_3) and amphetamine were synergistic in enhancing the weight loss of obese patients. Gwinup and Poucher (1967) compared weight loss in obese patients treated with triiodothyronine, thyroxine or with a placebo (Fig. 9–17). Doses of each hormone were gradually increased to tolerance. The patients receiving either thyroid preparation lost weight steadily, but the patients with placebo did not.

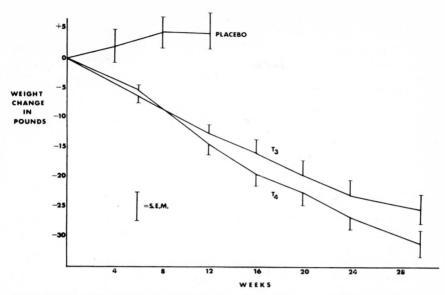

Figure 9–17.   Effect of triiodothyronine and thyroxine on weight loss. Each thyroid preparation was gradually increased to tolerance and produced more weight loss than placebo. (Reprinted from Gwinup, G. and Poucher, R.: Am. J. Med. Sci., *254*:416–420, 1967, with permission.)

In a widely quoted paper, Gordon, Goldberg and Chosy (1963) reviewed the metabolic features of obesity and extolled the virtue of a program which included a 1330 calorie diet in 6 feedings, use of polyunsaturated fats, triiodothyronine and intermittent injections of a mercurial diuretic. They failed to determine, however, whether the addition of T_3 and a mercurial diuretic produced more weight loss than the diet alone.

We re-examined this program to compare diet alone with T_3 and the mercurial diuretic. Twelve patients were hospitalized on the Clinical Research Center of the New England Center Hospital and placed on a program similar to the one described by Gordon, Goldberg and Chosy. After a careful dietary history, patients were fed an amount equivalent to their caloric intake as calculated from the diet history. They were then fasted for 48 hours and started on a 1320 calorie diet for 30 days. Group I, consisting of 6 patients, received the diet alone with no supplemental drugs. Group II received an injection of a mercurial diuretic on days 8, 18 and 28. Group III was treated with triiodothyronine beginning at 50 μg/day and increasing in dosage to a limit of 150 μg/day or until symptoms developed. They also received a shot of mercurial diuretic.

During the diet there were punctuated drops in weight on the day after administration of the mercurial diuretic. This was followed by a slowing of weight loss. Table 9–9 summarizes the data for all groups

TABLE 9–9. *Effect of Diet, Diuretics and*
Triiodothyronine on Weight Loss°

		WEIGHT LOSS	
GROUP	NUMBER OF PATIENTS	kg	percent of body weight
I	6	4.6±0.49*	4.3±.26*
II	4	5.5±0.70	4.9±.15
III	6	6.4±0.58	6.3±.52‡

*mean±SEM
‡p .01 compared with Group I
°Unpublished data from Bray, G. A., Glennon, J. A., Rüedi, B., Cheifetz, P. and Cassidy, C. E.

and shows that the 6 patients receiving the complete program (Group III) lost significantly more weight than either of the other groups of patients. This effect of triiodothyronine emerged from the data whether the results were expressed in terms of absolute weight loss or weight loss as a percentage of the initial weight.

These data support the observation of Gordon et al. (1963) and are in harmony with several other reports, which suggests that thyroid hormones tend to potentiate weight loss in obese subjects. Of particular interest are the studies of Kneebone (1968). He divided obese children into two groups based on the percentage of fall in plasma free fatty acids 30 minutes after oral glucose. Those children that failed to drop were labeled the "metabolic obese." This group responded poorly to diet alone, but had a significant loss of weight when T_3 was added to the dietary program (Gwinup and Poucher, 1967; Hollingsworth et al., 1970).

The mechanism for this enhanced weight loss during treatment with thyroid hormones resides in two effects: increased oxygen consumption and increased protein catabolism. Doses of triiodothyronine above 100 μg/day consistently increase metabolic rate of hospitalized obese patients (Bray et al., 1973). The effect is small but readily measured. Hollingsworth et al. (1970) gave T_3 to hospitalized obese patients and observed an increased rate of weight loss during the early phases of treatment. Oxygen consumption was also increased.

Thyroid hormones also increase nitrogen excretion (Ball et al., 1967; Bray et al., 1971, 1973; Kyle et al., 1966). Within the first days after hormone administration, there is increased loss of nitrogen with onset of a negative or more negative nitrogen balance. This effect persists for at least 30 days, although it reaches its peak within the first 10 days (Bray et al., 1971). Whether nitrogen balance returns to normal after long term treatment with small doses of thyroid hormone is not known.

Two recent studies have shown that the loss of nitrogen can be prevented. In one of these, anabolic steroids and growth hormone were used to prevent the loss of nitrogen induced by treatment with triiodothyronine (Bray et al., 1971). Prevention of the negative nitrogen balance with these drugs did not reduce the consumption of oxygen. Thus under these conditions all of the incremental calories came from the catabolism of fat. In the other report, the loss of nitrogen was prevented by increasing the dietary intake of protein (Lamki et al., 1973). The effects of 180 and 540 mg of thyroid on nitrogen balance were examined in 4 patients on a 600 or 1200 calorie diet. The rate of weight loss was comparable, using 180 mg of thyroid with 600-calorie intake or 540 mg of thyroid and 1200-calorie intake. The nitrogen balance was maintained in both groups, but the authors felt that the patients were happier on the higher dose of thyroid.

The contribution of fat and nitrogen to the enhanced catabolism during treatment with T_3 is shown in Figure 9–18 (Bray et al., 1973). Approximately two thirds of the increment in oxygen utilized during T_3 administration is related to the catabolism of fat and the remaining one third to the catabolism of protein. In terms of weight loss, however, more than two thirds of the increment is due to breakdown of lean body mass. As the initial burst of protein catabolism subsides, weight loss declines. The observations of Gordon et al. (1963), Kneebone (1968), and Gelvin et al. (1959) suggest that obese patients may respond differently to T_3 and thyroxine (T_4). To test this, we administered T_3, 200 μg/day, for 30 days followed by T_4, 800 μg/day, to two obese patients. The effects on oxygen consumption, nitrogen excretion and the excretion of potassium were comparable (Bray et al., 1971).

Data from a number of laboratories suggest that doses of T_3 in excess of 150 μg/day often do not produce the expected clinical symptoms of hypermetabolism in some obese patients (Bray, 1969b; Hollingsworth et al., 1970; Drenick and Fisler, 1970; Cornman and Alexander, 1965; Danowski et al., 1964). To evaluate this observation further, we utilized a randomized, double blind crossover design to

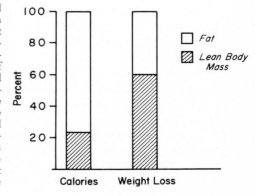

Figure 9–18. Contribution of fat and nitrogen to the caloric consumption and weight loss during treatment with triiodothyronine. The bars represent the distribution between endogenous fat and lean body mass of the incremental calories consumed during treatment with triiodothyronine. Metabolic expenditure (oxygen consumption) of six obese subjects was measured before and after treatment with triiodothyronine. Seventy five percent of this increment in caloric expenditure came from fat, but catabolism of fat accounted for only 40 percent of the weight loss.

treat 12 obese patients. They received triiodothyronine (T_3), 225 μg/day, or placebo for one month, then they received the other drug. All patients showed objective alterations in metabolism, including slight tachycardia and increased concentration of plasma tyrosine (Bray et al., 1973). (Tyrosine was used because it is increased by thyroid hormones.) Serum T_3 was increased, thyroxine decreased and the uptake of radioactive iodine by the thyroid gland was suppressed.

Each patient was evaluated twice during treatment with T_3 and twice while receiving placebo. An objective rating was used to assess symptoms. Half of the patients showed no symptoms during treatment with T_3. Using the objective measures, we noted that the asymptomatic patients (i.e., those who had had no symptoms on T_3) had less weight loss and a smaller rise in heart rate than those who had had symptoms with T_3. These findings suggest that, for evaluating unwanted side effects, clinical criteria are relatively insensitive to the metabolic consequences of treatment with thyroid hormones in some obese patients.

A second explanation for the few physiologic effects of T_3 may be found in the relations between turnover of thyroid hormones and their effects on tissues. Berson and Yalow (1954) showed that the degradation of organic iodine (D) was related to approximately three times the square of the PBI [$D = 2.94$ (PBI).^{2}] If the entire source of thyroid is exogenous and this dose is doubled, the PBI (or thyroxine) would be expected to increase by the $\sqrt{2}$ or 1.4. To double the PBI would thus require a fourfold increase in ingested hormone. The biologic effects of a twofold increase in ingested hormone will depend on tissue sensitivity. If the relationship is a linear one, doubling of the absorbed hormone would produce a 1.4 fold increase in PBI and a corresponding increase in biologic effect. If biologic effects are also related to the log dose of the circulating thyroid hormone, then doubling the absorbed dose of thyroxine would produce less than a 1.4 fold rise in biologic effect.

From the above discussion, it is clear that thyroid hormones induce a number of changes in obese patients which will tend to enhance their weight loss. Although some of these effects are desirable, others are not, and these unwanted effects have been used as arguments against the safety of thyroid hormone in the treatment of obesity. One useful effect is the stimulation of oxygen consumption with increased utilization of endogenous fuel. However, the acceleration of protein catabolism and increased nitrogen excretion is undesirable. Although approximately two thirds of the extra calories expended as a result of treatment with T_3 result from the catabolism of fat (Bray et al., 1973), the majority of the early weight loss results from catabolism of protein. Recent studies by Lamki et al. (1973) have suggested that increasing the protein content of the diet can overcome this catabolic effect. If this is so, then losses of nitrogen can be prevented and are no drawback to the safety of thyroid hormones in treating obesity.

A more potentially dangerous side effect is the action of thyroid hormone to modify the chronotropic and inotropic properties of cardiac muscle (Freedberg and Hamolsky, 1974). Although the mechanism for these effects is not known, it is clear that treatment with thyroid hormones in experimental animals (Van Liere and Sizemore, 1971) and probably in man (Staffurth and Morrison, 1968) will increase the mass of the heart. Since obesity itself increases the work of the heart as well as its size (Alexander, 1965), the added cardiac load imposed by treatment with thyroid hormones could be detrimental. Indeed, the deleterious cardiac effects of D-thyroxine (a pharmacologic isomer of the naturally occurring L-thyroxine) observed when D-thyroxine is used to lower serum lipids in patients with atherosclerosis have led to its withdrawal from the trial of agents used in the Coronary Drug Project. (Stamler, 1972).

This project dealt with patients who had already had a myocardial infarction, so the conclusions may not apply to other people. To assess the toxicity of L-thyroxine, Asher (1972) reviewed the records of 7286 patients who had been treated with "diet pills," including thyroid; 39 of these patients had died. Twenty died of noncardiac causes and 19 from cardiac causes. Hypertension existed in 13 of these patients. From his review Asher felt that diet pills did not increase death rate. Unfortunately, this report is retrospective and is based on death certificates with all of their limitations. A prospective study is badly needed.

Finally, any beneficial effect of treatment with thyroid hormone must be evaluated in terms of long term weight loss as compared with other modes of treatment which do not use thyroid hormones (Harvey, 1973). From the data in the literature, an average of 25 percent of patients treated with diet alone will maintain a weight loss of more than 20 pounds at the end of one year (Stunkard and McLaren-Hume, 1959; Bray, 1970). In a paper about obese patients treated with a combination of thyroid and anorectic drugs, Asher and Dietz claimed that 38 percent lost more than 20 pounds and 10 percent lost more than 40 pounds (Asher and Dietz, 1972) (Fig. 9–19). Lyon and Dunlop (1932) and Gwinup and Poucher (1967) found a greater weight loss with thyroid preparations than with placebo. Two further reports suggest that thyroid preparations enhance the effect of anorectic drugs and augment weight loss (Gelvin et al., 1959; Kaplan and Jose, 1970).

However, behavior modification as an approach to treatment would appear to be better than either drug treatment or dietary treatment (Penick et al., 1971; Stunkard, 1972). Two reports have followed up patients previously treated with T_3 (Glennon, 1966; Goodman, 1969). In both, T_3 was initiated in low doses and increased stepwise.

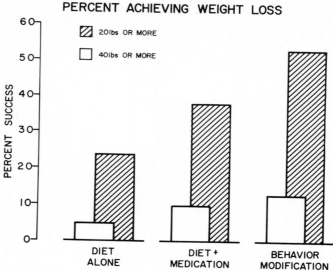

Figure 9–19. Comparison of weight loss by diet alone, diet with medication and behavior modification. The data from diet alone are those of Stunkard and McLaren-Hume (1959). The data on diet and medication are those of Asher and Dietz (1972) and the data on behavior modification are those of Penick et al. (1971). (See Chapter 8.) From Bray, G. A.; submitted for publication.

In Glennon's study the patients were started on treatment in the hospital. When they were re-evaluated two years later, 12 percent had maintained a weight loss of 20 pounds or more, and 6 percent had maintained a loss of more than 40 pounds; only one of 199 patients had approached her ideal weight. This outcome is no better than that achieved with diet alone. A similar conclusion was reached by Goodman (1969) who treated 55 patients in two groups. Four of 28 in one group had maintained their 20 pound weight loss and two had maintained a 40 pound weight loss for one year.

Although one can look at these data as an indictment of all forms of therapy in obesity, there is a positive side. By the use of techniques of nutritional modification, eating habits and patterns of exercise can, indeed, be altered by sympathetic clinical management without drugs in a significant number of patients. Indeed, at the present time treatment with behavioral modification appears to be superior to other nonsurgical forms of therapy such as diet alone or diet and drugs for obesity (Stunkard, 1972).

DRUGS WHICH UNCOUPLE OXIDATIVE PHOSPHORYLATION

A number of chemicals can uncouple oxygen utilization from the production of ATP (adenosine triphosphate) by the mitochondria. One of these is thyroid hormone. Although the major mechanism by which thyroid hormones stimulate oxygen consumption is probably not by uncoupling oxidative phosphorylation, this can occur at very high concentrations. Dinitrophenol, another compound which uncouples oxidative phosphorylation, has been used to treat obese patients. It was originally introduced for the treatment of obesity in 1933 (Tainter et al., 1933, 1935). It acts by uncoupling oxidative phosphorylation in the mitochondria, which allows food stuffs to be oxidized without coupling this process with the generation of adenosine triphosphate (ATP). For this reason, heat is produced but fewer high energy phosphate bonds are generated. The metabolic machinery thus runs at an accelerated rate to provide the needed amounts of ATP.

Dinitrophenol was given an enthusiastic trial as a treatment for obesity, but its toxicity outweighed its therapeutic value as an antiobesity agent (Simons, 1953). Tainter and his colleagues treated 170 patients with an average dose of 340 mg/day. All patients experienced warmth and sweating. The average weight loss was 1.4 lbs/wk, with an overall average of 17.1 lbs. Bayer and Gray (1935) and Simkins (1937) also reported substantial weight loss when obese patients were treated with dinitrophenol. Unfortunately, side effects were common and serious. Skin rash occurred in up to 20 percent of the patients. A peripheral neuropathy and decreased taste for sweet and salty foods indicated significant neurologic side effects (Simkins, 1937; Tainter et al., 1935). The appearance of cataracts and an occasional death led to discontinuation of this drug (Simons, 1953; Masserman and Goldsmith, 1934).

Aspirin is a third compound that uncouples oxidative phosphorylation (Smith and Dawkins, 1971). It increases the uptake of oxygen by lean individuals and obese patients (Bray, unpublished observations). The dose required to produce this effect is similar in obese and lean individuals and is in the range which also produces ringing in the ears (tinnitus) (20mg/dl). In addition, aspirin has many other effects which limit its use in obesity (Collier, 1969). The possibility of a nontoxic drug which could reduce the efficiency of metabolic processes remains an attractive avenue for pharmaceutical exploration.

HUMAN CHORIONIC GONADOTROPIN

The use of chorionic gonadotropin and diet as a treatment for obesity were suggested by Simeons (1954, 1956). His concept and methods were subsequently enlarged into a book entitled *Pounds and Inches: A New Approach to Obesity*. In his early clinical work on the treatment of Fröhlich's syndrome (see Chapter 5—Hypothalamic Obesity), Simeons observed that treatment with chorionic gonadotropin was associated with a loss of the ravenous appetite which the subjects had, and in many instances caused a change in body configuration. This change in configuration occurred without necessarily producing a change in body weight.

From this original observation, Simeons initiated treatment of obese patients with a program which consisted of a 500 calorie diet* and daily injections of 125 iu of chorionic gonadotropin for a series of 20 to 40 injections. With this method, Simeons reported weight losses of 20 to 30 pounds in 40 days (1954). As a theoretical framework for his observation that body configuration as well as weight loss occurred, Simeons suggested that there were two kinds of fat: one of which was normal and one abnormal. Chorionic gonadotropin, he argued, was responsible for mobilization of this abnormal fat and its conversion to normal fat for metabolism.

Chemistry and Physiology

Chorionic gonadotropin is formed by the placenta of some mammals. It is released into the serum and is excreted in the urine during pregnancy. The blood concentrations or urinary levels can be used as a diagnostic test for the presence of pregnancy and for some forms of abnormal pregnancy. The biologic functions of chorionic gonadotropin are similar to those of the luteinizing hormone (LH) secreted by the pituitary (see Chapter 7). These two hormones have a similar peptide configuration, but chorionic gonadotropin differs by having a number of additional carbohydrate residues which slow the rate at which it is metabolized. During pregnancy HCG functions to maintain the corpus luteum which produces the steroidal hormones, including progesterone. The chemical preparations of chorionic gonadotropin which are sold are impure and contain minute amounts of a number of other substances in addition to HCG. The drug has been approved for treatment of menstrual dysfunction and for use in threatened abortion, but has not been approved for treatment of obesity.

The effects of chorionic gonadotropin on the metabolism of adipose tissue from experimental animals has been examined in one study (Fleigelman and Fried, 1970). In these experiments chorionic gonadotropin was given to rats, and the activity of three enzymes was measured in adipose tissue, liver and muscle. After treatment with HCG, the activity of lactate dehydrogenase (LDH), glucose 6-phosphate dehydrogenase (G6PD) and glycerol 3-phosphate dehydrogenase (GPD) was reduced in adipose tissue. In liver, there was a reduction in activity of glucose 6-phosphate dehydrogenase but not in

---

*Two meals each consisting of 100 g of lean meat (veal, beef, chicken breast or fish which was grilled or broiled), a low calorie vegetable salad without oil, an apple or orange, and an unsweetened rusk.

the other enzymes, and in muscle the activity of glycerol 3-phosphate dehydrogenase was reduced but the other two enzymes were unchanged. Although these experimental studies have never been confirmed, they raise the interesting possibility that chorionic gonadotropin may have a direct effect on adipose tissue, or may affect it indirectly through stimulation of steroid production.

Clinical Use of HCG in Obesity

The safety of chorionic gonadotropin at the doses which are used for treatment of obesity has rarely been questioned (Gusman, 1969; Hutton, 1970; Lebon, 1961). In a study by Craig et al. (1963), basal metabolism, protein bound iodine (PBI), blood sugar, serum cholesterol and lipids remained unchanged during treatment with HCG. The major question is whether this agent has any effectiveness as a treatment for obesity. A number of clinical trials have been performed to answer this question, and several of them are summarized in Table 9–10. Most of the studies were randomized double blind trials but one was single blinded, one was unblinded, and one was a "modified" double blinded in which the meaning of "modified" was never adequately explained. Dietary intakes in all but the study by Frank (1964), were 550 calories; the study by Frank used 1030 calories.

The study by Carne et al. (1961) was among the most interesting because they performed two separate comparisons. First they compared 12 patients receiving injections of saline with 10 patients receiving chorionic gonadotropin. In the second study he compared a group of 7 patients who received no injection with a control group who received injections of saline. From his studies two conclusions emerged. First, that patients receiving injections lost more weight than those receiving no injections; and second, that injections of chorionic gonadotropin were no more effective than injections of saline. Indeed, none of the published studies except the one by Asher and Harper (1973) has suggested that chorionic gonadotropin was more effective than placebo.

Asher and Harper (1973) reported 5 studies. In 4 of them the dropout rate was high and the weight loss was less than the expected 20 pounds. In spite of these drawbacks, there was no suggestion that the patients who received HCG did better than the controls. The fifth study showed a greater dropout rate among the control patients than among those treated with HCG. The average weight loss was greater in the treated patients, with a probability of $p < .05$. This means that one time in 20, patients receiving HCG will lose more weight than controls even if HCG is ineffective.

Frank (1964) compared hunger ratings in his patients and could find no reduction in hunger among those receiving HCG. On the other hand, Asher and Harper (1973) suggested that HCG might reduce

TABLE 9–10. *Studies Using Human Chorionic Gonadotropin (HCG) to Treat Obesity*

AUTHOR	YEAR	NUMBER ON HCG°		NO. OF CONTROL SUBJECTS	TREATMENT OF CONTROLS	DIET (kcal/DAY)
Sohar	1959		34	13	Saline	500 to 600
Hastrup	1960		20	18	No injections	500
Carne	1961	Study 1	13	12	Saline	500
		Study 2	–	11	Saline	
			–	10	No injections	
Craig	1963		11	9	Saline diluent	550
Frank	1964		63	30	Saline	1030
Lebon	1966		23	24	Saline	500
Asher	1973		20	20	Saline	550

°HCG 125 IU/day except Frank who used 200 IU/day.
†Average weight loss in 21 days was 9.6 lb for placebo and 13.0 lb for HCG treated patients.

hunger. A review of the published studies provides little support for the concept that chorionic gonadotropin is an effective agent in the treatment of obesity. Few would argue, however, that adhering to a 500 calorie diet for 40 days would be expected to produce a weight loss approximating one half pound (200 grams) per day or more. Hastrup et al. (1960) gave injections of HCG to one group of hospitalized patients eating a 500 calorie diet and found no difference in weight loss and no difference in the reports of hunger when compared with patients on the same diet receiving no injections.

The claim by Gusman, (1969) and Asher and Harper (1973) that HCG may diminish appetite or make it easier to adhere to a 500 calorie diet remains unsubstantiated. In unpublished studies from our laboratory, the effect of chorionic gonadotropin on the metabolic rate of hospitalized obese patients has been examined. Neither metabolic rate nor the rate of weight loss was significantly altered in two obese patients who were eating a 450 calorie diet, whether or not chorionic gonadotropin was given. In summary then, injections of HCG have not been shown to have any role in the weight loss achieved by obese patients eating a 500 calorie diet.

TABLE 9–10. *Studies Using Human Chorionic
Gonadotropin (HCG) to Treat Obesity*

DESIGN	AVERAGE LOSS OF HCG	WEIGHT CONTROL	COMMENTS AND CONCLUSIONS
Single blind Injections at home	239.2 g/day	234.3 g/day	In 47 "successful trials" (those losing over 150 g/day) HCG had no effect.
Unblinded Inpatients treated 20 days	10.96 lb	12.49 lb	HCG had no effect on hospitalized patients.
Randomized double blind Randomized—(no injection group had 3 visits/week)	21.0 lb	19.0 lb 22.4 lb 17.7 lb	Injections were better than no injections, but HCG not better than saline.
Randomized—double blind	6.5 lb	8.8 lb	HCG had no demonstrable effect. Weight loss due to diet.
Double blind 3 injections/week	12.3 lb	11.5 lb	Changes in body measurements and ratings of hunger were the same in both groups. HCG had no effect.
Double blind	14.1 lb†	12.3 lb	HCG possibly effective.
Modified double blind (3 patients from each vial)	19.9 lb	11.05 lb	HCG possibly effective. Five of placebo group and none of HCG group received fewer than 21 injections.

GROWTH HORMONE

The physiology and chemistry of growth hormone have been reviewed in Chapter 7. This hormone is important during the processes of growth and differentiation. Its calorigenic effects, however, are less well known, although they have been described in careful studies on panhypopituitary subjects by Henneman et al. (1960). In experimental animals, growth hormone increases metabolic rate after thyroidectomy, indicating that its calorigenic effects are not mediated through the release of thyroid hormone. Because growth hormone is calorigenic and its concentration is low in obese patients (Chapter 7), it might be a useful hormone in the treatment of obesity. Administration of growth hormone to obese individuals at a dose of 5 mg per day produced a significant increase in metabolic rate (see Fig. 4–2). The rise in metabolic rate takes one to three days to occur, but thereafter basal metabolism remains elevated throughout the day.

While these studies on growth hormones were in progress, Josimovich and MacLaren (1962) and Friesen (1968) isolated a protein from the human placenta which was similar to human growth hormone in its immunologic properties and in some of its physiologic actions. Because this protein was present in much greater quantities than growth hormone, we decided to compare the effects of 400 mg of the purified placental protein (PPP — also called placental somatomammotropin or placental lactogen) with 5 mg of growth hormone.

Grossly obese subjects were treated for eight days, were withdrawn from all drug therapy for eight days, and then treated for a second period of eight days with 5 mg of growth hormone. For half of the patients, the growth hormone treatment was first, and for the other half the placental lactogen was first (Fig. 9–20). Growth hormone increased oxygen uptake and reduced the loss of nitrogen in all eight patients, but placental lactogen had no detectable effect. The mechanism for the rise in oxygen uptake during treatment with growth hormone has not been established (Bray, 1969a), but it does not depend on the secretion or presence of thyroid hormone. This effect might be mediated by the release of free fatty acids.

A rise in the concentration in the free fatty acids could stimulate oxygen utilization in a manner similar to that observed in heart muscle in the studies performed by Challoner and Steinberg (1966). Whatever its mechanism, the calorigenic effects of growth hormone and the lack of calorigenic effect of placental lactogen are of considerable interest. Challoner and Steinberg raised the possibility that calorigenic hormones which have no significant detrimental effect on nitrogen loss might indeed be prepared, or that a compound which release growth hormone might be developed.

GLUCAGON

The physiology of glucagon has been reviewed in Chapter 7. This peptide, which contains 39 amino acids, is produced by the alpha cells of the Langerhans and is primarily a hormone of "glucose need." Two observations suggest a potential use in the treatment of obesity. The first of these are the experiments of Sudsaneh and Mayer (1959), in which they demonstrated that injections of glucagon into normal rats diminished gastric mobility and decreased food intake. This was followed by one careful clinical study in which glucagon was associated with a reduction in food intake (Schulman et al., 1957).

In this study, 10 hospitalized patients received an injection of glucagon (1 mg) or placebo prior to their mealtime three times a day for one week. The study was a double blind, crossover in which half the patients received the placebo injection first while the other half received glucagon. Caloric intake decreased by an average of 440 kCal/day (p <.001) during the treatment with glucagon. Intake of all foods was reduced. There was also a significant difference in weight. During treatment with glucagon there was an overall loss of 0.45

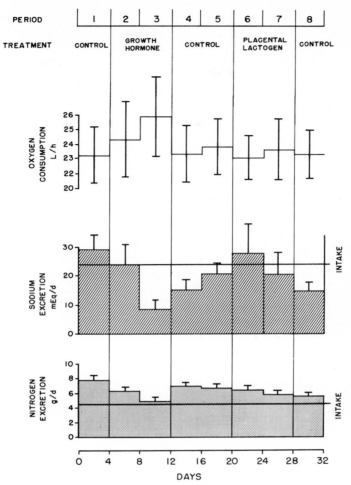

Figure 9-20. Effect on growth hormone and placental lactogen on obese patients. Eight obese women received placental lactogen (400 mg/day) or growth hormone (5 mg/day) for 2 periods of 4 days each. Growth hormone increased oxygen consumption and reduced nitrogen and sodium excretion, but placental lactogen did not.

pounds, and on placebo a gain of 3.4 pounds (p <.05). There are no studies using glucagon as an agent for treatment of obesity.

PROGESTERONE

Progesterone is a steroid produced by all steroid-producing tissues and is the principal hormone secreted by the ovary during the postovulatory phase of the menstrual cycle. This hormone increases the rate of breathing and, by so doing, produces a mild respiratory alkalosis. For this reason, it was tried in obese patients with alveolar hypoventilation (see Chapter 6). Lyons and Huang (1968) showed that during treatment with this compound there was a significant increase in ventilatory capacity, and a reduction in the respiratory acidosis associated with alveolar hypoventilation in obese patients. However, this effect has not been confirmed in other laboratories and its usefulness is therefore open to question.

MISCELLANEOUS AGENTS

Biguanides

Metformin and phenformin are hypoglycemic drugs used in the treatment of diabetes mellitus. The mechanism by which they lower blood sugar is unknown. When these drugs were given to obese diabetic patients, some authors noted that the treated patients lost more weight than patients treated with the sulfonylurea drugs (Clark and Duncan, 1968; Duncan et al., 1969; Stowers and Bewsher, 1969). Other trials, however, have failed to confirm this effect. Hart and Cohen (1970) used a crossover, double blind design to compare phenformin and placebo. Weight loss was greater in the first three months than in the second three months of this six month trial, but there was no significant effect of phenformin on the 50 patients who were studied. Munro et al. (1969) found a marginally greater effect which was statistically significant for the first 12 weeks, but not during the final 4 weeks of treatment.

Strong and Lawson (1970) compared the effects of metformin and fenfluramine. There was a slightly greater weight loss with the lower dose of metformin, but patients on the higher dose had no more weight loss than the placebo treated patients. In the same study, fenfluramine had a significant effect on weight loss. In studies on this action of metformin, Pederson (1965) and Pederson and Olesen (1968) demonstrated that this drug increased weight loss in hospitalized patients maintained on a constant dietary intake, but that when the drug was discontinued there was a rebound with weight returning to the predicted line of weight loss. They suggested that the drug might be acting to increase fluid loss in the treated patients. Finally, Czyzk et al. (1968) demonstrated that the biguanides may decrease intestinal absorption of glucose in both men and animals. This effect may have significance related to our discussion of agents affecting intestinal absorption.

Agents Which Impair Intestinal Absorption

The success of intestinal bypass operations in the treatment for obesity has led to the search for oral agents which might produce a medically reversible form of altered intestinal absorption (see Chapter 10). As noted above, biguanides impair the absorption of glucose. The evidence reviewed in Chapter 2 shows that there are glucose receptors in the intestinal mucosa. The work of Soulairac (1967) showed that the experimental manipulations which depress glucose absorption also depress food intake. The possibility of inhibiting food intake by interfering with intestinal absorption of glucose thus merits intensive pharmaceutical investigation.

Another approach to manipulating intestinal absorption has focused on the possibility of producing decreased fat absorption and steatorrhea, (Goldsmith et al., 1960; Bray and Gallagher, 1968). Several groups of investigators have demonstrated that neomycin increases the loss of fat in the stools. In doses of 6 to 12 grams, this drug consistently produces steatorrhea (Faloon et al., 1966). Hvidt and Kjeldsen (1963) have demonstrated that a dose as low as 3 grams per day can impair fat absorption in 5 out of ten patients. This principle may be applicable to the treatment of obesity, but this particular drug is limited by the fact that doses of neomycin which are associated with steatorrhea produce morphologic alteration in the intestinal mucosa. Because obesity is a chronic condition, the possibility that irreversible alteration in intestinal absorption might occur limits the use of these agents, (Dobbins et al., 1968).

Cholestyramine is a second drug which produces steatorrhea. This ion-exchange resin binds bile acids in the intestine and leads to increased fecal excretion of fat. In studies to examine the relationship between cholestyramine and fecal fat excretion, we hospitalized two grossly obese patients in the Clinical Research Center (Fig. 9–21). Each patient was maintained on a 1200 calorie diet in which 80 percent of the calories were provided as fat. Cholestyramine in doses of 36 grams per day was administered to each of these patients for 9 days. There was a significant increase in fat excretion during the period of treatment with cholestyramine, but the loss of fat in the stools was disappointingly low.

Campbell, Juhl and Quaade (1970) have similarly demonstrated that 30 grams of cholestyramine daily can increase the fecal fat excretion by threefold in six obese patients. In one unpublished study, the effectiveness of cholestyramine was evaluated in an obesity clinic. Patients failed to lose significant amounts of weight because of the large quantity of relatively unpleasant tasting resin required to produce the desired effect. Thus, at present, the available agents for decreasing fat absorption and producing malabsorption have not proven to be effective in dealing with the problem of obesity.

Feeding indigestible fats is another approach to inducing reversible malabsorption. The triglyceride of stearic acid, for example, is insoluble, poorly absorbed and would be difficult to dissolve. Better success, however, has been noted with hexaglyceride in which 6 fatty

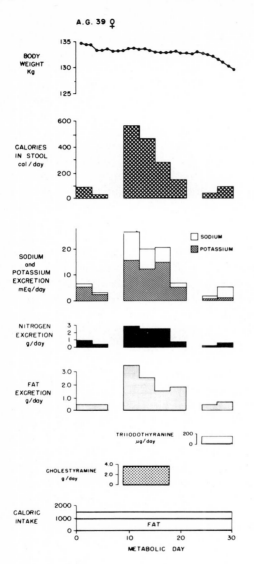

Figure 9–21. Effect of cholestyramine on body weight and fecal fat of one obese patient. Cholestyramine 36 g/day produced a disappointingly small rise in fecal fat excretion.

acids are esterified with a cyclic hexa-alcohol. This structure can be made to taste and behave like the usual fats except that they cannot be digested. Thus they appear in the stools as undigested fat. This approach obviously merits intensive evaluation.

Digitalis

For many years digitalis was used in the treatment of obesity, (Bram, 1940). It was originally introduced to diminish the heart rate of patients receiving thyroid hormone. In a careful study by Asher and Dietz, (1972) on office patients, digitalis was shown to be without effect on heart rate and to have no effect in enhancing rate of weight loss. Thus there is no indication for using digitalis as a primary treatment in obesity. Similarly the use of diuretics for obese patients in the absence of detectable edema or congestive heart failure seems unwarranted.

Bulk Fillers

Methylcellulose has been used for the suppression of appetite because it swells in the stomach. This agent, however, swells relatively slowly and it is thought unlikely that it would diminish appetite significantly. Thus these agents are better laxatives than anorexiants. In one trial by Duncan et al. (1969), this agent produced relatively little weight loss in refractory obese patients when compared with placebo or with phenmetrazine. Badham (1953) in a letter to *Lancet*, however, suggested that this agent might be helpful in a weight losing regimen. However, his study had no control and is thus open to question. A reliable study remains to be conducted. One early report suggested that belladonna alkaloids might reduce food intake but this has not been confirmed (Greene, 1940).

L-Dopa

This substance is an intermediate in the synthesis of dopamine, norepinephrine and epinephrine (see Fig. 9–1). Because L-Dopa can enter the brain, it has been used to provide a precursor for dopamine in the treatment of Parkinsonism, a neurologic disorder. When dose levels get too high, nausea is one of the undesirable side effects of this drug. Quaade (1974) has explored the possibility that this drug might produce nausea in obese patients and thus be a useful drug in treating obesity. The obese patients who were treated did not lose a significant amount of weight.

Hydroxycitrate

The final agent for discussion is hydroxycitrate (Sullivan et al., 1974). (-)-Hydroxycitrate, one of the isomers of this compound, is a potent inhibitor of citrate-cleavage enzyme which catalyzes the conversion of citrate to acetyl-CoA and oxaloacetate. This enzymatic conversion stands at a crucial position in the synthesis of fatty acids. When this compound was fed to animals in nontoxic doses for 11 to 30 days, it caused a significant reduction in food intake and body weight. At present this compound has not been tried in human beings, but it offers a new avenue for future exploration.

REFERENCES

Adlersberg, D. and Mayer, E.: Results of prolonged medical treatment of obesity with diet alone, diet and thyroid preparations and diet and amphetamine. J. Clin. Endocrinol., 9:275–284, 1949.

Albrecht, F. K.: The use of benzedine sulfate in obesity. Ann. Intern. Med., 21:983–989, 1944.

Alexander, J. K.: Chronic heart disease due to obesity. J. Chronic. Dis., 18:895–898, 1965.

Alfaro, R. D., Gracanin, V. and Schlueter, E.: A clinical pharmacologic evaluation of diethylpropion. Lancet, 80:526–530, 1960.

Anden, N. E.: Effects of amphetamine and some other drugs on central catecholamine mechanisms. In: Amphetamines and related compounds; Proc. Mario Negri Instit. Pharmacol. Res. Italy; (Costa, E. and Garattini, S. eds.,) New York, Raven Press, pp. 447–462, 1970.

Angrist, B., Shopsin, B., Gershon, S. and Wilk, S.: Metabolites of monoamines in urine and cerebrospinal fluid, after large dose amphetamine administration. Psychopharmacol., 26:1–9, 1972.

Asher, W. L.: Mortality rate in patients receiving "diet pills." Curr. Ther. Res., 14:525–539, 1972.

Asher, W. L.: Voranil: A new anorexigenic. In: Treating the Obese. (Asher, W. L. ed.) New York, Medcom Press, p. 132–136, 1974.

Asher, W. L. and Harper, H. W.: Effect of human chorionic gonadotropin on weight loss, hunger and feeling of well-being. Am. J. Clin. Nutr., 26:211–218, 1973.

Asher, W. L. and Dietz, R. E.: Effectiveness of weight reduction involving "diet pills." Curr. Ther. Res., 14:510–524, 1972.

Axelrod, J.: Amphetamine: metabolism, physiological disposition and its effects on catecholamine storage. In: Amphetamines and Related Compounds. Proc. Mario Negri Instit. Pharmacol. Res., Italy; (Costa, E. and Garattini, S., eds.) New York, Raven Press, pp. 207–216, 1970.

Badham, J. N.: Methylcellulose for obesity. Lancet, 2:1316, 1953.

Ball, M. F., Kyle, L. H. and Canary, J. J.: Comparative effects of caloric restriction and metabolic acceleration of body composition in obesity. J. Clin. Endocrinol., 27:273–278, 1967.

Bayer, L. M. and Gray, H.: Obesity treatment by diet, thyroid and dinitrophenol; results on 106 outpatients. Am. J. Med. Sci., 189:86–91, 1935.

Beckett, A. H. and Brookes, L. G.: The effect of chain and ring substitution on the metabolism, distribution and biological action of amphetamines. In: Amphetamines and Related Compounds. Proc. Mario Negri Instit. Pharmacol. Res., Italy. (Costa, E. and Garattini, S. eds.) New York, Raven Press, pp. 109–120, 1970.

Benoit, F. L. and Durrance, F. Y.: Radiothyroxine turnover in obesity. Am. J. Med. Sci., 249:647–653, 1965.

Beregi, L. G., Hugon, P., LeDouarec, J. C., Laubie, M. and Duhault, J.: Structure-activity relationship in CF_3 substituted phenethylamines. In: Amphetamines and Related Compounds. Proc. Mario Negri Instit. Pharmacol. Res., Italy. (Costa, E. and Garattini, S., eds.) New York, Raven Press, p. 21–61, 1970.

Berneike, K. H.: Further studies on the medical treatment of obesity with Preludin. Med. Klin., 50:494–495, 1955.

Berry, R. L.: Obesity treatment of complicated and uncomplicated cases with chlorphentermine hydrochloride. Indust. Med. Surg., 34:490–492, 1965.

Berson, S. A. and Yalow, R. S.: Quantitative aspects of iodine metabolism. Exchangeable organic iodine pool, and the rates of thyroidal secretion, peripheral degradation and fecal excretion of endogenously synthesized organically bound iodine. J. Clin. Invest., 33:1533–1552, 1954.

Bethell, M. F.: Toxic psychosis caused by Preludin. Br. Med. J., 1:30–31, 1957.

Biel, J. H.: Structure-activity relationship of amphetamine and derivatives. In: Amphetamines and Related Compounds; Proceedings of the Mario Negri Institute for Pharmacological Research, Italy. (Costa, E. and Garattini, S., eds.) New York, Raven Press, pp. 3–19, 1970.

Bizzi, A., Bonaccorsi, A., Jespersen, S., Jori, A. and Garattini, S.: Pharmacological studies on amphetamine and fenfluramine. In: Amphetamines and Related Compounds; Proc. Mario Negri Instit. Pharmacol. Res./Italy. (Costa, E. and Garattini, S., eds.) New York, Raven Press, pp. 577–595, 1970.

Bliss, P. B., Kirk, C. J. C. and Newall, R. G.: The effect of fenfluramine on glucose tolerance, insulin, lipid and lipoprotein levels in patients with peripheral arterial disease. Postgrad. Med. J., 48:409–413, 1972.

Boileau, P. A.: Control of weight gain during pregnancy: use of diethylpropion hydrochloride. Appl. Ther., 10:763–765, 1968.

Boothby, W. M. and Sandiford, I.: Summary of the basal metabolism data on 8614 subjects with special reference to the normal standards for estimation of the basal metabolic rate. J. Biol. Chem., 54:783–803, 1922.

Bose, A.: Low calorie intake in post-operative convalescence. Trial with diethylpropion as an adjunct. Clin. Trial., 6:167, 1969.

Boxer, E. I., Chalmers, R. B., Craddock, D., Davies, D. J., Stewart, J. M., Sydenham, J. T. and Wheatley, D.: Two new anorexian drugs. Practitioner, 187:214–218, 1961.

Bram, I.: Digitalis in dietary treatment of obesity. Report of 140 cases. Med. Rec., 151:131–132, 1940.

Bray, G. A.: Calorigenic effect of human growth hormone in obesity. J. Clin. Endocrinol. Metab., 29:119–122, 1969a.

Bray, G. A.: The myth of diet in the management of obesity. Am. J. Clin. Nutr., 23:1141–1148, 1970.

Bray, G. A., Raben, M. S., Londono, J. and Gallagher, T. F., Jr.: Effects of triiodothyronine, growth hormone and anabolic steroids on nitrogen excretion and oxygen consumption of obese patients. J. Clin. Endocrinol., 33:293–300, 1971.

Bray, G. A., Schwartz, M., Rozin, R. R. and Lister, J.: Relationships between oxygen consumption and body composition of obese patients. Metabolism, 19:418–429, 1970.

Bray, G. A.: Effect of diet and triiodothyronine on the activity of sn-glycerol-3-phosphate dehydrogenase and on the metabolism of glucose and pyruvate by adipose tissue of obese patients. J. Clin. Invest., 48:1413–1422, 1969b.

Bray, G. A., Melvin, K. E. W. and Chopra, I. J.: Effect of triiodothyronine on some metabolic responses of obese patients. Am. J. Clin. Nutr., 26:715–721, 1973.

Bray, G. A., and Gallagher, T. F.: Suppression of appetite by bile acids. Lancet, 1:1066, 1968.

Burland, W. L.: Review of experience with fenfluramine. In: Obesity in Perspective. Fogarty International Center Series on Preventive Medicine, Vol. II, Part II. (Bray, G. A. ed.) Washington, D.C., U.S. Government Printing Office. 1976, pp. 429–440.

Campbell, U. D., Juhl E. and Quaade, F.: Treatment of obesity with cholestyramine. Nord. Med., 84:1628–1629, 1970.

Carlsson, A.: Amphetamine and brain catecholamines. In: Amphetamines and Related Compounds. Proc. Mario Negri Instit. Pharmacol. Res., Italy. (Costa, E. and Garattini, S., eds.), New York, Raven Press, pp. 289–300, 1970.

Carne, S.: The action of chorionic gonadotrophin in the obese. Lancet, 2:1282–1284, 1961.

Cass, L. J.: Evaluation of phendimetrazine bitartrate as an appetite suppressant. Can. Med. Assoc. J., 84:1114–1116, 1962.

Challoner, D. R. and Steinberg, D.: Oxidative metabolism of myocardium as influenced by fatty acids and epinephrine. Am. J. Physiol., 211:897–902, 1966.

Clarke, B. F. and Duncan, L. J. P.: Comparison of chlorpropamide and metformin treatment on weight and blood glucose response of uncontrolled obese diabetics. Lancet, 1:123–126, 1968.

Clein, L. J. and Benady, D. R.: Case of diethylpropion addiction (letter). Br. Med. J., 2:456, 1962.

Collier, H. O. J.: A pharmacological analysis of aspirin. Adv. Pharmacol. Chem. Ther., 7:333–405, 1969.

Copinschi, G., Wegienka, L. C., Hane, S. and Forsham, P. H.: Effect of arginine on serum levels of insulin and growth hormone in obese subjects. Metabolism, 16:485–491, 1967.

Cornman, D. and Alexander, F.: Effects of l-triiodothyronine alone in the treatment of obesity. Fed. Proc., 24:189, 1965 (abs).

Craig, L. S., Ray, R. E., Waxler, S. H. and Madigan, H.: Chorionic gonadotrophin in the treatment of obese women. Am. J. Clin. Nutr., 12:230–234, 1963.

Croughs, W., Visser, H. K. A. and Woldring, M. G.: Studies of thyroxine secretion and degradation rate in children with different thyroidal functional states. Comparison of thyroid function in children and adults. J. Pediatr., 67:343–352, 1965.

Cunningham, G. L. W.: Diethylpropion in the treatment of obesity. J. Coll. Gen. Pract., 39:347–349, 1963.

Czyzk, A., Tawecki, J., Sandowski, J. and Ponikowska, I.: Effect of biguanides on intestinal absorption of glucose. Diabetes, 17:492–498, 1968.

Danowski, T. S., Sarver, M. E., D'Ambrosia, R. D. and Moses, C.: Hydrocortisone and/or desiccated thyroid in physiologic dosage. X. Effects of thyroid hormone excesses on clinical status and thyroid indices. Metabolism, 13:702–716, 1964.

Decina, L. and Tanyol, H.: Treatment of obesity with a new anorexiant, diethylpropion without special stress on diet. N.Y. State, J. Med., 60:2702–2705, 1960.

DeFelice, E. A., Bronstein, S. and Cohen, A.: Double blind comparison of placebo and 42–548, a new appetite suppressant in obese volunteers. Curr. Ther. Res., 11:256–262, 1969.

Dobbins, W. O., III, Herrero, B. A. and Mansbach, C. M.: Morphologic alterations associated with neomycin induced malabsorption. Am. J. Med. Sci., 255:63–77, 1968.

Domino, E. F., Albers, J. W., Potvin, A. R., Repa, B. S. and Tourtellotte, W. W.: Effects of d-amphetamine on quantitative measures of motor performance. Clin. Pharmacol. Ther., 13(2):251–257, 1972.

Drenick, D. J. and Fisler, J. L.: Prevention of recurrent weight gain with large doses of thyroid hormones. Curr. Ther. Res., 12:570–576, 1970.

Duckman, S., Chen, W. and Weir, J. H.: Double blind evaluation of chlorphentermine hydrochloride versus placebo in postpartum weight control. Curr. Ther. Res., 10:619–625, 1968.

Duncan, L. J., Clarke, B. F. and Munro, J. F.: The effect of biguanide treatment on body weight in diabetics and non-diabetics. Postgrad. Med. J., 45:13, 1969.

Edison, G. R.: Amphetamines: A dangerous illusion. Ann. Intern. Med., 74:605–610, 1971.

Edwards, D. A. W. and Swyer, G. I. M.: Comparative values of dextroamphetamine sulphate, dried thyroid gland and placebo in the treatment of obesity. Clin. Sci., 9:115–126, 1950.

El-Khodary, A. Z., Ball, M. F., Oweiss, I. M. and Canary, J. J.: Insulin secretion and body composition in obesity. Metabolism, 21:641–655, 1972.

Ersner, J. S.: The treatment of obesity due to dietary indiscretion (over-eating) with Benzedine Sulfate. Endocrinology, 27:776–780, 1940.

Faloon, W. W., Paes, I. C., Woolfolk, D., Nankin, H., Wallace, K. and Haro, E. N.: Effects of neomycin and kanakycin upon intestinal absorption. Ann. N.Y. Acad. Sci., 132:879–887, 1966.

Feinstein, Alvan R.: The treatment of obesity, an analysis of methods, results and factors which influence success. J. Chronic Dis., 11:349–393, 1960.

Fineberg, S. K.: An appraisal of anorexiants in the treatment of obesity. J. Am. Geriat. Soc., 20:576–579, 1972.

Fineberg, S. K.: Evaluation of anorexigenic agents. Studies with chlorphentermine. Am. J. Clin. Nutr., 11:509–516, 1962.

Fleigelman, R. and Fried, G. H.: Metabolic effects of human chorionic gonadotropin (HCG) in rats. Proc. Soc. Exp. Biol. Med., 135:317–319, 1970.

Follath, F., Burkart, F. and Schweizer, W.: Drug-induced pulmonary hypertension? Br. Med. J., 1:265–266, 1971.

Follows, O. J.: A comparative trial of fenfluramine and diethylpropion in obese hypertensive patients. Br. J. Clin. Pract., 25:236–238, 1971.

Frank, B. W.: The use of chorionic gonadotropin hormone in the treatment of obesity. Am. J. Clin. Nutr., 14:133–136, 1964.

Freed, S. C. and Mizel, M.: The use of amphetamine combinations for appetite suppression. Ann. Intern. Med., 36:1492–1497, 1952.

Freedberg, A. S. and Hamolsky, M. W.: Effects of thyroid hormones on certain nonendocrine organ systems. In: Handbook of Physiology, Section 7: Endocrinology, Volume III Thyroid (Geiger, S. R., Ed.) Am. Physiol. Soc. Washington, D.C., 1974, pp. 435–468.

Friesen, H. G., Suwa, S. and Pare, P.: Synthesis and secretion of placental lactogen and other proteins by the placenta. Rec. Prog. Hor. Res., 25:161–188, 1968.

Gadek, R. J., Feldman, H. S. and Lucariello, R. J.: Study of l-phenyl-2-aminopropane alginate (levonor), New anorectic. J.A.M.A., 167:433–437, 1958.

Galton, D. J. and Bray, G. A.: Metabolism of α-glycerol phosphate in human adipose tissue in obesity. J. Clin. Endocrinol. Metab., 27:1573–1580, 1967.

Garattini, S.: Recent advances in the pharmacology of anorectic agents. *In:* Recent Advances in Obesity Research: I. Proceedings of the First International Congress on Obesity. London, Newman Publishing, 1975, pp. 354–367.

Garattini, S., Bonaccorsi, A., Jori, A. and Samanin, R.: Appetite suppressant drugs: past, present and future. *In:* Obesity: Causes, Consequences and Treatment. (Lasagna, L. ed.), New York, Medcom Press, 1974, pp. 70–80.

Garrow, J. S., Belton, E. A. and Daniels, A.: A controlled investigation of the glycolyptic action of fenfluramine. Lancet, 2:559–561, 1972.

Gelvin, E. P., Kenigsberg, S. and Boyd, L. J.: Results of addition of liothyronine to a weight-reducing regimen. J.A.M.A., 170:1507–1512, 1959.

Gelvin, E. P. and McGavack, T. H.: Dexedrine and weight reduction, N.Y. State J. Med., 49:279–282, 1949.

Gelvin, E. P., McGavack, T. H. and Kenigsberg, S.: Alpha-(2-Piperidyl)-benzhydro-hydrochloride. (Pipradrol) as an adjunct in the dietary management of obesity. N.Y. State J. Med., 55:2336–2338, 1955.

Gelvin, E. P., McGavack, T. H. and Kenigsberg, S.: Phenmetrazine in the management of obesity. Am. J. Digest, Dis., 1:155–159, 1956.

Glennon, J. A. and Brech, W. J.: Serum protein bound iodine in obesity. J. Clin. Endocrinol., 25:1673–1674, 1965.

Glennon, J. A.: Weight reduction–An enigma. Arch. Intern. Med., 118:1–2, 1966.

Glowinski, J.: Effects of amphetamine on various aspects of catecholamine metabolism in the central nervous system of the rat. *In:* Amphetamines and Related Compounds; Proc. Mario Negri Instit. Pharmacol. Res., Italy. (Costa, E. and Garattini, S., eds.), New York, Raven Press, pp. 301–316, 1970.

Goldrick, R. B., Havenstein, N. and Whyte, H. M.: Effect of caloric restriction and fenfluramine in weight loss and personality profile of patients with long standing obesity. Aust. N.Z. J. Med., 3:131–141, 1973.

Goldsmith, G. A., Hamilton, J. G. and Miller, O. N.: Lowering of serum lipid concentrations: mechanisms used by unsaturated fats, nicotinic acid and neomycin: Excretion of strerols and bile acids. Arch. Intern. Med., 105:512–517, 1960.

Goodman, E. L. and Housel, E. L.: The effect of d-amphetamine sulfate in the treatment of the obese hypertensive patient. Am. J. Med. Sci., 227: 250–254, 1954.

Goodman, N. G.: Triiodothyronine and placebo in the treatment of obesity. A study of fifty-five patients. Med. Ann. D. C., 38:658–662, 1969.

Gordon, E. S., Goldberg, M, and Chosy, G. J.: A new concept in the treatment of obesity. J.A.M.A., 186:156–166, 1963.

Götestam, K. G. and Gunne, L. M.: Subjective effects of two anorexigenic agents, fenfluramine and AN 448 in amphetamine-dependent subjects. Br. J. Addict., 67:39–44, 1972.

Greene, J. A.: Effect of belladonna on appetite of patients with obesity and with other diseases. J. Lab. Clin. Med., 26:477–478, 1940.

Groppetti, A., Misher, A., Naimzada, M., Revuelta, A., Costa, E.: Evidence that in rats l-benzyl-β-methoxy-3-trifluoromethyl-phenethylamine (SK & F 1-39728) dissociates anorexia from central stimulation and actions on brain monoamine stores. J. Pharmacol. Exp. Ther., 182:464–473, 1972.

Gross, J. and Pitt-Rivers, R. H.: Physiological activity of 3:5:3'-L-triiodothyronine. Lancet, 1:593–594, 1952.

Gusman, H. A.: Chorionic gonadotropin in obesity: further clinical observations. Am. J. Clin. Nutr., 22:686–695, 1969.

Gwinup, G. and Poucher, R.: A controlled study of thyroid analogs in the therapy of obesity. Am. J. Med. Sci., 254:416–420, 1967.

Hadler, A. J.: Weight reduction with phenmetrazine: a double-blind study. Curr. Therap. Res., 9:462–467, 1967a.

Hadler, A. J.: Studies of aminorex: A new anorexigenic agent. J. Clin. Pharmacol., 7:296–302, 1967b.

Hadler, A. J.: Sustained action phendimetrazine in obesity. J. Clin. Pharmacol., 8(2):113–117, 1968.

Hadler, A. J.: Mazindol, a new non-amphetamine anorexigenic agent. J. Clin. Pharmacol., 12:453–458, 1972.

Hampson, J., Loraine, J. A. and Strong, J. A.: Phenmetrazine and dexamphetamine in the management of obesity. Lancet, 1:1265–1267, 1960.

Harris, S. C., Ivy, A. C. and Searle, L. M.: The mechanism of amphetamine-induced loss of weight. J.A.M.A., *134*:1468–1475, 1947.

Hart, A. and Cohen, H.: Treatment of obese non-diabetic patients with phenformin. A double-blind crossover trial. Br. Med. J., *1*:222–24, 1970.

Harvey, R. F.: Thyroxine "addicts." Br. Med. J., *2*:35–36, 1973.

Hastrup, B., Nielsen, B. and Skouby, A. P.: Chorionic gonadotropin and the treatment of obesity. Acta Med. Scand., *168*:25–57, 1960.

Heil, G. and Ross, S.: Chemical agents affecting appetite. *In:* Obesity in Perspective. Fogarty International Center Series on Preventive Medicine, Vol. II, Part II. (Bray, G. A. ed.) Washington, D.C., U.S. Government Printing Office. 1976, pp. 409–418.

Henneman, P. H., Forbes, A. P., Moldawerm, M., Dempsey, E. F. and Carroll, E. L.: Effects of human growth hormone in man. J. Clin. Invest., *39*:1223–1228, 1960.

Henry, R. C.: Weight reduction pills. J.A.M.A., *201*:895–896, 1967.

Hirsh, L. S.: Reducing appetite in treating obesity; a rational use for propadrine hydrochloride. Ohio State Med. J., *36*:742–743, 1940.

Hoebel, B. G.: Satiety: Hypothalamic stimulation, anorectic drugs and neurochemical substrates. *In:* Hunger: Basic Mechanisms and Clinical implications (Novin, D., Wyrwicka, W. and Bray, G. A., eds.), New York, Raven Press, 1976, pp. 33–50.

Hoebel, B. G., Cooper, J., Kamin, M. C. and Willard, D.: Appetite suppression by phentolamine in humans. Obesity Bar. Med., *4*:192–197, 1975a.

Hoebel, B. G., Krauss, I. K., Cooper, J. and Willard, D.: Body weight decreased in humans by phenylpropanolamine taken before meals. Obesity Bar. Med., *4*:200–206, 1975b.

Hollingsworth, D. R., Amatruda, T. T., Jr. and Scheig, R.: Quantitative and qualitative effects of l-triiodothyronine in massive obesity. Metabolism, *19*:934–945, 1970.

Hung, W., Gancayco, G. P. and Heald, F. P.: Thyroxine metabolism in obese adolescent males. Pediatrics, *36*:877–881, 1965.

Hutton, J. H.: Chorionic gonadotrophin and obesity. Am. J. Clin. Nutr., *23*:243–244, 1970.

Hvidt, S. and Kjeldsen, K.: Malabsorption induced by small doses of neomycin sulphate. Acta Med. Scand., *173*:699–705, 1963.

Jackson, I. M. D. and Whyte, W. G.: Chlorphentermine SA in the treatment of obesity and the effect of weight loss on steroid excretion. Br. Med. J., *5459*:453–455, 1965.

Jelliffe, R. W., Hill, D., Tatter, D. and Lewis, E.: Death from weight-control pills. A case with objective postmortem confirmation. J.A.M.A., *208*:1843–1847, 1969.

Johnston, L. C. and Bernstein, L. M.: Body composition and oxygen consumption of overweight, normal and underweight women. J. Lab. Clin. Med., *45*:109–118, 1955.

Jones, H. S.: Diethylpropion dependence. Med. J. Aust., *1*:267, 1968.

Jordan, M. J. and Bader, G. M.: Use of diethylpropion combined with a supplement for safe and effective weight control in pregnancy. Surgery, *112*:663–6, 1961.

Josimovich, J. B. and MacLaren, J. A.: Presence in the human placenta and term serum of a highly lactogenic substance immunologically related to pituitary growth hormone. Endocrinology, *71*:209–220, 1962.

Kahan, A. and Mullins, A. G.: Dangers of Preludin. Br. Med. J., *1*:1355, 1958.

Kalb, S. W.: Amphetamine (Benzedrine) sulfate and thyroid extract in the treatment of obesity: observations on 500 cases. J. Med. Soc. N.J., *39*:74–75, 1942a.

Kalb, S. W.: The effect of amphetamine (benzedrine) sulfate, propadrine hydrochloride and propadrine hydrochloride in combination with sodium delvinal on the appetite of obese patients. J. Med. Soc. N.J., *39*:584–586, 1942b.

Kaplan, N. M. and Jose, A.: Thyroid as an adjuvant to amphetamine therapy of obesity. A controlled double-blind study. Am. J. Med. Sci., *260*:105–111, 1970.

Kaufmann, N. A. and Blondheim, S. H.: Action of fenfluramine. Lancet, *1*:104, 1973.

Kneebone, G. M.: Drug therapy: An effective treatment of obesity in childhood. Med. J. Aust., *2*:663–665, 1968.

Kyle, L. H., Ball, M. F. and Doolan, P. D.: Effect of thyroid hormone on body composition in myxedema and obesity. N. Engl. J. Med., *275*:12–17, 1966.

Lamki, L., Ezrin, C., Koven, I. and Steiner, G.: l-thyroxine in the treatment of obesity without increase in loss of lean body mass. Metabolism, *22*:617–622, 1973.

Lasagna, L.: Attitudes toward appetite suppressants. J.A.M.A., *225*:44–48, 1973.

Laurian, L., Oberman, Z. and Herzberg, H.: Free fatty acids in obese subjects treated with anorexigenic drugs (phenmetrazine). Israel J. Med. Sci., *4*:311–314, 1968.

Lawlor, R. B., Trivedi, M. C. and Yelonsky, J. O.: A determination of the anorexigenic potential of dl-amphetamine, d-amphetamine, l-amphetamine and phentermine. Arch. Int. Pharmacodyn., *179*:401–407, 1969.

Lawson, A. A. H., Roscoe, P., Strong, J. A., Gibson, A. and Peattie, P.: Comparison of fenfluramine and metformin in treatment of obesity. Lancet, *2*:437–441, 1970.

Lebon, P.: Treatment of overweight patients with chorionic gonadotrophin: follow-up study. J. Am. Ger. Soc., *14*:116–125, 1966.

Lele, R. D., Joshi, V. R. and Nathwani, A. N.: A double-blind clinical trial of fenfluramine. Br. J. Clin. Pract., *26*:79–82, 1972.

LeRiche, W. H.: Phentermine produces weight loss comparable to that produced by d-amphetamine. Canad. Med. Assoc. J., *82*:467–470, 1960.

LeRiche, W. H. and Van Belle, G.: Study of phendimetrazine bitartrate as an appetite suppressant in relation to dosage, weight loss and side effects. Canad. Med. Assoc. J., *87*:29–31, 1962.

LeRiche, W. H. and Csima, A.: A long-acting appetite suppressant drug studied for 24 weeks in both continuous and sequential administration. Canad. Med. Assoc. J., *97*:1016–1020, 1967.

Lesses, M. F. and Myerson, A.: Human autonomic pharmacology XVI. Benzedrine sulfate as an aid in the treatment of obesity. N. Engl. J. Med., *218*:119–124, 1938.

Levin, J., Trafford, J. A. P., Newland, P. M. and Bishop, P. M. F.: Chlorphentermine in the management of obesity. Practitioner, *191*:65–69, 1963.

Londono, H. J., Gallagher, T. F., Jr. and Bray, G. A.: Effect of weight reduction, triiodothyronine and diethylstilbestrol on growth hormone in obesity. Metabolism, *18*:986–992, 1969.

Lucey, C. and Hadden, D. R.: Chlorphentermine. A new "appetite suppressant." A cross-over double blind trial. Ulster Med. J., *31*:181–4, 1962.

Lyon, D. M. and Dunlop, D. M.: The treatment of obesity. A comparison of the effects of diet and of thyroid extract. Q. J. Med., *1*:331–352, 1932.

Lyons, H. A. and Huang, C. T.: Therapeutic use of progesterone in alveolar hypoventilation associated with obesity. Am. J. Med., *44*:881–888, 1968.

Martel, A.: Preludin (phenmetrazine) in the treatment of obesity. Canad. Med. Assoc. J., *76*:117–120, 1957.

Martin, W. R., Sloan, J. W., Sapira, J. D. and Jasinski, D. R.: Physiologic, subjective and behavioral effects of amphetamine, methamphetamine, ephedrine, phenmetrazine and methylphenidate in man. Clin. Pharm. Therap., *12*:245–258, 1971.

Masserman, J. H. and Goldsmith, H.: Dinitrophenol: its therapeutic and toxic actions in certain types of psychobiologic underactivity. J.A.M.A., *102*:523–525, 1934.

Means, J. H.: The basal metabolism in obesity. Arch. Intern. Med., *17*:704–710, 1916.

Miller, A. T. and Blyth, C. S.: Estimation of lean body mass and body fat from basal oxygen consumption and creatinine excretion. J. Appl. Physiol., *5*:73–78, 1952.

Mossberg, H. O.: Obesity in children. Acta Paediatr. Scand. (*Suppl. 2*)*35*:1–122, 1948.

Munro, J. F., MacCuish, A. C., Wilson, E. M. and Duncan, L. J. P.: Comparison of continuous and intermittent anorectic therapy in obesity. Br. Med. J., *1*:352–354, 1968.

Munro, J. F., MacCuish, A. C., Marshall, A., Wilson, E. M. and Duncan, L. J. P.: Weight reducing effect of diguanides in obese non-diabetic women. Br. Med. J., *2*:13–15, 1969.

Natenshon, A. L.: Clinical evaluation of new anorexic agent, phenmetrazine hydrochloride (preludin). Am. Pract. Digest. Treat., *7*:1456–1459, 1956.

Nathanson, M. H.: The central action of beta-aminopropylbenzene (benzedrine) clinical observations. J.A.M.A., *108*:528–531, 1937.

Nelson, R. A., Anderson, L. F., Gastineau, C. F., Hayles, A. B. and Stamnes, C. L.: Physiology and natural history of obesity. J.A.M.A., *223*:627–630, 1973.

Nicoloff, J. T. and Drenick, E. J.: Altered peripheral thyroxine metabolism in severe obesity. Clin. Res., *14*:148, 1966. (Abs).

Nielsen, I. M. and Dubnick, B.: Pharmacology of chlorphentermine. *In*: Amphetamines and Related Compounds. Proc. Mario Negri Instit. Pharmacol. Res., Italy. (Costa, E. and Garattini, S. eds.), Raven Press, New York, pp. 63–73, 1970.

O'Connor, C. A. and Brodbin, P.: Fenfluramine in obesity. Br. J. Clin. Pract., *24*:118, 1970.

Oddie, T. H., Meade, J. H., Jr. and Fisher, D. A.: An analysis of published data on thyroxine turnover in human subjects. J. Clin. Endocrinol. Metab., *26*:425–436, 1966.

Patel, N., Mock, D. C., Jr. and Hagans, J. A.: Comparison of benzphetamine, phenmetrazine, d-amphetamine and placebo. Clin. Pharmacol. Ther., 4(3):330–333, 1963.

Pedersen, J.: The effect of metformin on weight loss on obesity. Acta Endocrinol. (Kbh), 49:479–486, 1965.

Pedersen, J. and Olesen, E. S.: Observations on the mechanisms of increased weight loss during metformin administration in obesity. Acta Endocrinol. (Kbh), 57:683–688, 1968.

Penick, S. B., Filion, R., Fox, S. and Stunkard, A. J.: Behavior modification in the treatment of obesity. Psychosom. Med., 33:49–55, 1971.

Pinder, R. M., Brogden, R. N., Sawyer, P. R., Speight, T. M. and Avery, G. S.: Fenfluramine—A review of its pharmacological properties and therapeutic efficacy in obesity. Drugs, 10:241–323, 1975.

Pinter, E. J. and Pattee, C. J.: Some data on the metabolic function of the adrenergic nervous system in the obese and during starvation. J. Clin. Endocrinol., 28:106–110, 1968.

Poindexter, A.: Appetite suppressant drugs: a controlled clinical comparison of benzphetamine, phenmetrazine d-amphetamine and placebo. Curr. Ther. Res., 2:354–363, 1960.

Premachandra, B. N., Perlstein, I. B. and Blumenthal, H. T.: Thyroid autoimmunity, thyroxine transport and angiopathy in human obesity in physio-pathology of adipose tissue. (Vague, J. and Denton, R. M., eds.), Excerpta Medica Foundation Amsterdam, pp. 289–301, 1969.

Putman, J. J.: Cases of myxedema and acromegalia treated with benefit by sheep's thyroids: recent observations respecting the pathology of the cachexias following disease of the thyroid; clinical relationships of Graves's Disease and acromegalia. Am. J. Med. Sci., 106:125–148, 1893.

Quaade, F.: Untraditional treatment of obesity. In: Obesity Symposium (Burland, W. L., Samuel, P. and Yudkin, J. eds.), Edinburgh, Churchill Livingstone, 1974, pp. 338–352.

Rabinowitz, J. L. and Myerson, R. M.: The effects of triiodothyronine on some metabolic parameters of obese individuals. Blood ^{14}C-glucose replacement rate, respiratory $^{14}CO_2$, the pentose cycle, the biological half-life of T_3 and the concentration of T_3 in adipose tissue. Metabolism, 16:68–75, 1967.

Rauh, J. L. and Lipp, R.: Chlorphentermine as an anorexigenic agent in adolescent obesity. Report of its efficacy in a double study of 30 teenagers. Clin. Pediat., 7:138–140, 1968.

Resnick, M. and Joubert, L.: A double blind evaluation of an anorexiant, a placebo and diet alone in obese subjects. Can. Med. Assoc. J., 97:1011–1015, 1967.

Ressler, C.: Treatment of obesity with phenmetrazine hydrochloride, a new anorexiant. J.A.M.A., 165:135–138, 1957.

Ressler, C.: Liothyronine in the management of obesity. N.Y. State J. Med., 59:615–621, 1959.

Ressler, C. and Schneider, S. H.: Clinical evaluation of phendimetrazine bitartrate. Clin. Pharmacol. Ther., 2:727–732, 1961.

Rivlin, R. S.: Riboflavin metabolism. N. Engl. J. Med., 283:463–472, 1970.

Roberts, E.: The treatment of obesity with an anorexigenic drug. Ann. Intern. Med., 34:1324–1330, 1951.

Robillard, R.: Preludin treatment of obesity in diabetes mellitus: Preliminary report. Can. Med. Assoc. J., 76:938–940, 1957.

Robins, A. H.: Pondimin-fenfluramine hydrochloride. 1973 Manual.

Rosenberg, B. A.: A double-blind study of diethylpropion in obesity. Am. J. Med. Sci., 242:201–206, 1961.

Rosenberg, P.: The use of mood ameliorating agents in the treatment of psychogenic obesity. Am. Pract. Digest. Treat., 4:818–820, 1953.

Rosenthal, G. and Solomon, H. A.: Benzedrine sulfate in obesity. Endocrinology, 26:807–812, 1940.

Rossum, J. M. van and Simons, F.: Locomotor activity and anorexogenic action. Psychopharmacologia, 14:248–254, 1969.

Runyan, J. W., Jr.: Observations on the use of phendimetrazine, a new anorexigenic agent, in obese diabetics. Curr. Ther. Res., 4:270–275, 1962.

Russek, H. I.: Control of obesity in patients with angina pectoris: a double blind study with diethylpropion hydrochloride. Am. J. Med. Sci., 251:461–464, 1966.

Samuel, P. D. and Burland, W. L.: Drug treatment of obesity. *In:* Obesity in Perspective. Fogarty International Center Series on Preventive Medicine, Vol. II, Part II. (Bray, G. A. ed.) Washington, D.C., U.S. Government Printing Office. 1976, pp. 419–428.

Sandoz-Wander, Inc.: Sanorex (Mazindol): A new anorexiant—A monograph, 1973.

Schapiro, M. M. and Bogran, N.: Dietless weight loss with benzphetamine (Didrex): a controlled comparison with phenmetrazine and placebo. Curr. Ther. Res., 2:333–345, 1960.

Schulman, J. L., Carleton, J. L., Whitney, E. and Whitehorn, J. C.: Effect of glucagon on food intake and body weight in man. J. Appl. Physiol., 11:419–421, 1957.

Scoville, B. A.: Review of amphetamine-like drugs by the Food and Drug Administration. *In:* Obesity in Perspective. Fogarty International Center Series on Preventive Medicine, Vol. II, Part II. (Bray, G. A. ed.) Washington, D.C., U.S. Government Printing Office, 1976, pp. 441–443.

Scriba, P. C., Richter, J., Horn, K., Breckebans, J. and Schwartz, K.: Zur Frage der Schilddrusenfunktion bei Apdipositas. Klin. Woch., 45:323–324, 1967.

Seaton, D. A., Rose, K. and Duncan, L. J. P.: Sustained action chlorphentermine in the correction of refractory obesity. Practitioner, 193:698–702, 1964.

Sedgewick, J. P.: A treatment for refractory obesity using fenfluramine without dietary restriction. Br. J. Clin. Pract., 24:251–252, 1970.

Silverman, M.: Subacute delirious state due to "Preludin" addition. Br. Med. J., 1:696–697, 1959.

Silverman, M. and Okun, R.: The use of an appetite suppressant (diethylpropion hydrochloride) during pregnancy. Curr. Ther. Res., 13:648–653, 1971.

Silverstone, J. T. and Stunkard, A. J.: The anorectic effect of dexamphetamine sulphate. Br. J. Pharmacol., 33:513–522, 1968.

Silverstone, J. T., Turner, P. and Humperson, P. L.: Direct measurement of the anorectic activity of diethylpropion (Tenuate Dospan). J. Clin. Pharmacol., 8:172–179, 1968.

Simeons, A. T. W.: Chorionic gonadotropin in geriatrics. J. Am. Geriat. Soc., 4:36–40, 1956.

Simeons, A. T. W.: The action of chorionic gonadotrophin in the obese. Lancet, 2:946–947, 1954.

Simkin, B. and Wallace, L.: A controlled clinical trial of benzphetamine (Didrex) in the management of obesity. Curr. Ther. Res., 2:33–38, 1960.

Simkins, S.: Dinitrophenol and desiccated thyroid in the treatment of obesity: A comprehensive clinical and laboratory study. J.A.M.A., 108:2110–2193, 1937.

Simons, E. W.: Mechanisms of dinitrophenol toxicity. Biol. Rev., 28:453–479, 1953.

Smart, J. V., Sneddon, J. M. and Turner, P.: A comparison of the effects of chlorphentermine, diethylpropion and phenmetrazine on critical flicker frequency. Br. J. Pharmacol., 30:307–316, 1967.

Smith, M. J. H. and Dawkins, P. D.: Salicylates and enzymes. J. Pharm. Pharmacol., 23:729–744, 1971.

Sohar, E.: A forty-day 550 calorie diet in the treatment of obese outpatients. Am. J. Clin. Nutr., 7:514–518, 1959.

Soulairac, A.: Control of carbohydrate intake. *In:* Handbook of Physiology. Chapter 28, pp. 387–398, 1967.

Staffurth, J. S. and Morrison, N. D. W.: Heart size in thyrotoxicosis. Postgrad. Med. J., 44:885–890, 1968.

Stamler, J.: The coronary drug project: findings leading to further modifications of its protocol with respect to dextrothyroxine. J.A.M.A., 220:996–1008, 1972.

Steel, J. M. and Briggs, M.: Withdrawal depression in obese patients after fenfluramine treatment. Br. Med. J., 3:26–27, 1972.

Steel, J. M., Munro, J. F. and Duncan, L. J. P.: A comparative trial of different regimens of fenfluramine and phentermine in obesity. Practitioner, 211:232–236, 1973.

Stewart, D. A., Bailey, J. D. and Patell, H.: Tenuate dospan as an appetite suppressant in the treatment of obese children. Appl. Ther., 12:34–36, 1970.

Stowers, J. M. and Bewsher, P. D.: Studies of the mechanism of weight reduction by phenformin. Postgrad. Med. J., 45:13–19, 1969.

Strong, J. A. and Lawson, A. A. H.: Double blind crossover trial of fenfluramine and metformin in the treatment of obesity. *In:* Amphetamines and Related Compounds. Proc. Mario Negri Instit. Pharmacol. Res. Italy; (Costa, E. and Garattini, S., eds.) New York, Raven Press, 1970, pp. 673–691.

Stunkard, A. J.: New therapies of the eating disorders: Behavior modification of obesity and anorexia nervosa. Arch. Gen. Psychiatry, 26:391–398, 1972.

Stunkard, A., Rickels, K. and Hesbacher, P.: Fenfluramine in the treatment of obesity. Lancet, 1:503–505, 1973.

Stunkard, A. J. and McLaran-Hume, M.: The results of treatment for obesity. Arch. Int. Med., 103:79–85, 1959.

Sudsaneh, S. and Mayer, J.: Relation of metabolic events to gastric contractions in the rat. Am. J. Physiol., 197:269–273, 1959.

Sullivan, A. C., Triscari, J. and Hamilton, J. G.: Effect of (-)-hydroxycitrate upon the accumulation of lipid in the rat. Lipids, 9:129–134, 1974.

Tainter, M. L., Stockton, A. B. and Cutting, W. C.: Use of nitrophenol in obesity and related conditions. A progress report. J.A.M.A., 101:1472–1475, 1933.

Tainter, M. L., Stockton, A. B. and Cutting, W.: Dinitrophenol in the treatment of obesity: Final report. J.A.M.A., 105:332–336, 1935.

Tang, A. H. and Kirch, J. D.: Appetite suppression and central nervous system stimulation in the Rhesus monkey. Psychopharmacologia, 21:139–146, 1971.

Truant, A. P., Olon, L. P. and Cobb, S.: Phentermine resin as an adjunct in medical weight reduction: A controlled, randomized double-blind prospective study. Curr. Ther. Res., 14:726–738, 1972.

Turtle, J. R. and Burgess, J. A.: Hypoglycemic action of fenfluramine in diabetes mellitus. Diabetes, 22:858–867, 1973.

Ulrich, H.: Narcolepsy and its treatment with benzedrine sulfate. N. Engl. J. Med., 217:696–701, 1937.

Van Liere, E. J. and Sizemore, D. A.: Regression of cardiac hypertrophy following experimental hyperthyroidism in rats. Proc. Soc. Exp. Biol. Med., 136:645–648, 1971.

Waal-Manning, H. J. and Simpson, F. O.: Fenfluramine in obese patients on various antihypertensive drugs: Double-blind controlled trial. Lancet, 2:1392–1395, 1969.

Weidenhamer, J. E.: l-triiodothyronine as adjunctive therapy in the management of obesity. Am. Pract. Digest. Ther., 8:419, 1957.

Wichelow, M. J. and Butterfield, W. J. H.: Effects on fenfluramine on peripheral glucose metabolism in man. In: Amphetamines and Related Compounds; Proc. Mario Negri Instit. Pharmacol. Res., Italy. (Costa, E. and Garattini, S., eds.) New York, Raven Press, 1970, pp. 611–618.

Williams, J.: Trial of a long acting preparation of diethylpropion in obese diabetes. Practitioner, 200:411–414, 1968.

Wood, L. C. and Owen, J. A.: Clinical evaluation of a new anorexigenic drug, aminoxaphen, in obese diabetics. J. New Drugs, 5:181–185, 1965.

CHAPTER 10

SURGICAL APPROACHES TO THE TREATMENT OF OBESITY

GASTROINTESTINAL BYPASS

HISTORICAL BACKGROUND

The gastrointestinal bypass is the one surgical approach to obesity which has met with measured success. This technique was introduced in several institutions in the early 1950's. The first operation was reported by Kremen et al. (1954) who had performed a jejunoileostomy on an obese patient who subsequently lost a considerable amount of weight. This was followed by the application of jejunocolic anastomoses to the treatment of obesity. In 1963 Payne, DeWind and Commons reported a series of 11 patients in whom they had anastomosed 15 inches of jejunum to the transverse colon. Diarrhea with loss of electrolytes in the diarrheal fluid were unsatisfactory sequelae of this operation. To reduce these complications, several surgeons increased the length of the jejunum to 20 or 25 inches (Sherman, 1965; Lewis et al., 1966; Shibata et al., 1967).

Over 70 patients with a jejunocolic anastomosis have been reported in the medical journals (Payne et al., 1963; Woods and Chermos, 1963; DeMuth and Rottenstein, 1964; Sherman, 1965; Lewis, Turnbull and Page, 1966; Troncelletti, 1966; Bondar and Pisesky, 1967; Kaufman and Weldon, 1967; Shibata, MacKenzie and Long, 1967; Maxwell, Richards and Albo, 1968; Delena et al., 1970; Shagrin et al., 1971). Weight loss varied with length of the jejunum. With 15 inches of jejunum, the patients had lost 48 percent of body weight in one year. When the upper intestinal segment was lengthened to 20 inches, the patients lost 31 percent of their previous weight in 12 months. At 25 inches, weight loss was even slower—26 percent at 12

411

months (Shibata et al., 1967). Problems with this operation include: severe electrolyte losses (Payne et al., 1963; DeMuth and Rottenstein, 1964; Shibata et al., 1967), liver failure (Delena et al., 1970; Bondar and Pisesky, 1967; Drenick et al., 1970), and at least 17 deaths.

The high mortality and severe side effects terminated the use of the jejunocolic bypass. In its place two different kinds of jejunoileostomy and a gastric bypass have been introduced.

INTESTINAL SHORT CIRCUIT OPERATIONS

Operative Procedure

This operation can be subdivided into the two types shown in Fig. 10–11. In one operation the end of the distal segment of the jejunum is attached to the side of the ileum near the ileocecal valve. This procedure was originally proposed by Sherman (1965), and the first large series was reported by Payne and DeWind (1969). The other operation was first performed by Kremen et al. (1954) on one patient, but was introduced on a large scale by Scott et al. (1970) and by Salmon (1971). In both operative procedures the distal cut end of the jejunum must be closed and securely attached to the omentum to prevent intussception. With the end-to-end operation, the defunctionalized ileal end is anastomosed to the colon for drainage of the gastrointestinal secretion (Fig. 10–1).

Two major considerations are involved in the decision about which operation to select. These are: (1) the technical difficulties related to the weight of the patient, and (2) the length of the jejunal and ileal intestinal segment to be selected. Technically, performance of an end-to-side operation should be simpler than an end-to-end procedure, since only one anastomosis is involved. The jejunum is attached to the side of the ileum and the severed jejunal segment is closed and anchored securely to the omentum. The technical problems with performing an end-to-end operation are greater because two separate anastomoses are necessary. The first of these is the anastomosis between jejunum and ileum to provide continuity for the intestinal tract. The second is the anastomosis between the severed ileal end and the colon to allow discharge of the gastric secretions from the defunctionalized bowel.

Weight loss with either operation appears to depend primarily on the length of the functional intestinal segment left in continuity. Operations where more than 25 inches of intestine is left in continuity produce very slow weight loss. Figure 10–2 plots the weight loss one year or more after an intestinal bypass operation in patients having varying lengths of jejunum and ileum anastomosed end-to-side (Weismann, 1973). With a total length of 25 inches, it did not seem to

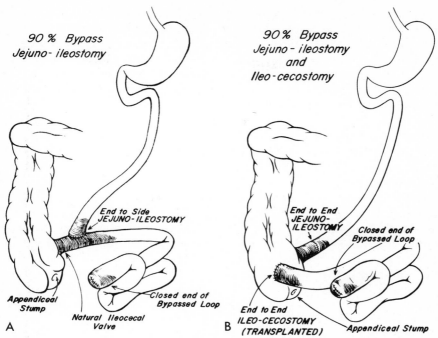

Figure 10–1.   Two types of jejunoileostomy. *A*, End-to-side jejunoileostomy originally pioneered by Dr. Payne. End-to-end jejunoileostomy and end-to-side ileocecostomy for drainage of the defunctionalized bowel. In the end-to-end jejunoileostomy now done at Harbor General Hospital we do the secondary ileal anastamosis to the transverse colon or to the sigmoid.

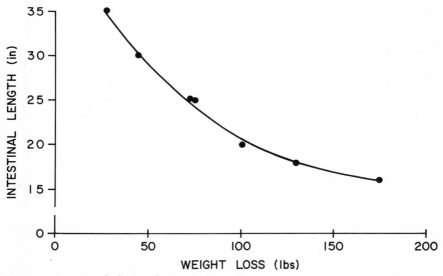

Figure 10–2.   Weight loss and intestinal length. Operations with more than 35 inches left in continuity produce very little weight loss. (Adapted from Weismann, R. E.: Am. J. Surg., *125*:437–446, 1973, with permission.)

matter whether 20 to 15 inches of jejunum were anastomosed to 5 and 10 inches of ileum respectively, since weight loss was nearly identical. Payne et al. (1973) have concluded from their clinical studies with varying lengths of intestinal segments that 14 inches of jejunum and 4 inches of ileum are the preferred dimensions. Scott et al. (1973) have examined the metabolic and nutritional consequences of anastomosing end-to-end 12 inches of jejunum to 6 to 12 inches of ileum. They concluded that weight loss is greater with the shorter segment, but that more nutritional problems develop when the ileum is short. They recommend that the shorter ileal segment be reserved for patients weighing over 350 lbs.(160 kg), and that an ileal segment of 8 inches be used for lighter patients.

The error in measurement of intestinal length is also a reason for differences in weight loss. Bachman and Hallberg (1974) have measured intestinal length of 56 obese patients and 32 normal weight patients. When measured early in the operation, the intestine averaged 10 percent longer than when measured later. At comparable times in the operation, the intestine was longer in the obese than in the nonobese controls (Table 10–1). Patients whose obesity began in childhood had significantly shorter intestines than individuals with adult onset obesity (Bachman and Hallberg, 1974). Two of the 31 patients operated on at Harbor General Hospital had lost over 100 lbs on a low calorie diet during the 6 months before surgery. At operation, their intestine measured just over 4 m, which suggests that dietary intake may be a major factor in controlling intestinal length. In a study using the end-to-end technique, Quaade et al. (1974) showed that reduction of the ileal segment by one centimeter led to a significantly greater weight loss. From these several studies, we conclude that the degree of weight loss is mainly a function of the length of intestine.

The minimum weight attained and the tendency to regain weight also vary between the two types of operation. With the end-to-side operation, there is some retrograde reflux of intestinal contents into the bypassed segment (Quaade et al., 1971). With hypertrophy of the intestine which is thought to occur after this operation, the reabsorption of nutrients refluxed into the defunctionalized bowel

TABLE 10–1.   *Intestinal Length in Lean and Obese Patients**

SEX	NUMBER		BODY WEIGHT (kg)		INTESTINAL LENGTH (m)	
	Obese	*Nonobese*	*Obese*	*Nonobese*	*Obese*	*Nonobese*
Male	13	12	149.7	69.2	8.24	6.98
Female	43	20	137.2	61.5	7.34	6.16

*Adapted from Bachman and Hallberg: Acta Chir. Scand., *140*:47–63, 1974, with permission.

might be enhanced. The degree of reflux might also be enhanced by the slow rate of gastric emptying and the slow transit time for a barium meal through the small intestine, which occurs in the postoperative period in patients with an end-to-side operation (Quaade et al., 1971).

With an end-to-end anastomosis, the secretions from the defunctionalized loop enter directly into the colon, and reflux of nutrient solutions into this loop is much less likely. Therefore, some patients with an end-to-side anastomosis will plateau in body weight at a higher level and may ultimately regain some weight as more of the nutrients entering the defunctionalized bowel are reabsorbed. Thus in deciding which operative procedure to select, the smaller number of technical problems in performing an end-to-side operation must be weighed against the possibilities of a smaller weight loss and of regaining weight.

Clinical Features

Over 900 patients who have had jejunoileostomy as treatment for obesity have been reported in medical journals, and an additional 490 cases have been described in personal communications to the author. The discussion which follows will compare the data on 31 patients who have been operated on at Harbor Hospital (in collaboration with Dr. John Benfield and Dr. Michael Peter) with the data on 230 additional patients who have been operated on in the southern part of Los Angeles County by 6 other surgeons (Benfield et al., unpublished observations) and with the results from other published cases (Buchwald et al., 1974; Moxley et al., 1974; Payne, et al., 1973; Brown et al., 1974; O'Leary et al., 1974; Shibata et al., 1971; Juhl et al., 1971; Quaade et al., 1971; Scott et al., 1973; Baber et al., 1973; Solow et al., 1974; Weismann, 1973; Hunt, personal communication; Salmon, 1971; Holzbach et al., 1974; Kantor, 1970; Drenick et al., 1970; Shagrin et al., 1971; Dickstein and Frame, 1973; Benfield et al., unpublished observations; Bray et al., 1975; Morgan and Moore, 1967; Starkloff et al., 1974; Scott et al., 1969; Fikri and Cassella, 1973; Gazet, et al., 1974).

The criteria and indications for selecting patients to undergo an intestinal bypass procedure have been summarized by Loren DeWind (1974) and are listed below.

CRITERIA AND INDICATIONS FOR INTESTINAL BYPASS TREATMENT OF GROSSLY OBESE PATIENTS

Weight more than 100 pounds over standard for height, sex and age
Failure of other forms of treatment for obesity
Presence of one or more of the following:
   Hypertension
   Pickwickian syndrome

Diabetes mellitus
Congestive heart failure
Infertility
Degenerative arthritis of hips, knees or feet
Hyperlipidemia
Stable adult life pattern
Acceptance of expected hazards as indicated by signing an informed consent
Agreement to undergo revision if needed and to avoid pregnancy for 6 to 12
    months after surgery
Availability of the following:
    Experienced team of internist and surgeon
    Good laboratory and intensive care facilities
Absence of the following:
    Renal failure
    Serious myocardial disease
    Inflammatory bowel disease
    Pulmonary embolization
    Cirrhosis of the liver or active hepatitis

The reason for such criteria is obvious. The risks to life brought on by obesity are rarely immediate, but the risks of operative mortality from a major operation are immediate.

Thus without a clear understanding of the risks involved in the surgery and without criteria which will minimize the inclusion of patients who are in a lower risk category, physicians and surgeons may be needlessly exposing patients to injury. To minimize this problem we provide each patient with a description of the operation and its risks, complications and benefits. A copy of these instructions is appended to this chapter. To safeguard the rights of the patient, all potential candidates should receive a thorough and complete explanation of the risks and benefits. For patients who want the viewpoint of other patients, we urge them to contact the Intestinal Bypass Society and, if possible, to visit a local chapter meeting.

It is important that the physician performing the procedure be willing to take care of the patient as long as is necessary postoperatively. Since we do not yet know the full extent of the complications which may occur, and since the surgeon produces an "iatrogenic" disease to replace the obesity, he is committed to providing indefinite availability of medical care for any patient who is operated on. This can best be done when the operation is undertaken as a "team"effort and involves surgical, medical and psychiatric staff (Benfield and Bray, 1975).

The age of the patients undergoing this procedure in our series ranged from 19 to 39 years, with only one over 30 (Bray et al., 1975). Among the 230 patients from south Los Angeles, the average age was 35, with a range from 14 to 69 (Benfield et al., 1974). Nineteen were

---

Intestinal Bypass Society, P.O. Box 6913, St. Louis, Mo. 63123

weight of the patient, the degree of intestinal bypass and the operative procedure selected.

After the first year body weight is lost at a slower rate ranging between ½ pound and 2½ pounds per week. This rate declined further with time until a new plateau level is reached. This plateau is dependent upon the decline in the patient's caloric needs as he loses weight and the adaptation of the intestinal tract to absorb more nutrients. In most series the patient's weight plateaus between 68 and 114 kg (150 and 250 pounds) or after losing 30 to 50 percent of initial body weight. However, an occasional patient fails to lose a significant amount of weight following the initial operation. This would appear to result from an inadequate bypass and such patients often undergo a revision of their jejunoileostomy.

Diarrhea

All patients who have had a jejunoileostomy for obesity have diarrhea, but it is less important to them than might be anticipated. In the early postoperative period, liquid stools might range from 8 to 15 or more per day. The major difficulty associated with the diarrhea is the rectal irritation and the tendency to develop hemorrhoids. By 2 to 6 weeks after the operation, however, the number of bowel movements decreases to between 4 and 15, and by the end of six months it has decreased further to 2 to 6 (Benfield et al., 1976). Buchwald et al., (1974) noted that 80 percent of their patients were having only 2 to 4 stools at the end of one year after the operation. Among the patients reported by Salmon (1971), 36 percent did not have diarrhea at the end of the first six months postoperatively. However, a significant 25 percent had diarrhea one year later, and 13 percent still had diarrhea two years after the operation (Salmon, 1971). Fikri and Casella (1973) had to lengthen the original bypass because of intractable diarrhea in 4 of 52 patients.

In general the diarrhea can be controlled by one of three measures. In the early period all of our patients responded to diphenoxylate (Lomotil) for the control of diarrhea, but few needed this medication after 4 to 6 weeks. Separating the intake of water from the ingestion of food will also help reduce the intestinal transit time and thus reduce the diarrhea. Finally several of our patients have used a psyllium seed extract (Metamucil) to help with the diarrhea. Although this preparation is designed to relieve constipation, it can act to absorb water in the intestine if it is swallowed as a slurry with only a small amount of water.

If the diarrhea persists with large numbers of watery stools, the possibility of serious complications may be increased. This is illustrated by the use of a 38 year old woman who was referred to us after two episodes of hypocalcemic tetany which had been treated at another hospital. She had weighed 220 pounds at the time of her initial end-to-end jejunoileostomy. Her weight had declined steadily in the postoperative period, but her diarrheal stools persisted. When she was admitted to our hospital, she was having up to 20 liquid bowel movements each day. After a thorough evaluation it was decided that a reanastomosis was indicated, and she was taken to the operating room where a loop of the defunctionalized intestine was found to have herniated through the omentum. The jejunoileal bypass appeared to be functioning well. How herniation of the defunctionalized loop could produce persistent diarrhea, if indeed this was the case, remains a mystery.

Postoperative Surgical and Metabolic Problems

Complications associated with this surgery can be divided into two groups: those which arise directly from the operation itself and those metabolic changes which occur in the early and late postoperative course. Table 10–3 summarizes the frequency of various complications among 18 groups of patients reported in medical journals. The number of such complications is in the numerator of each fraction, and the total number of cases in which this complication was reported is in

TABLE 10–3. *Complications of Jejunoileostomy in Treatment of Obesity*

COMPLICATIONS	OCCURRENCE	PERCENTAGE	RANGE
Major			
Early			
Operative mortality	46/1499	3.1	0 to 6.5
Pulmonary emboli	11/545	2.0	1 to 6
Wound infection	50/641	7.8	2 to 10
Gastrointestinal hemorrhage	9/294	3.1	0 to 6
Renal failure	5/140	2.8	0 to 3
Tetany or severe electrolyte imbalance	15/346	4.3	0 to 9
Severe nausea and vomiting	5/140	2.8	
Later			
Urinary calculi	29/913	3.2	3 to 30
Liver disease	22/954	2.3	0 to 14
Anemia	6/263	2.3	0 to 3
Acute cholecystitis	6/86	7.0	0 to 7
Intestinal obstruction	11/526	1.9	0 to 3.5
Megacolon	4/83	4.8	
Minor			
Diarrhea			100
Minor electrolyte abnormalities			40 to 80
Hypoproteinemia			40 to 100
Vomiting			10 to 80
Polyarthritis	7/324	2.2	0 to 6
Hair loss	5/140	3.5	0 to 100
Vitamin deficiency		>80	
Malnutrition		>80	
Reanastomosis	21/569	3.7	

the denominator. The range of values are the highest and lowest estimates available from the various series. The overall mortality was 3.1 percent for the series of 1500 patients, with a range of 0 to 11.5 percent. This range exists as a result of several variables: (1) the experience of the surgical and medical team (2) the degree of obesity among the patients, and (3) whether or not complicating diseases are prominent in the series of patients.

A number of major problems may occur in the early postoperative period which are associated with significant morbidity or death. Pulmonary embolism has been reported in five series (Payne et al., 1973; Buchwald et al., 1974; Weismann, 1973; Salmon, 1971; Fikri and Casella, 1973). We have not observed this problem in our patients, although one of them has had severe thrombophlebitis postoperatively. Infection in the operative wound with its thick layers of fat is not a surprising occurrence, and has been the most frequent postoperative complication other than seromucoid drainage from the wounds. Evisceration has been a problem in some series (Salmon, 1971; Baber et al., 1973), but can usually be prevented if the wound has been securely closed with wire sutures (Benfield et al., 1976).

Gastrointestinal hemorrhage has occurred in one of our patients and in several series (Buchwald et al., 1974; Payne, 1973; Scott et al., 1973; Baber et al., 1973). Our patient developed massive intestinal bleeding from erosive gastritis while she was recovering from halothane-induced jaundice. Renal failure and severe nausea and vomiting can occur, and in one series had a frequency of 2.8 percent (DeWind, 1974). Two of the later complications are also surgical in nature. Intestinal obstruction due to intussusception or to adhesive bands has been reported in 1.9 percent of the patients. (Payne, 1973; Baber et al, 1973; Hunt, personal communication; Benfield et al., 1976; Fikri and Casella, 1974).

PSEUDO-OBSTRUCTIVE MEGACOLON.   This complication has recently come to light (Fikri and Casella, 1974). This presents as intermittent abdominal swelling and distension, and usually occurs one, two or more years after the operation. We initially thought that one of our patients who had developed this problem had a partial volvulus of the sigmoid colon. However, repair of this presumed defect produced only a short remission (Barry et al., 1975; Bray et al., 1976).

The dilated segment of intestine occurs just beyond the anastomosis of the defunctionalized bowel, and can involve either the distal ileum or the colon. Thus megacolon can occur with either the end-to-side or end-to-end operation. This pseudo-obstructive complication is worsened by eating, and it can be relieved by antibiotics for variable periods of time. Suppression of intestinal anaerobics with metronidazole diminishes the swelling promptly. However, overgrowth with aerobic intestinal bacteria may lead to recurrence. Antibiotic treatment of the aerobes will then reduce the symptoms, but long term resolution has not yet been achieved. For some patients this complication may necessitate reanastomosis. In our experience, pseudo-obstructive megacolon is the most common complication of jejunoileostomy. It has occurred within a year and a half in more than 25 percent of the patients who were operated on at the Harbor General Hospital (Barry et al., 1975; Benfield et al., 1976).

MALNUTRITION.   Malnutrition is one price for the weight loss produced by jejunoileostomy. The surgery is clearly designed to produce malabsorption of various nutrients, including calories, and thus to produce weight loss. Hypoproteinemia occurs in many patients and is more profound in patients whose functional intestine is 18 inches long than in patients with 24 inches of functioning bypass (Scott et al., 1973). Among our patients serum albumin declined from 4.3 g/dl preoperatively to 3.6 g/dl postoperatively. An explanation for the decline in albumin has been suggested by the increased excretion of fecal nitrogen and the reduced concentrations of amino acid in the serum (Scott et al., 1971; Moxley et al., 1974). All of the essential amino acids except methionine declined during the first four months after the jejunoileostomy. The largest declines were 38 percent for lysine and valine and 34 percent for leucine. The absorption of amino acids from the gastrointestinal tract was also impaired. The pattern observed in the early postoperative period is similar to the findings in malnourished children with Kwashiorkor. Since amino acids absorbed from the gastrointestinal tract are the major source of amino acids for the synthesis of protein, it is not surprising that hypoalbuminemia develops.

Loss of hair has been noted by all of our patients and in various journal reports after an intestinal bypass (Buchwald et al., 1974). The degree of hair loss is variable, and its regrowth beginning between 6 and 12 months after the operation is probably a sign that amino acid absorption has increased.

Pregnancy occurring during the period of protein deficiency may have serious implications for the fetus. Maternal malnutrition during pregnancy is associated with a decrease in the formation of new cells, particularly brain cells. Thus malnutrition during the fetal period can be associated with some degree of mental retardation in the infant. There are reports of 11 pregnancies in women who had undergone a jejunocolic or jejunoileal bypass for obesity (Everett et al., 1974; Barrow et al., 1969; Wills, 1971; Payne, 1963). The birth weights of all infants were less than those of children previously born to these women. In the patient reported by Everett et al. (1974) detailed metabolic studies showed that the patient who had become pregnant 7 months after the jejunoileostomy was malnourished during gestation. Her excretion of fecal fat was markedly elevated (71.5 g/day) and the absorption of D-xylose was depressed. The low birth weight of the infant (2495 g) and the development of acidosis in the infant shortly after birth are both thought to have resulted from the malnourished state of the mother and infant.

Malnutrition is also manifested by the changes in absorption of fecal fats and in the reduced absorption of fat soluble vitamins. Scott et al. (1971) have reported preoperative and postoperative measurements of fat absorption in 7 patients. In 3 of these patients the preoperative excretion of fat in the stools was elevated (12.8 to 17 g/24hours) but not in the other 4. In all 7 patients the postoperative values were significantly higher than the preoperative measurements, with the highest value being 121 g/day. O'Leary et al. (1974) have also documented steatorrhea after an intestinal bypass. We have obtained sequential measurements of fecal fat excretion of 11 of our patients. Three of these patients had values above 7 g of fat per day in their stools before jejunoileostomy. In the first month postoperatively the absorption of fat declined in all patients, with 22 to 91 percent of the orally administered fat appearing in the feces. With the passage of time, there was a reduction in the quantity of fat appearing in the stools. By six months the values ranged from 4 to 60 g/24hours and by 18 months the excretion was further reduced.

The increased excretion of fat in the stools in the period of malnutrition probably results from decreased ileal absorption of bile acids. It is now well established that the absorption of fats from the intestine involves two processes. The first is the cleavage of triglycerides into fatty acids and monoglycerides by the pancreatic lipase. The second process is the formation of micelles which are composed of fatty acids, monoglycerides and bile salts. In this form the fatty acids can be absorbed into the intestinal mucosa, where they are re-esterified to form triglycerides. They are then packaged into chylomicrons or secreted directly into the portal circulation (this occurs only if the fatty acids in the triglyceride are less than 12 carbons in length). The bile salts are in turn absorbed in the ileum to be returned to the intestinal circuit through the biliary tract. Loss of the ileal surface after a jejunoileostomy reduces the absorption of bile salts and impairs the formation of micelles. Thus the procedure reduces the intestinal absorption of fatty acids.

The compensatory mechanisms in the liver increase the production of bile salts from cholesterol and plasma cholesterol drops. Payne (personal communication) found that the cholesterol declined from 227 mg/dl before operation to 169 mg/dl postoperatively. Scott et al. (1971, 1973) found that cholesterol dropped rapidly within the first 1 to 5 months and then tended to stabilize. In most of these patients the postoperative values ranged between 100 and 164 mg/dl, with the majority being below 120 mg/dl. In our patients cholesterol also dropped sharply in the first few months after intestinal bypass. The preoperative value was 182 mg/dl. During the immediate postoperative period this declined to 109 mg/dl and then tended to stabilize close to 100 mg/dl. There was no tendency to rise with time, even though the absorption of fecal fat was increasing. Serum carotene and serum triglycerides also decline after jejunoileostomy (Scott et al., 1973; Sandstead, 1976). In our patients the preoperative carotene was 90 mg/dl, which declined to 21 mg/dl postoperatively.

The state of malnutrition is also manifested as vitamin deficiencies. Absorption of vitamin B_{12} is uniformly impaired because the ileal surface from which it is absorbed is drastically reduced. Among our patients the absorption of vitamin B_{12} fell from 18.7 percent of the administered dose (normal greater than 10 percent) to a low of 2.9 percent postoperatively. With the passage of time there was a gradual improvement. By 18 months after the operation many of the patients were within the normal range, and some had even returned to the preoperative level. Vitamin A and vitamin E, two other fat soluble vitamins, are also reduced in the plasma of patients who have undergone a jejunoileostomy (Scott et al., 1971, 1973).

Finally, malnutrition and malabsorption are manifested by the loss of electrolytes in the stools and by the decreased absorption of D-xylose. Serum potassium is frequently reduced and potassium supplements are needed by most patients in the early postoperative period. In our patients potassium declined from 4.2 mEq/l, before operation to an average low of 3.6 mEq/l after operation. However, in only two patients did it fall below 3 mEq/l, and one of these patients became symptomatic, with weakness which was corrected by potassium supplementation. With the passage of time, however, this requirement for potassium had disappeared. Magnesium was below 1.5 mEq/l in only one patient (Swenson et al., 1974). Plasma calcium concentrations in all of our patients declined, but none has had tetany and none has required therapy, in contrast with some other reports (Buchwald et al., 1974; DeMuth and Rottenstein, 1964).

One unusual patient deserves mention. She was referred to us 4 months after her intestinal bypass because of mild elevation in her bilirubin. Her weight at the time of operation had been 306 pounds (140 kg), and at the time of referral to us she weighed 220 lbs (100 kg). She refused to have her intestines reanastomosed, although there were some early fibrotic changes on the liver biopsy obtained by needle aspiration. With long term follow-up her liver gradually improved, but we noticed that her serum calcium remained between 10.1 and 10.9 mg/dl. Her serum albumin was consistently at or just below normal, indicating the presence of mild hypercalcemia. A diagnosis of hyperparathyroidism was made, and her neck was explored. A parathyroid adenoma was found and removed. Postoperatively she has required supplemental calcium and vitamin D.

A schematic diagram of the sequence of events in the early and late postoperative period is presented in Figure 10-6. This figure has been divided into three parts. The first six months are the period of

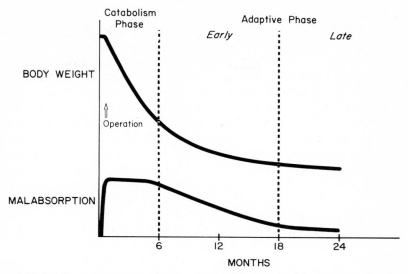

Figure 10–6. Postoperative response to intestinal bypass. Malabsorption and malnutrition are maximal initially and gradually subside as the intestine adapts. When this happens weight loss slows and a new steady weight occurs.

maximal malnutrition, maximal weight loss and the period of greatest intestinal malabsorption. Between 6 and 18 months there are gradual adaptations in intestinal absorption and in eating patterns. The extent to which supplementation of nutrients is needed after this period is at present unknown (see below).

URINARY CALCULI.   Urinary calculi have been reported with a frequency varying between 0.3 percent and 30 percent. They have been reported in 12 of 156 patients by Payne (1973), in 7 of 31 patients by O'Leary et al. (1974), in 5 of 230 patients from Los Angeles, and in 3 of the 31 patients operated on at the Harbor General Hospital (Bray et al., 1976). Metabolic studies have been performed in several patients with postoperative renal stones (O'Leary et al., 1974; Dickstein and Frame, 1973).

O'Leary et al. (1974) found that the renal stones were composed of calcium oxalate in 4 of 7 patients. Oxalate excretion was 66 to 91 mg/day (normal, 19 to 44) in four patients who were hospitalized and given a constant 1700 calorie diet. Oxalate excretion declined during the period of adaptation to the 1700 calorie diet. Urinary calcium, citrate and magnesium excretion were lower than normal in patients who formed stones, but the glyoxalate excretion was higher. The excretion of oxalate in the urine was not altered by feeding either taurine or cholestyramine.

Dickstein and Frame (1973) have reported 11 patients with renal stones, 9 of whom had undergone a jejunocolic anastomosis, and two of whom had had a jejunoileostomy. Calcium oxalate stones were documented in 6 of these 11 patients. The interval between operation and the detection of renal stones varied from 24 days to 6 years, with an average of 20 months. Among those with renal stones, the excretion of oxalate averaged 51 mg/24 hours compared with 27.5 mg/24 hours for a group of patients with an intestinal bypass who did not have renal stones. Calcium excretion and urinalysis were not different between the groups. Neither the rate of weight loss nor the frequency of the diarrhea was related to the development of renal stones. Infection and dehydration were not thought to be significant factors. Dietary intake of oxalate may well be important, and we put our patients on a diet low in oxalates (Benfield et al., 1976).

POLYARTHRITIS.   A polyarthritis with migratory arthralgias has been described in 0 to 6 percent of the patients with intestinal bypass operations (see Table 10–3) (Buchwald et al., 1974; Payne and De-Wind, 1973; Shagrin et al., 1971; Hess, 1974). We have had two patients develop this problem. Shagrin et al. have reported 7 patients with "rheumatoid-like polyarthritis and polyarthralgia." These patients had all undergone a jejunocolostomy (see above), but the syndrome of polyarthritis has also been observed in patients who have had a jejunoileostomy.

All 7 of the patients reported by Shagrin et al. (1971) had a tensynovitis involving the wrists. The fingers were involved in 5 patients, and the knees and ankles in 3 patients. The symptoms were of short duration in 5 of the patients but were more persistent in the other 2. Rheumatoid factor, antinuclear factor and lupus erythematous (LE) cells were absent from the plasma. In discussing these patients Shagrin et al. noted the relationship between diseases of the joints and such inflammatory diseases of the intestine as ulcerative colitis, regional enteritis and Whipple's disease. They suggested that the altered intestinal physiology which accompanies the jejunocolic (or jejunoileal) anastomosis may underlie the precipitation of joint disease. For those with mild symptoms, the use of salicylates and rest were effective treatment but for the other two, corticosteroids were needed.

LIVER DISEASE.   Liver disease is one of the most difficult postoperative complications of the intestinal bypass. The majority of obese patients have abnormalities of the liver at the time of intestinal bypass. Table 10–4 summarizes from several studies the histologic finding of various degrees of fat in the liver. Only 16 percent (53 out of 328) of the patients had normal liver biopsies, with the majority showing moderate to marked fatty infiltration. Kern et al. (1973) observed a higher frequency of histologic abnormalities in males than in females (62 percent versus 27 percent). The degree of abnormality also increased in the heavier patients, but was not related to age. Buchwald et al. (1974) have noted the increased severity of histologic changes in

TABLE 10–4. *Distribution of Fatty Liver in Obese Patients*

| | | GROUP | | | |
| | | I | II | III | IV |
AUTHOR	TOTAL NUMBER OF PATIENTS	NORMAL LIVER	<25	*Percent Fat in Liver* 25 to 50	>50
Zelman (1952)	19	2	7	8	2
Drenick et al. (1970)	30	0	28	2	
Shibata et al. (1971)	7	2	3	2	0
Salmon (1971)	33	12	17	—	4
Kern et al. (1973)	151	9	60	30	52
Holzbach et al. (1974)	11	0	6	3	2
Buchwald et al. (1974)					
Preoperative	77	28	24	9	16
Postoperative 1 year		4	16	18	24
2 years		1	5	7	3

In Zelman's study ratings were 0, 1, 2 or 3. In Drenick's study 28 patients had some fat, but less than 50 percent; they were assigned to Group II. In Salmon's study, the moderate group were assigned to Group II and the marked to Group IV. In Holzbach's study minimal abnormalities were assigned to Group II, moderate to Group III and marked to Group IV.

males, and that there is a definite correlation with the degree of over-weight. Excess body weight was 207 percent above normal for the patients with normal liver biopsies, and 254 percent above normal in the patients whose biopsies were more than 50 percent fat.

In a study of the triglyceride content in liver biopsies, Holzbach et al. (1974) showed that there was a significant increase in quantity of fat in biopsies read as marked fatty infiltration, but that the tri-glyceride content of the biopsies with minimal and moderate fatty infiltration was the same. In this study the degree of hepatic lipid did not correlate with the degree of obesity, a finding which differs from the conclusions of Kern et al. (1973) and Buchwald et al. (1974). Zelman (1952) has examined in detail the histologic features of 19 needle biopsies from obese patients. None of the biopsies was completely normal. Using the criteria of cellular degeneration, focal necrosis, retention of bile pigment, fat vacuolization, liver cell regeneration, periportal cellular infiltration and periportal fibrosis, all biopsies were normal (by at least one of these criteria), and there was an average of 3.1 abnormalities per patient.

Liver function tests may also present a range of results in obesity. Retention of Bromsulphalein (BSP) occurs in all of the patients reported by Zelman (1952), and 13 of 14 reported by Westwater and Fainer (1958). The rise in BSP observed during fasting probably reflects the effect of fasting itself (Barrett, 1971) rather than the effects of the obesity (Rozental et al., 1967). Fifty percent of the patients reported by Zelman (1952) showed abnormalities in other serum proteins, and some had abnormally high levels of cholesterol. Westwater and Fainer (1958) also reported abnormalities in the cephalin flocculation and thymol turbidity tests, two tests which measure functional properties of plasma proteins.

The effects of weight loss produced by hypocaloric diets or by total starvation on hepatic function and histology have been reported by Rozental et al. (1967) and by Drenick et al. (1970). Both studies conducted tests both before and after weight loss by the two methods mentioned. During the early phase of weight loss there was a transient increase in the extent of hepatocellular degeneration and focal necrosis (Drenick et al., 1970). In the early phase of weight loss by total starvation, Rozental et al (1967) also observed more fibrosis, and a distinct fine pericellular fibrillar collagen. However, in the two patients who were starved the longest, there was a definite diminution in the quantity of fat. This decrease in fat after pronounced weight loss would be consistent with the finding of normal liver histology among 14 patients who had maintained normal weight for an average of 17 months. In conclusion, it would appear that the hepatic abnormalities which are so common on liver biopsies at the time of surgery would regress if weight loss were produced and maintained by dietary methods (Bray et al., 1976).

After jejunoileostomy, hepatic function and hepatic architecture both deteriorate to some degree in the catabolic phase, and this may continue into the phase of adaptation (Fig. 10–6). The levels of serum glutamic oxaloacetic transaminase (SGOT), alkaline phosphatase and serum glutamic pyruvic transaminase (SGPT) all rise in the early postoperative period (Scott et al., 1973; Moxley et al., 1974). Preoperatively only one of our patients had an abnormal SGOT (over 50 units). Postoperatively 70 percent rose above this upper limit of normal, with a mean maximal value of 116 units.

The pattern of rise was also interesting. The peak level of 116 ± 28 units was reached in the first postoperative month. Thereafter it declined to reach nearly normal levels by six months postoperatively. The rise in alkaline phosphatase was somewhat slower. Preoperatively about half of our patients had values at or just above the upper limits of normal. After operation a peak value of twice normal was reached by the second month, but this gradually declined toward the preoperative normal levels by 6 to 9 months. Juhl et al. (1971) have also reported a rise in serum aspirate transaminase above normal limits in patients with end-to-end jejunoileostomy. A rise in BSP was also observed but, as noted above, this may well reflect starvation rather than the state of the liver (Barrett, 1971).

Deterioration in the histologic pattern has also been observed. Salmon (1971) found some degree of increased fatty infiltration in almost all patients, but only one of this series of 120 patients developed jaundice. Thompson and Meyerowitz (1970) reported that 7 patients had improvement in their liver biopsies 15 to 18 months after intestinal bypass, while 4 others were worse, and one showed no change. In the study reported by Holzbach et al. (1974) none of the biopsies was histologically improved, while 5 remained the same and 6 had become worse. The largest groups of patients with liver biopsies are that reported by Buchwald et al. (1974), Schwartz (personal communication) and Kern et al., (1973).

It was reported that one year after surgery only 4 of 62 patients had normal liver biopsies, compared with 28 of 77 before bypass surgery. At two years only 1 out of 16 patients had a normal liver biopsy, and 3 biopsies still contained more than 50 percent fat. Two years after an intestinal bypass weight loss is essentially stable, yet there was little sign of improvement in the histologic picture of the liver. In one patient that we have biopsied 7 years after an end-to-side intestinal bypass there was still a significant quantity of fat. The hepatic response to weight loss and weight maintenance after an intestinal bypass procedure is thus very different from the effects of weight loss produced by a hypocaloric diet or by starvation. In the latter forms of treatment, liver histology returns to normal; this happens, but slowly, in patients who have had an intestinal bypass.

Although the liver improves very slowly, rarely does it deteriorate to the point of hepatic failure and death. When this happens, however, it usually occurs within the first six months after operation. In one of our male patients hepatic failure developed within the first three months, accompanied by rapid onset of coma and death. At autopsy his liver showed marked fatty change with cirrhosis. In 2 other patients who have been referred to us, jaundice and hepatic failure developed within five months after surgery. One of them died and at autopsy had a liver weighing just over 600 grams. The other patient was reanastomosed. Her postoperative course was difficult; the concentration of bilirubin reached 26 mg/dl, and hepatic coma appeared. Gradually, however, she has improved.

Brown et al. (1974) have described the sequence of events as follows,

The earliest detectable functional abnormality is a decrease in the uptake of technetium sulfa colloid by the Kupffer cells of the liver. Next, BSP dye retention develops followed by hypoalbuminemia and hypokalemia. Mild elevation of the SGOT, SGPT, and alkaline phosphatase may occur at this time (the sequence up to this point has been observed in many patients who do not become jaundiced or develop hepatic failure). Accompanying these findings are fluid retention with weight gain, peripheral edema and often ascites. Next, hyperbilirubinemia of the conjugated type occurs. At this point, mild hypoprothrombinemia may occur.

Determination of serum SGOT and SGPT monthly may be helpful. If they remain elevated or rise after 3 months, if albumin drops to low levels, or if the bilirubin rises, the patient should have hepatic scans with both technetium sulfa colloid and rose bengal. A liver biopsy should also be seriously considered.

Several hypotheses have been proposed to explain the appearance of moderate or severe liver disease after an intestinal bypass operation. These include: protein deficiency, a deficiency of choline, inadequate absorption of essential fatty acids, formation and absorption of excess quantities of lithocholic acid, deficiency of vitamin E or the formation of toxic bacterial products. The studies of Bondar and Pisesky (1967) strongly implicate the defunctionalized bowel. They resected 80 percent of the small intestine in 2 dogs who were both alive and well 16 months later. In animals with an end-to-side anastomosis in which the defunctionalized loop was left in situ, all dogs died of electrolyte imbalance and liver failure within 6 months.

In another experiment McClelland et al. (1970) showed that irrigation of the defunctionalized loop of the bypass with either predigested gelatin or with medium chain triglycerides would prevent the death of the animals. When the loop was irrigated with Sulfathalidine or methylcellulose, however, the animals died. In these and other animal studies, lean dogs have been the principal subjects of study. The difference in hepatic response to injury between dogs and man, and the use of normal weight dogs (when intestinal bypasses are most frequently used to treat obese human beings) leaves these experimental results open to question (Buchwald et al., 1974).

Sherr et al. (1974) have recently shown that high concentrations of bile acids may be one factor in the impairment of hepatic function. Other deleterious agents also appear to be necessary.

Restoration of intestinal continuity would appear to be mandatory in the face of progressive hepatic failure. Reanastomosis may also be necessary for intractable loss of electrolytes. Patients will occasionally request reanastomosis. Among 596 patients, 21 (3.7 percent) were reanastomosed. Revision with shortening or lengthening of the intestine may also be necessary. Two of our patients have required such a revision because they failed to lose weight after the initial operation.

Beneficial Effects

The positive rewards from a successful intestinal bypass procedure fall into two categories; psychosocial and medical. The psychosocial consequences of intestinal bypass have been reported by Solow et al. (1974) and by Brewer et al. (1974). Castelnuovo-Tedesco and Schiebel (1976) have evaluated the patients who were operated on at the Harbor General Hospital to minimize any hazard that might result from the removal of the psychological defense mechanisms provided by massive obesity. None of our patients has gotten worse psychologically in the postoperative period, and most patients are better.

Solow et al. (1974) reported 29 patients, of whom 12 were psychologically impaired before surgery. The psychiatric diagnoses in these 12 included schizophrenia (3), neurosis (5), and personality disorder (4). Postoperatively, 23 patients reported that they were more active both physically and socially. As a group they were less self-conscious and thus had less hesitation in leaving the house to engage in activities. Mood was improved in 22 patients and in 27 self-esteem had risen. Body image improved in 23 patients. Because of the marked physical changes, two marriages ended in failure and in a third, the woman had several extramarital affairs. The patients who were psychologically impaired before the operation behaved afterwards as the well-adjusted group behaved.

Among the series of psychological tests which Solow used, only those rating depression and self-esteem showed significant improvement after surgery. The authors conclude by stating that, "The findings in this study fail to support the view that behavioral abnormalities regularly accompany substantial reduction of adipose tissue in the obese," (Solow et al.,1974).

Kalucy et al. (1975) reported on 12 patients 2 years post bypass. They observed that self-acceptance improved, the patients were happier, and that the eating patterns became normal postoperatively. These individuals continued to act as though they were still large, but they no longer felt ugly and disgusting. Although there was a gradual reduction in body image postoperatively, the decrease was slower than the decline in body weight.

The data by Solow et al. (1974) are in essential agreement with the observations on patients who were operated on at the Harbor General Hospital, and indicate that psychosocial rewards may indeed by significant for the successful patient.

The medical benefits of intestinal bypass are summarized below.

BENEFICIAL EFFECTS OF INTESTINAL BYPASS

Permanent weight loss
Lower cholesterol
Lower triglycerides
Improved joint function
Decreased insulin requirement in diabetes
Improved pulmonary function and work tolerance
Reduction in blood pressure
Improved self-esteem
Improved body image
Economic rehabilitation

There is little doubt that blood pressure will be reduced, insulin requirements decreased and cholesterol and triglycerides lowered (Scott et al., 1973; Buchwald et al., 1974; Fikri and Casella, 1973). Half (11/20) of the hypertensive patients operated on by Fikri and Casella became normotensive. Insulin requirements decreased in all five patients and could be discontinued in two. Whether life expectancy is increased is unknown.

From the data reported by Marks (see Chapter 6), one could argue that the reduction in body weight with the decrease in risk factors would be associated with prolonged life. However, we do not yet know what the long term consequences of intestinal malabsorption and malnutrition may be on hepatic function or on the maintenance of normal function of other organ systems. The performance of this operation must still be considered an investigational procedure.

Management of the Bypass Patient

From the schematic diagram shown in Figure 10–6, the importance of careful follow-up during the first 6 months is clear. The rate of weight loss is greatest during this time, and the risk of developing severe liver trouble is at its highest. Table 10–5 outlines some of the procedures and intervals of follow-up which we recommend. Patients are told to avoid hot dry climates for 6 to 9 months. They are advised not to become pregnant. Careful evaluation of hepatic function and electrolyte concentration is carried out at 2 to 4 week intervals for the first 6 months.

We provide each patient with a high protein diet and a list of high potassium foods (Appendix 10–1) which we encourage them to eat. We also give them a list of foods which are high in oxalate (Appendix 10–2) which they should avoid. If additional potassium is needed, we usually avoid solutions of 10 percent KCl, since this produces nausea in many patients. K-Lyte or K-ciel (potassium chloride) are much better tolerated. Diarrhea is controlled for 4 to 6 weeks with diphenoxy-

TABLE 10–5. *Outline of Medical Management
in the Postoperative Period*

	FREQUENCY OF VISITS	TESTS	TREATMENT MAY INCLUDE
Catabolic phase 6 to 9 months	2 to 4 weeks	SGPT SGOT Potassium (K^+) Calcium (Ca^{++}) Magnesium (Mg^{++}) Albumin Liver scan or biopsy (if indicated)	Vitamin B_{12} by injection Potassium supplements Multi-vitamins Folate Antidiarrheal drugs Protein or calcium supplements
Early adaptation 6 to 18 months	1 to 3 months	SGPT	Vitamin B_{12} by injection Protein and calcium supplements
Late adaptation after 18 months	6 to 12 months	Schilling Test D-xylose Albumin	Vitamin B_{12} injections every 1 to 3 months if Schilling remains low

late (Lomotil). It is not usually needed after this. Hemorrhoids can be a severe problem requiring steroid cream and surgical treatment in some instances. As recovery from the malnutrition develops with adaptation of the intestine to absorb more nutrients, the body can build up its own stores.

In the period of adaptation which probably lasts up to 18 months or more, follow-up is necessary with injections of vitamin B_{12} on a 1 to 6 month schedule. After 18 months a Schilling test should be useful to determine whether additional treatment with vitamin B_{12} is necessary. The use of calcium or magnesium supplements is dictated by laboratory findings. We have put most patients on ferrous sulfate because serum iron is often low. The possibility of long term liver problems must be kept in mind, and it is desirable to perform periodic liver biopsies or to obtain liver scans until these functions begin to return to normal.

GASTRIC BYPASS OPERATIONS

The gastric bypass which was developed by Mason and his collaborators at the University of Iowa has two variants (Mason and Ito, 1967, 1969; Printen and Mason, 1973; Printen, 1974, personal communication). When a gastric bypass is performed, 90 percent of the stomach is left in continuity with the duodenum. The remaining 10 percent is anastomosed to the jejunum. The technical complexities of this operation led to attempts to use a simpler gastroplasty in which a 1 to 1.5 cm channel is left connecting a smaller upper segment of the stomach to a larger lower segment (see Printen and Mason, 1973, for details of operation). Difficulty with ulceration of the gastric channel has led to general abandonment of the gastroplasty.

At present over 435 operations using gastric bypass have been performed at the University of Iowa. Early in the postoperative period patients note a decreased intake of food and early satiety with each meal. There is a slow steady weight loss which averages between 2 and 2.5 pounds per week. The median weight loss for the first year after surgery is 47 kg (104 pounds) in 41 patients (range 0 to 90.5 kg). The results were less satisfactory in another study where the median weight loss at one year was 24 kg (53 pounds) in 17 patients (7 kg to 89 kg) (Printen and Mason, 1973). A plateau in body weight is usually reached between 20 and 26 months after the operation. Table 10–6 summarizes the results with this operation. The operative mortality in this series is now 3 percent (Printen, 1974, personal communication). The overall mortality with the first 130 gastric bypass operations was 4.6 percent and the mortality with 56 gastroplasties was 2 percent. This level of mortality is close to that observed with the jejunoileostomy (Table 10–3).

Marginal ulcers (1.4 percent) and wound infections have been the

TABLE 10–6. *Results with Gastric Bypass as a Treatment for Obesity**

RESULT	PERCENTAGE OF OCCURRENCE
Deaths	3
Marginal ulcer	1.4
Wound infection	10
Obstruction	0
Perforation	0
Anemia	0.2
Electrolyte abnormalities	0
Abnormal liver tests	0
Liver biopsies	Improved

*Printen, personal communication (1974).

other two significant problems. The numerous metabolic problems which have been so troublesome for patients who have a jejunoileal anastomosis have not been observed with this operative approach to obesity. In particular renal stones, hepatic failure and severe disturbances of electrolytes have not been encountered. Moreover, the state of marked malnutrition observed during the rapid weight loss after a jejunoileostomy is apparently avoided by this operation. From this brief review, it is clear that this operation deserves more extensive evaluation by other surgeons.

LIPECTOMY OR PANNICULATOMY

Lipectomy or panniculatomy is the removal of skin and subcutaneous fat. Numerous patients have undergone this surgical procedure in an effort to reduce obesity. In general, this operation has met with only limited success in the obese patient because most patients tend to regain any weight which is removed. The major use of this operation is in plastic repair for patients who have already lost a large amount of weight after an intestinal bypass or after prolonged dietary therapy. In one such operation, Meyerowitz et al. (1973) removed 38.5 kg of fat and skin. Kral and Sjostrom (1975) have removed 15 percent of the total number of fat cells from 2 patients, and nearly 25 percent from a third.

Our experience with 3 patients typifies the more conservative results in this area. These 3 patients were young girls who had lost 150 to 200 pounds (68 to 90 kg) by caloric restriction during metabolic studies at the Clinical Research Center. After discharge from the hospital, they maintained their body weight for nine to twelve months at essentially the same level that they had at the time of their discharge from the hospital. With this indication that their dietary habits had been altered, we agreed to remove part of the abdominal panniculus.

The quantity of skin and adipose tissue removed from each patient ranged beween 3 and 6 kilograms (6.6 to 13.2 pounds). The size of individual adipocytes in the removed fat was measured and the total number of fat cells in the piece of the removed panniculus was calculated. Total body fat and number of fat cells were also estimated. By our calculation this procedure had removed about 1 percent of the total adipocytes in the body.

In the postoperative period, all three regained the weight which they lost. There was, however, an important difference in the distribution of weight. The area from which adipose tissue was initially removed in the lower abdomen remained much thinner than the adjacent areas above or below. That is, the reaccumulation of triglyceride in fat cells seemed to occur in areas other than those where the abdominal panniculus had been removed. These data would be consistent with the current view that the total number of adipose cells in the human body is fixed shortly after puberty and does not increase. If it were possible to remove a large enough number of adipose cells in an adult, the degree of obesity might indeed be reduced. However, short of total panniculectomy, this seems an unlikely approach for long term success.

LATERAL HYPOTHALAMIC LESIONS

The hypothalamus in man, as in the experimental animal, is thought to have at least two areas involved in regulating food intake (see Chapter 2). The ventromedial hypothalamic center is presumably involved in regulation of body mass. In humans injury to this area is often followed by obesity and the hypothalamic syndrome (see Chapter 5). In experimental animals the lateral hypothalamus integrates food seeking behavior, and destructive lesions in this area reduce food intake. In man lateral hypothalamic tumors also produce decreased food intake and weight loss. Theoretically, therefore, it should be possible to destroy the lateral hypothalamus and thus decrease food intake as a way of treating obesity.

This techique has been tried, but the results were disappointing (Quaade, 1974). An electrode was introduced unilaterally into the lateral hypothalamus. It was advanced slowly until a region was found in which stimulation elicited hunger. A lesion was made at this point. Unilateral lesions of this sort did not alter to any significant degree the body weight in 3 subjects on whom it was tried. The hazards of this approach are clear. An irreversible lesion might produce permanent aphagia, resulting in starvation and death. This technique cannot be recommended.

JAW-WIRING

Limiting the ingestion of food has taken many forms (see Chapters 8 and 9), the most recent of which is the use of wires to connect the upper and lower jaws (Garrow, 1974; Laskin, 1974). The procedure is similar to operations which stabilize the mandible after a fracture. Wires are connected from the base of the teeth on the upper jaw to the lower jaw. This prevents opening the jaws and limits food intake to liquids. If the patient restricts the liquid intake to hypocaloric levels, he will lose weight. One patient we have seen, however, drank large quantities of high caloric foods and lost no weight.

The major risks of this procedure are injury to the teeth and the possibility of aspiration. If the wires are left on longer than 8 to 10 weeks, the risk of losing teeth from the upper or lower jaw increases significantly. Thus most patients have had the wires in place for less than 3 months.

When the jaws are wired together, only liquids can be readily ingested. Similarly internal secretions are more difficult to expectorate. The risk of aspirating, particularly if vomiting occurs, is a serious potential hazard. Any patient undergoing this procedure should understand this risk and be willing to carry small wire cutters at all times which can be used to snip the wires in an emergency. One patient who came to us after the wires had been removed told of cutting the wires on one occasion when she became nauseated while riding on a roller coaster. Thus with proper instruction, this procedure can be carried out with little risk. However, it is of short term value if the patient has not learned to modify his eating behavior.

APPENDICES TO CHAPTER 10

Apricots, Apricot nectar	Milk—all types
Bananas	Nectarines
Bran Cereals	Oranges and orange juice
Broccoli	Papaya
Buttermilk	Peaches, fresh
Cantaloupe	Pomegranate
Coconut, fresh or pkg.	Potatoes, white
Dried fruit (no figs)	Prunes and prune juice
Dried peas, beans and lima beans	Salt substitute
Grapefruit and juice	Sunflower seeds
Honeydew melon	Tangerines
Lite-Salt	Tomatoes and tomato products
Mangos	V-8 Juice
Meat—all kinds—lean	Yogurt, low fat

These foods are highest in potassium content for average size portions of food.

APPENDIX 10–2. *Foods High in Oxalate*

Artichokes	Green onions
Beets	Gooseberries
Beet greens	Nuts—all kinds
Blackberries	Okra
Carrots	Parsley
Celery	Pepper
Chocolate—all kinds	Peppers, sweet and green
Coca cola	Plums
Cocoa	Poppy seeds
Concord grapes	Potatoes, sweet
Cranberries	Raspberries
Currants	Rhubarb
Dandelion greens	Spinach
Endive	Strawberries
Figs, fresh, dried and preserved	Swiss chard
Fruit peels	Tea—all kinds
Gelatin	Yams

ADVICE TO PATIENTS
UNDERGOING INTESTINAL BYPASS

(Reprinted from Bray, George A. and Bethune, John E.: Treatment and Management of Obesity, Hagerstown, Harper and Rowe, 1974, pp. 141–144, with permission.)

You will undergo a rather drastic operation designed to limit the absorption of excess calories from your intestinal tract. You will note some or all of the following symptoms afterwards:

Diarrhea. This may be severe, with frequent watery movements up to 20 times daily. It will usually be most severe after your largest meal, and most commonly occur in the evening and early night time hours. This is expected and must be tolerated. Normally, it declines over several weeks to 5 to 7/day and eventually to 2 to 5/day.

Soreness of the rectal area. The passage of chemicals and partly digested food causes this. It is more troublesome to some patients than to others. It gradually gets better unless you have a hemorrhoid problem. Hemorrhoids may require treatment later.

Gassy distention and rumbling. This is variable and unpredictable. It may not occur until several months after surgery.

Loss of appetite. This is common in the early weeks after surgery, and normal appetite usually returns in about six to eight weeks. Your taste for foods may change and you may crave certain things. Within reason this is not harmful.

General physical weakness. This is usually not profound, but you may notice lethargy, lack of ambition, sluggishness, and some discouragement. This can last several weeks.

Pains in the abdomen or side. These may or may not be serious. If more than just passing cramps, they should be reported to the doctor. They may signal a twist in the intestine or passage of a kidney stone.

Unexpected complications of surgery. Although very uncommon, some patients have not healed their internal or external incisions during hospitalization. Some have had bleeding from the intestine, infection, clots on the lung or a heart attack, and some have succumbed from the operation.

Within the first few days or weeks after surgery, certain adaptations of the body are necessary and must occur. The most important of these are listed here and form the basis for the recommendations which follow.

The shortened intestine cannot handle the same quantity of food you have usually eaten. It may enlarge with time to hold larger amounts of food.

The absorption of liquids by the intestine is markedly limited, and most of what you drink will go right through, especially if liquids are taken rapidly.

The lower intestine is now reached by food and liquid far sooner than before the operation and may be shocked by contact with cold or hot liquids (chiefly cold).

The digestive juices are rapidly poured into the large intestine and produce severe irritation when they reach the rectal area.

The absorption of certain essential minerals, chiefly potassium, calcium and sometimes magnesium, as well as bicarbonate, is markedly hampered.

With lowered food absorption, the body stores of fat are mobilized, and must go to the liver to be metabolized into a form from which the body can derive energy. The liver is under severe stress, for it must store and dispose of this fat load, and change it chemically so that the muscles can use it for fuel.

The kidneys are supplied with far less water than normal. This results in lower urine output at the same time that large amounts of water run through the intestine. Under these conditions, kidney stones may form.

There are other changes occurring in the body, the causes of which are not well understood. It is possible that you may have symptoms or complications not discussed here. It is important that you understand the investigative nature of this procedure, and that the medical profession may not yet have all the answers to every problem that may arise.

RECOMMENDATIONS FOR THE INTESTINAL BYPASS PATIENT

From our experience we are prepared to make a number of suggestions about diet, daily life pattern, and medication which should be followed carefully. These directions will help to minimize your discomfort and disability. You must realize, however, that no two cases are alike, and sometimes problems will arise even when you do everything "right."

(1) For the first six weeks after surgery you should carefully avoid eating or drinking anything colder than room temperature. You will have a craving for cold drinks and very cold foods such as ice cream. Cold food and drink shocks the newly formed food pathway so it cannot absorb necessary minerals, and washes food elements through which should be absorbed.

(2) You must eat some food every day, even though you have no appetite and feel nauseated. Complete failure to eat stresses the lever severely and prevents replacement of vital minerals and chemicals which cannot be replaced completely even by intravenous therapy.

(3) You must avoid drinking large quantities of liquid with meals. A little milk on cereal, a cup of soup and a cup of coffee, tea or milk are permissible but, in general, the meal should be taken quite dry.

(4) Fluid intake should be spread out over waking hours, but not within a one half hour period before or a one hour period after meals. It would be permissible, for example, to drink three or four ounces of water every half hour according to your thirst, but not to drink one or two quarts at a time every two or three hours.

(5) Foods high in potassium should be taken with each mean. Examples are bananas, dried dates, cantaloupe and most fruits, as well as meats. Other high potassium foods may be found on lists available from your doctor or the Heart Association.

(6) Alcohol in all forms must be avoided for at least one year. The liver metabolism is severely stressed by alcohol, and even small amounts may result in severe liver damage. In addition, alcohol produces effects on the brain which result in bizarre and unpredictable behavior, with danger to yourself or others.

(7) You should avoid standing or sitting for long periods in the hot sun, or visiting the desert during the first year. Severe dehydration can occur rapidly from moderate perspiration.

If any of these instructions are not clear, the doctor will be able to clarify them for you by phone or on a regular office visit. If you find a certain technique or way of life that eases some of the problems, we are always happy to learn about it and will pass it along to others.

I hereby certify that I have received a copy of the attached AD-VICE AND RECOMMENDATIONS, and that I have read same and agree to follow them to the best of my ability, if selected as a candidate for an intestinal shunt procedure for the control of obesity.

SIGNED_____

DATE _____

WITNESS _____

REFERENCES

Baber, J. C., Jr., Hayden, W. F. and Thompson, B. W.: Intestinal bypass operations for obesity. Am. J. Surg., 126:769–772, 1973.

Backman, L. and Hallberg, D.: Small intestinal length. An intraoperative study in obesity. Acta Chir. Scand., 140:57–63, 1974.

Barrett, P. V. D.: Hyperbilirubinemia of fasting. J.A.M.A., 217:1349–1353, 1971.

Barron, J., Frame, B. and Bozalis, J. R. A.: A shunt operation for obesity. Dis. Colon Rectum, 12:115, 1969.

Barry, R. E., Benfield, J. R., Nicell, P. and Bray, G. A.: Colonic pseudo-obstruction: A new complication of jejunoileal bypass. Gut., 16:903–908, 1975.

Benfield, J. R., Greenway, F. L., Bray, G. A., Barry, R. E., Leehago, J., Mena, I. and Schedewie, H.: Is jejunoileal bypass for obesity justified? Surg. Gynecol. Obstet. In press 1976.

Benfield, J. R. and Bray, G. A.: Is obesity a surgical disease? Western J. Med., 123:396–398, 1975.

Bondar, G. F. and Pisesky, W.: Complications of small intestinal short-circuiting for obesity. Arch. Surg., 94:707–716, 1967.

Bray, G. A., Barry, R. E., Benfield, J., Castelnuovo-Tedesco, P. and Rodin, J.: Food intake and taste perferences for glucose and sucrose decrease after intestinal bypass surgery. In: Hunger: Basic Mechanisms and Clinical Implications, (Novin, D., Wyrwicka, W. and Bray, G. A., eds.), New York, Raven Press, 1976, pp. 431–439.

Bray, G. A., Passaro, E., Castelnuovo-Tedesco, P., Barry, R. E., Drenick, E. and Benfield, J.: Intestinal bypass operation as a treatment for obesity. Ann. Intern. Med. In press 1976.

Brewer, C., White, H. and Baddeley, M.: Beneficial effects of jejunoileostomy on compulsive eating and associate psychiatric symptoms. Brit. Med. J., 4:314–315, 1974.

Brown, R. G., O'Leary, J. P. and Woodward, E. R.: Hepatic effects of jejunoileal bypass for morbid obesity. Am. J. Surg., 127:53–58, 1974.

Buchwald, H., Lober, P. H. and Varco, R. L.: Liver biopsy findings in seventy-seven consecutive patients undergoing jejunoileal bypass for morbid obesity. Am. J. Surg., 127:48–52, 1974.

Castelnuovo-Tedesco, P. and Schiebel, D.: Studies of superobesity. II. Psychiatric appraisal of surgery for superobesity. In: Hunger, Basic Mechanisms and Clinical Implications. (Novin, D., Wyrwicka, W., and Bray, G. A., eds.) New York, Raven Press, 1976, pp. 459–471.

Castelnuovo-Tedesco, P. and Schiebel, D.: Studies of superobesity. II. Psychiatric appraisal of jejuno-ileal bypass surgery. Am. J. Psychiatry, 133:26–31, 1976.

Deleña, S. A., Fechner, R. E., Brown, H. and Shelton, E. L., Jr.: Reversible fatty liver with fibrosis following jejunocolic shunt. South. Med. J., 63:399–402, 1970.

DeMuth, W. E. and Rottenstein, H. S.: Death associated with hypocalcemia after small bowel short-circuiting. New. Engl. J. Med., 270:1239–1240, 1964.

DeWind, L. T.: Jejunoileal bypass surgery for obesity. In: Treatment and Management of Obesity. (Bray, G. A. and Bethune, J. E., eds.); Harper and Row, Hagerstown, 1974, pp. 132–140.

Dickstein, S. S. and Frame, B.: Urinary tract calculi after intestinal shunt operations for the treatment of obesity. Surg. Gynecol. Obstet., 136:257–260, 1973.

Drenick, E. J., Simmons, F. and Murphy, J. F.: Effect on hepatic morphology of treatment of obesity by fasting, reducing diets, and small bowel bypass. N. Engl. J. Med., 282:829–834, 1970.

Everett, R. B., Crosby, W. M., Welsh, J. D. and Thompson, J. B.: Pregnancy after jejunoileal bypass for obesity. Surg. Gynecol. Obstet., 139:215–216, 1974.

Fikri, E. and Cassella, R. R.: Jejunoileal bypass for massive obesity. Results and complications in fifty-two patients. Ann. Surg., 179:460–464, 1973.

Garrow, J. S.: Dental splinting treatment of hyperphagic obesity. P. Nutr. Soc., 33(2):A29, 1974.

Gazet, J. C., Pilkington, T. R. E., Kalucy, R. S., Crisp, A. H. and Day, S.: Treatment of gross obesity by jejunal bypass. Brit. Med. J., 4:311–313, 1974.

Hess, R. J.: Polyarthritis after small bowel bypass. J. Oklahoma State Med. Assoc., 67:283–285, 1974.

Holzbach, R. T., Wieland, R. G., Lieber, C. S., DeCarli, L. M., Koepke, K. R. and Green, S. G.: Hepatic lipid in morbid obesity assessment at and subsequent to jejunoileal bypass. N. Engl. J. Med., 290:296–299, 1974.

Juhl, E., Christoffersen, P., Baden, H. and Quaade, F.: Liver morphology and biochemistry in eight obese patients treated with jejunoileal anastomosis. N. Engl. J. Med., 285:543–547, 1971.

Kalucy, R. S., Solow, C., Hartman, M., Crisp, A. H., McGuinness, B. and Kalucy, E. C.: Self reports of estimated body widths in female obese subjects with major fat loss following ileo-jejunal bypass surgery. In: Advances in Obesity Research. I. Proc. of 1st International Congress on Obesity, Oct. 9–11, 1974, London, Newman Publishing Ltd., 1975, pp. 331–332.

Kantor, S.: Drastic cures for obesity. Lancet, 2:52, 1970.

Kaufmann, H. J. and Weldon, H. W.: Intussusception: A late complication of small-bowel bypass for obesity. J.A.M.A., 202:1147–1148, 1967.

Kern, W. H., Heger, A. H., Payne, J. H. and DeWind, L. T.: Fatty metamorphosis of the liver in morbid obesity. Arch. Pathol., 96:342–346, 1973,

Kral, J. G. and Sjostrom, L. V.: Surgical reduction of adipose tissue hypercellularity. In: Advances in Obesity Research. I. Proc. 1st International Congress on Obesity, London, Newman Publishing Ltd., 1975, pp. 327–330.

Kremen, A. J., Linner, J. H. and Nelson, C. H.: Experimental evaluation of nutritional importance of proximal and distal small intestine. Ann. Surg., 140:439–448, 1954.

Laskin, D. M.: Oral surgeons face a weighty problem. J. Oral Surg.,September, 1974.

Lewis, L. A., Turnbull, R. B. and Page, T. H.: Effects of jejunocolic shunt on obesity serum lipoproteins, lipids and electrolytes. Arch. Intern. Med., 117:4–16, 1966.

Mason, E. E. and Ito, C.: Gastric bypass in obesity. Surg. Clin. North Am., 47:1345–1351, 1967.

Mason, E. E. and Ito, C.: Gastric bypass. Ann. Surg., 170:329–339, 1969.

Maxwell, J. G., Richards, R. C. and Albo, D., Jr.: Fatty degeneration of the liver after intestinal bypass for obesity. Am. J. Surg., 116:648–652, 1968.

McClelland, R. N., DeShazo, C. V. and Heimbach, D. M.: Prevention of hepatic injury after jejunoileal bypass by supplemental jejunostomy feedings. Surg. Forum, 21:368–370, 1970.

Meyerowitz, B. R., Gruber, R. P., Laub, D. R.: Massive abdominal panniculectomy. J.A.M.A., 225:408–409, 1973.

Morgan, A. P. and Moore, F. D.: Jejunoileostomy for extreme obesity: Rationale, metabolic observations and results in a single case. Ann. Surg., 166:75–82, 1967.

Moxley, R. T., III, Pozefsky, T. and Lockwood, D. H.: Protein nutrition and liver disease after jejunoileal bypass for morbid obesity. N. Engl. J. Med., 290:921–926, 1974.

O'Leary, J. P., Thomas, W. C., Jr. and Woodward, E. R.: Urinary tract stone after small bowel bypass for morbid obesity. Am. J. Surg., 127:142–147, 1974.

Payne, J. H., DeWind, L. T. and Commons, R. R.: Metabolic observations on patients with jejunocolic shunts. Am. J. Surg., 106:273–289, 1963.

Payne, J. H. and DeWind, L. T.: Surgical treatment of obesity. Am. J. Surg., 118:141–147, 1969.

Payne, J. H., DeWind, L. T., Schwab, C. E. and Kern, W. H.: Surgical treatment of morbid obesity. Sixteen years of experience. Arch. Surg., 106:432–437, 1973.

Printen, K. J. and Mason, E. E.: Gastric surgery for relief of morbid obesity. Arch. Surg., 106:428–431, 1973.

Quaade, F.: Stereotaxy for obesity. Lancet, 1:267, 1974 (letter).

Quaade, F.: Untraditional treatment of obesity. In: Obesity Symposium Proceedings of the Servier Research Institute Symposium held December, 1973. (Burland, W. L., Samuel, P. and Yudkin, J. eds.), London, 1974, pp. 338–352.

Quaade, F., Juhl, E., Feldt-Rasmussen, K. and Baden, H.: Blind-loop reflux in relation to weight loss in obese patients treated with jejunoileal anastomosis. Scand. J. Gastroenterol., 6:537–541, 1971.

Rozental, P., et al.: Liver morphology and function tests in obesity and during total starvation. Am. J. Dig. Dist., 12:198–208, 1967.

Salmon, P. A.: The results of small intestine bypass operations for the treatment of obesity. Surg. Gynecol. Obstet., 132:965–979, 1971.

Sandstead, H. H.: Jejunoileal shunt in obesity. In: Obesity in Perspective. Fogarty International Center Series on Preventive Medicine, Vol. II, Part II. (Bray, G. A. ed.) Washington, D.C., U.S. Government Printing Office. 1976, pp. 459–471.

Scott, H. W., Jr. and Law, D. H., IV: Clinical appraisal of jejunoileal shunt in patients with morbid obesity. Am. J. Surg., 117:246–253, 1969.

Scott, H. W., Jr., Law, D. H., IV, Sandstead, H. H., Lanier, V. C., Jr. and Younger, R. K.: Jejunoileal shunt in surgical treatment of morbid obesity. Ann. Surg., 171:770–782, 1970.

Scott, H. W., Jr., Sandstead, H. H., Brill, A. B., Burko, H. and Younger, R. K.: Experience with a new technique of intestinal bypass in the treatment of morbid obesity. Ann. Surg., 174:560–572, 1971.

Scott, H. W., Jr., Dean, R., Shull, H. J., Abram, H. S., Webb, W., Younger, R. K. and Brill, A. B.: New considerations in use of jejunoileal bypass in patients with morbid obesity. Ann. Surg., 177:723–735, 1973.

Shagrin, J. W., Frame, B. and Duncan, H.: Polyarthritis on obese patients with intestinal bypass. Ann. Intern. Med., 75:377–380, 1971.

Sherman, C. D., Jr., May, A. G. and Nye, W. et al.: Clinical and metabolic studies following bowel by-passing for obesity. Ann. N.Y. Acad. Sci., 131:614–622, 1965.

Sherr, H. P., Padmanabhan, P. Nair, J. J. White, J. G. Banwell and Lockwood, D. H.: Bile acid metabolism and hepatic disease following small bowel bypass for obesity. Am. J. Clin. Nutr., 27:1369–1379, 1974.

Shibata, H. R., Mackenzie, J. R. and Long, R.: Metabolic effects of controlled jejunocolic bypass. Arch. Surg., 95:413–428, 1967.

Shibata, H. R., MacKenzie, J. R. and Huang, S.: Morphologic changes of the liver following small intestinal bypass for obesity. Arch. Surg., 103:229–237, 1971.

Solow, C., Silberfarb, P. M. and Swift, K.: Psychosocial effects of intestinal bypass surgery for severe obesity. New. Engl. J. Med., 290:300–305, 1974.

Starkloff, G. B., Wolfe, B. M. and Ramach, K. R.: Management of complications following intestinal bypass for morbid obesity. Mo. Med., 71:119–121, 1974.

Swenson, S. A., Lewis, J. W. and Sebby, K. R.: Magnesium metabolism in man with special reference to jejunoileal bypass for obesity. Am. J. Surg., 127:250–255, 1974.

Thompson, R. H., Jr. and Meyerowitz, B. R.: Liver changes after jejunoileal shunting for massive obesity. Surg. Forum, 21:366–370, 1970.

Troncelliti, M. A.: Ileal bypass. Hosp. Top., 44:117–120, 1966.

Weismann, R. E.: Surgical palliation of massive and severe obesity. Am. J. Surg., *125*:437–446, 1973.

Westwater, J. O. and Fainer, D.: Liver impairment in the obese. Gastroenterol., *34*:686–693, 1958.

Wills, C. E., Jr.: Obstetrical delivery after jejunoileostomy for obesity. J. Med. Assoc. Ga., *60*:39, 1971.

Wood, L. C. and Chremos, A. N.: Treating obesity by "short-circuiting" the small intestine. J.A.M.A., *186*:63, 1963.

Zelman, S.: The liver in obesity. A.M.A. Arch. Intern. Med., *90*:141–156, 1952.

INDEX

447